PSYCHOSURGERY

To Maty

and

To William Morrison Carroll

PSYCHOSURGERY

A Scientific Analysis

Mark A. J. O'Callaghan
BA, BSc, MSc
Clinical Psychologist, Department of Psychology,
University of Birmingham
District Psychology Services, Department of Psychology,
Hollymoor Hospital, Birmingham, England

and

Douglas Carroll
BSc, PhD
Lecturer in Psychology, Department of Psychology,
University of Birmingham, Birmingham, England

MTP PRESS LIMITED
International Medical Publishers

Published by
MTP Press Limited
Falcon House
Lancaster, England

British Library Cataloguing in Publication Data
O'Callaghan, Mark A. J.
Psychosurgery.
1. Psychosurgery
I. Title II. Carroll, Douglas
617'.481 RD594

ISBN-13: 978-94-010-9705-5 e-ISBN-13: 978-94-010-9703-1
DOI:10.1007/ 978-94-010-9703-1

Softcover reprint of the hardcover 1st edition 1982

Filmset by Northumberland Press Ltd, Gateshead

Contents

Acknowledgements

It has taken us over three years to complete this book. The variety and complexity of the issues surrounding psychosurgery have simply defied a hasty analysis. However, we hope that our time and energies have been well spent and that the product is both reasonable and readable.

Over the three years a host of people have, either wittingly or unwittingly, lent their assistance, support and even encouragement. At the risk of giving offence, we have had to be selective; a complete list of credits would run into several pages. First of all, we owe much to our colleagues and friends in the Departments of Psychology at the University of Birmingham and Hollymoor Hospital; we can envisage few better working environments. Second, we are deeply indebted to the various libraries at the University of Birmingham (the Barnes Medical Library, the Education Library, the Main Library and the Inter-Library Loan Service) and their unerringly helpful librarians; this debt extends also to the British Lending Library and the other libraries both in Britain and elsewhere that have contributed through the Inter-Library Loan Service. Third, a legion of typists have laboured painstakingly on our manuscript through the various stages of its development; they include Jill Bolton, Marie Chalmers, Shaheen Chowdrey, Sue Garvey, Barbara Hudson, Beverley Humphries, Lesley Leigh, Halina O'Callaghan and Edna Stanley. Fourth, illustrations are the careful work of Edward and Maureen Fellows of the Department of Physical Metallurgy, University of Birmingham. Fifth, we would like to acknowledge Dr. B. Barraclough for quotations from the Report of the Royal College of Psychiatrists' Research Committee (1977). Sixth, we would like to thank special friends for their tolerance, patience and indulgence over the past three years. These most important people are Anne, Christopher and Liam Carroll, Gail and Mike Phillips, Ioanna Nicolaidou, Helen Smith, and Matthew O'Callaghan.

Finally, while each of us assumed initial responsibility for individual chapters (M. O'C. undertook Chapters 1–7, D. C. Chapters 8–12), our close collaboration throughout, and the various, and at times drastic, revisions undertaken ensured that all chapters represent an integration of our thinking and a product of our joint industry. Our ultimate contributions to the book, then, were for all intents and purposes equal, and the order of authorship reflects only the initial division of labour.

Introduction

Of all the therapies that comprise psychiatric practice, the use of brain surgery to modify behaviour is the most contentious. That such behavioural neurosurgery, or psychosurgery, provokes opposition is far from surprising. The paramount status of the brain seems to belie mechanical intervention. The irreversible nature of the intervention seems to aggravate the outrage. Thus, opponents of the practice contend that psychosurgical procedures constitute a grievous assault on the integrity of the personality. Its proponents, on the other hand, confidently testify that it is a valid and efficacious form of treatment for many seemingly intractable psychiatric disorders. Argument and counterargument have pursued the practice since its initial upsurge in the 1940s, although the decline in its popularity in the 1960s occasioned a temporary cease-fire. However, the recent resurgence of psychosurgery has ensured that it is once again a matter of controversy.

In the United Kingdom the characteristically subdued tenor of the debate frequently obscures the popularity of the practice and the commitment of its opposition. A recent application by the Royal College of Psychiatrists to the Medical Research Council for funds to mount a large controlled trial of psychosurgical procedures was turned down. Several opposition lobbyists might claim some credit for the proposal's lack of success. The Schizophrenia Association of Great Britain clearly and publicly expressed their disapproval of the trial. The Patient's Protection Law Committee presented Parliament with a petition condemning the Royal College's submission. The most significant opposition activity to date in the United Kingdom was the formulation of a bill, for presentation before the House of Commons, to curtail psychosurgical operations, sponsored by Joyce Butler (1977). The bill, formally titled the *Medical Experimentation Act*, sought to:

> protect patients and others from being subjected to medical experiments upon them without their consent; and to prohibit experiments in the case of certain other persons, and to provide for penalties; and for purposes connected therewith. (p. 1)

In the United States similar legislative restraints have been sought. Dr. Peter Breggin's (1972) presentation to the Congressional Record, *The Return of Lobotomy and Psychosurgery*, was seen by many as a milestone in this campaign. Generally, the American debate has been much more public than its British counterpart. The fray has not been confined mainly within the pages of academic outlets. More readily accessible presentation of the arguments has ensured a sensitized American public.

While the opponents of psychosurgery are united in their primary aim, diverse rationales underlie this opposition. Distinct critical approaches can be discerned. Some, like Dr. Breggin, view psychosurgery as merely the most salient example of the many ideologically oppressive procedures that characterize present psychiatric practice. Such opinion has attracted the label "antipsychiatry." Others are more circumscribed in their opposition: the efficacy and validity of psychosurgery is what they specifically challenge. In fact, representatives of this approach contend that the antipsychiatrists jeopardize the opposition case by relying on emotive description and polemic rather than on scientific objectivity and careful scholarship.

Certainly, the proponents of psychosurgery possess little regard for the antipsychiatric lobby. As Mark and Ordia (1976) exemplified:

> Antipsychiatrists have not advanced scientifically valid arguments against the neurosurgical treatment of patients with abnormal aggression; most of the members of the movement are not board-certified in clinical neurology or neurosurgery. Their lack of information about the brain, coupled with the unfortunate results of their own campaign against the diagnosis and treatment of mentally ill patients, has disqualified them as credible critics. (p. 728)

Indeed, the contributions of both opponents and advocates of psychosurgery frequently offer little in the way of objective and scientific analyses. Clearly, only by avoiding the tempting pitfalls of subjectivity and polemic can any evaluation of psychosurgery acquire sufficient status to seriously influence the debate. So much of it at present is characterized by misrepresentation, misunderstanding and downright ignorance.

Even the boundaries of the activities subsumed by the term "psychosurgery" do not attract a consensus. Mark and Ordia argued that psychosurgery has become "a catchword intended to stir up emotions and produce irrational and harmful obstruction in the path of patients seeking treatment" (p. 725). For present purposes we shall abide by the definition given by Alan A. Stone (1975), Professor of Psychiatry and Law at Harvard University, in the Massachusetts Task Force Report on psychosurgery. Stone defined psychosurgery as:

> ... any procedure which, by direct or indirect access to the brain, removes or destroys or interrupts the continuity of the brain tissue that is histologically normal (i.e. tissue that is normal as seen under a microscope, though its physiological functions or properties might obviously be abnormal) for the purpose of altering behavior or treating a psychiatric illness. We include as psychosurgery the implantation of electrodes for either of these purposes, even without subsequent electrocoagulation. We do not include neurosurgical procedures designed to diagnose or treat intractable physical pain or epilepsy where these conditions are clearly demonstrable. Nor do we include any other neurosurgical procedures used to diagnose or treat organic brain conditions even though such procedures may also involve destruction of normal brain tissue. (pp. 27–28)

Stone's definition is adopted because it is clear and precise and because it proved acceptable to all shades of opinion represented by the Task Force. However, it must be conceded that some outsiders would not accept Stone's exclusions. The use of surgery for the treatment of intractable pain, epilepsy and Parkinsonism has been designated as neurosurgery by some but included under the rubric of psychosurgery by others. Finally, it is important to note that it is not the techniques and physiological foci of surgical exercises *per se* which qualify them as examples of psychosurgery. The same procedures and foci characterize neurosurgery. It is the explicit intention of the surgery to promote behavioural change that is crucial.

Psychosurgery, then, is brain surgery conducted explicitly to amend specific aspects of human behaviour. The success, scientific validity and social implications of such an enterprise comprise the subject of this book.

The opening chapter traces the historical precursors of psychosurgery and charts the major landmarks in its more recent development. Chapter 2 describes the technical aspects of psychosurgery. Details of the common and more esoteric operative procedures are provided; the operative methods and brain areas of surgical interest are discussed.

The next five chapters offer a detailed review of evidence relating to the efficacy of psychosurgical procedures. Chapter 3 provides a quantitative overview of the pertinent experimental and case studies. For the reader's convenience, the results of the various operative procedures are organized in tables. In Chapters 4–7, these studies receive critical scrutiny. Chapter 4 considers the make up of the populations selected for psychosurgical intervention. The selection criteria are evaluated, together with general problems in psychiatric diagnosis and prognosis. In this chapter the handful of so-called controlled studies of psychosurgery are subjected to critical scrutiny. In Chapter 5, adverse operative sequelae receive comprehensive documentation and discussion. Chapter 6 examines the anatomical precision of psychosurgical lesions. In Chapter 7, the scientific validity and status of psychosurgical experiments are specifically examined. Concern here is with the sophistication and power of the experimental designs conventionally employed. In addition, the rigour and validity of the assessment procedures used to gauge the behavioural consequences of psychosurgical operations also receive close attention.

Chapter 8 evaluates the theoretical foundations of psychosurgery. The neuropsychological models of brain functional organization underlying psychosurgical practices are uncovered and their tenets examined in the light of prevailing neuropsychological data and theory.

The next three chapters are concerned with the ethical, legal and social issues that surround psychosurgery. Chapter 9 focusses on the ethical issues. The reason for psychosurgery's prominence in ethical discourse are explored, as is the interaction of its scientific and ethical status. Problems attending consent are also rehearsed. Chapter 10 deals with the regulation of psychosurgical procedures. The various prescriptions that have been offered for policing and controlling psychosurgery are evaluated. Recommendations are made. In Chapter 11, the sociopolitical implications of psychosurgery are discussed. The charge that psychosurgery is politically rather than medically inspired is examined.

The final chapter offers brief summary and conclusions.

1

Historical introduction

The observation of a rectangular hole in a prehistoric skull (Figure 1.1) by the American anthropologist E. G. Squier (1877) during a visit to the Cuzco district of Peru between 1863 and 1865, and the subsequent report on it by the French anthropologist and anatomist Paul Broca (1867), firmly established that an operation on the head of a living human had been carried out in prehistoric times. That the aperture had been man-made was fairly evident, and that it had beeen anything but deliberate was highly unlikely. Further, Broca's observation of signs of infection in the porous structure of the bone surrounding the opening established that the patient had survived the operation, even if only temporarily. This then was the first confirmed instance of the prehistoric surgical procedure of trephining performed on the head of a living human.

Trephining (trepanning, trephination or trephanation) is an operation whereby an aperture (called a trephine hole) is made in the skull by the removal of a piece of bone (sometimes known as a bone button or roundel). Brothwell (1972), of the British Museum, noted the difficulty of establishing whether such holes were man-made and the result of deliberate surgical intervention, or the consequence of accident or injury. It is also difficult to establish whether they occurred before, during or after death. The appearance of tool marks and evidence of either contemporary bone infection (osteitis), as indicated by a halo of pitting in the surrounding skull, or of subsequent healing are considered necessary. Healing, according to Brothwell, is indicated

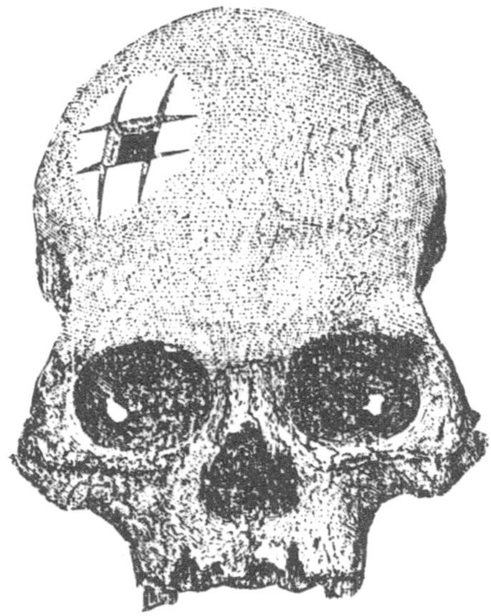

Figure 1.1 The prehistoric skull found by Squier at Cuzco, the first established case of the prehistoric operation of trephining (from: Squier, 1877)

"if the edges of the hole are rounded and the exposed diploic spaces of the spongy inner table show signs of closing or have closed" (p. 128). Based on this, Brothwell suggested that over 50% of the known cases of trephining demonstrated complete healing. One skull, also from the Cuzco region of Peru, has as many as seven healed trephine holes.

The skull certainly shows that the Peruvian practitioners were extremely adroit at these operations. Although the technical aspects of the operations were unsophisticated, these surgeons were sufficiently skilled to avoid causing extensive injury such as severing the meningeal vessels (vessels of the membranes that surround the brain) or incising the dura mater (the outermost of the three layers of the meninges) during the course of the operation. Walker (1951) observed, "the Incas developed trepanning to a commonly practised skilled art" (p. 5). However, as Piggott (1940) noted, the practice was observed in prehistoric Europe as well, and it appears to have been practised in many areas of the world (Brothwell, 1972). Nevertheless, probably the earliest known pictorial representation of trephining comes from a Peruvian huaco or clay pitcher found and described by Macedo (1917). This shows a surgeon operating upon a patient with a tumi, a cutting instrument, probably in this case made of stone. Usually a bronze tumi was used (Figure 1.2), such as that found, according to Asenjo (1963), by Antze. This particular bronze tumi actually depicts an operation.

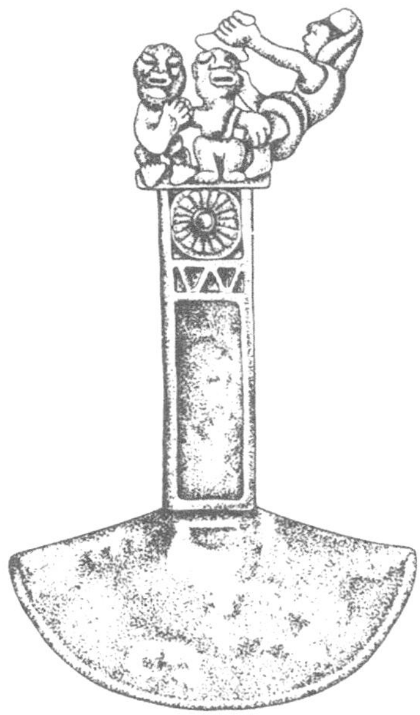

Figure 1.2 The bronze cutting instrument, known as Antze's tumi, which depicts the operation of trephining (from: Asenjo, 1963). Courtesy of Charles C. Thomas, Publisher, Springfield, Illinois

The frontal areas were the most common site for operation, followed by the parietal lobe and then the occipital lobe. The reasons for surgery, however, are not always readily apparent. Brothwell (1972) listed four suggestions as to their purpose: to obtain roundels for use as amulets; as surgical treatment of an injury, especially a skull fracture; as a treatment for headaches, epilepsy and other illnesses; or to promote longevity. Certainly in some cases it is clear that surgery coincided with brain disorders and was therefore presumably intended as treatment (cf. Oakley *et al.*, 1959).

Since then, brain surgery has commonly been used to treat deleterious cerebral abnormalities and has developed from being a "commonly practised skilled art" of prehistoric times into contemporary neurosurgery:

> The pioneering days are over. Neurosurgery is an accepted part of medical practice, more widely available than ever before and expanding. (Jennett, 1964, p. vii)

Certainly, in terms of underlying scientific rationale and technological sophistication, brain surgery has come a long way since early adventures in trephining. However, much of this advance has been extremely recent. Even fairly contemporary precursors of present-day surgical activities attracted widespread charges of quackery. As Garrison (1924) illustrated –

> In the sixteenth and seventeenth centuries it was a common byword to describe a person mentally unbalanced as having "a stone in his head". The therapeutic imposture consisted in making a superficial incision in the scalp, and palming a stone or stones, which were cast into a convenient basket at stated intervals during the patient's struggles. (p. 303)

One of the paintings composed sometime between 1475 and 1480, by the Flemish artist Hieronymus Bosch, shows such an operation. The Gothic inscription that adorns the painting reads as follows:

MEESTER SNIJT DIE KEIE RAS
MEJNE NAME IS LUBBERT DAS
(MASTER CUT OUT THIS STONE
MY NAME IS LUBBERT DAS)

The stone (Keie) mentioned here is the stone of madness, which was commonly thought (by individuals such as Lubbert Das – a name denoting a fool) to underlie insanity. The artist depicts this Master as a charlatan by making him wear a funnel instead of a hat. The funnel was one of the favourite symbols of trickery in the painter's repertoire, a symbol he often used to denote alchemy.

Clearly both psychosurgery and neurosurgery can boast an historically impressive but scientifically ambiguous pedigree. However, although neurosurgery has been scientifically elevated from the quackery of the past, many contemporary critics contend that psychosurgery is still characterized by such arbitrary and erratic practices.

The first testament of a surgical procedure clearly meeting our definition of psychosurgery was probably given by Ruggiero Frugardi of Palermo, one of the Salerno School in Italy in the twelfth century. The text of the relevant passage given below is taken from the manuscript held in Florence:

> *De mania et melancolia*
> *Ad maniam uel melancoliam in summitate capitis incidatur cutis in modum crucis et craneum perforetur, ut material exhalet ad exteriora.*
>
> (Concerning mania and melancholy
> For mania and melancholy the skin at the top of the head should be incised in a cruciate fashion and the skull perforated to allow matter to escape.)

The first modern account of psychosurgery to be published was by Dr. Gottlieb Burckhardt (1891), who was the Director of an Institution for the insane at Prefargier, Switzerland. Burckhardt reported that for two years he had been trying to find a new means of treating otherwise incurable psychoses. Referring to his decision to operate, Burckhardt noted that "None of the cases operated upon was of traumatic origins, the indications for the operation were therefore purely psychiatric" (p. 463). Drawing on the results of animal experiments at the time and his own clinical observations, Burckhardt suggested that the psychotic behaviour displayed by some of his more uncontrollable patients was due, in part, to some malfunction of the brain. Thus, severing connections between certain brain areas should provide relief. The results were not impressive, however, for only one patient demonstrated a clear subsequent attenuation of psychotic symptoms, while one died and another developed epilepsy following the operation. The others showed no clear or substantial remission of psychotic symptoms but were reported as being easier to handle. Burckhardt remained optimistic. Greater attention to such surgical approaches would, he argued, undoubtedly bring better results. He concluded his report:

> But I will not allow myself to be discouraged, and hope that my colleagues won't also, and instead will use my experience and will themselves tread the path of cortical extirpation and achieve ever better and more satisfactory results. (p. 548)

Burckhardt's results, however, did not encourage any widespread enthusiasm for the psychosurgical method of treatment, and it was only many years later that Puusepp (1937) reported that he also had operated on three manic-depressive patients, in 1910, at the Psycho-Neurological Institute in St. Petersburg, Russia. He severed the nerve connections between the parietal and frontal lobes. He was not impressed with the results, noting that "the success of the operation was rather poor, so that I no longer continued operations of this sort" (p. 14). Despite this setback, Puusepp did return to psychosurgery after the publication of Moniz's apparently more successful results in the mid-1930s. Until that time, then, Burckhardt's and Puusepp's early enterprises clearly had little impact, and for the first third of this century, interest in psychosurgery was minimal. However, accumulating data from surgical experiments on the brain of non-human animals were to rekindle enthusiasm.

The animal experiments in the 1930s that renewed interest in psychosurgery were the latest in the long line stretching far back into the last century. Their purpose was to elucidate the function of the frontal areas of the cerebral cortex. These are highly developed regions in man and the main distinguishing features of the human brain. The functions of the frontal areas of the brain were shrouded in mystery. They attracted the label "silent areas", since they could not be clearly anchored to any definite functions connected with the processing of sensory information or the movement of skeletal muscles. Stimulation or injury of the frontal areas in humans revealed few obvious sensory or motor effects. Early examples of such injury testify to the subtleties of the behavioural effects observed.

One of the most dramatic cases of injury to the frontal areas of the brain was reported by Harlow, initially in 1848.

A dramatic accident befell Phineas Gage, a foreman of a construction gang working for the Rutland & Burlington Railroad in Vermont. On September 13, 1848, he was engaged in a routine blasting job. This involved placing a charge of blasting powder and a fuse in a hole and tamping (or packing it down) with an iron rod prior to adding sand. While engaged in this exercise, Gage was momentarily distracted. The tamping-iron struck the rock and ignited the powder, causing an explosion. The tamping-iron (a round smooth rod, 3 feet 7 inches in length and $1\frac{3}{4}$ inches in diameter, weighing $13\frac{1}{4}$ pounds) was driven into the air like a missile towards Gage's face. The iron passed right through Gage's left cheek and emerged from the top of his head (Figure 1.3), finally descending some distance away, smeared with brain. Gage was knocked to the ground by the explosion. He emitted a few convulsive twitches but in a few minutes was sufficiently recovered to speak. His men picked him up and carried him a short distance to an oxcart. He sat upright in the cart and was driven three-quarters of a mile to an hotel. Gage got out of the cart himself. He was able to climb a long flight of stairs in the hotel.

Dr. Williams attended Gage until Dr. Harlow arrived. They both examined the patient. Harlow reported that he was able to insert an index finger into either end of the aperture in Gage's head. Despite such an injury, Harlow noted that Gage's physical recovery was fairly rapid. However, Harlow (1866–1868) reported more insidious changes in Gage following the accident:

> The equilibrium or balance, so the speak, between his intellectual faculties and animal propensities, seems to have been destroyed. He is fitful, irreverent, indulging at times in the grossest profanity (which was not previously his custom), manifesting but little deference for his fellows, impatient of restraint or advice when it conflicts with his desires, at times pertinaciously obstinate, yet capricious and vacillating, devising many plans of future operation, which are no sooner arranged than they are abandoned in turn for others appearing more feasible. A child in his intellectual capacity and manifestations, he has the animal passions of a strong man. Previous to his injury, though untrained in the schools, he possessed a well-balanced mind, and was looked upon by those who knew him as a shrewd, smart business man, very energetic and persistent in executing all his plans of operation. In this regard his mind was radically changed, so decidedly that his friends and acquaintances said he was "no longer Gage". (pp. 339–340)

Gage remained capricious and vacillating. Apparently he could not hold down a responsible job; instead he tried his hand at various jobs in various countries. He even exhibited himself and the tamping-iron to earn money. In 1861, twelve and a half years after the accident, Gage died in San Francisco. Just prior to his death, he suffered a series of convulsions. Unfor-

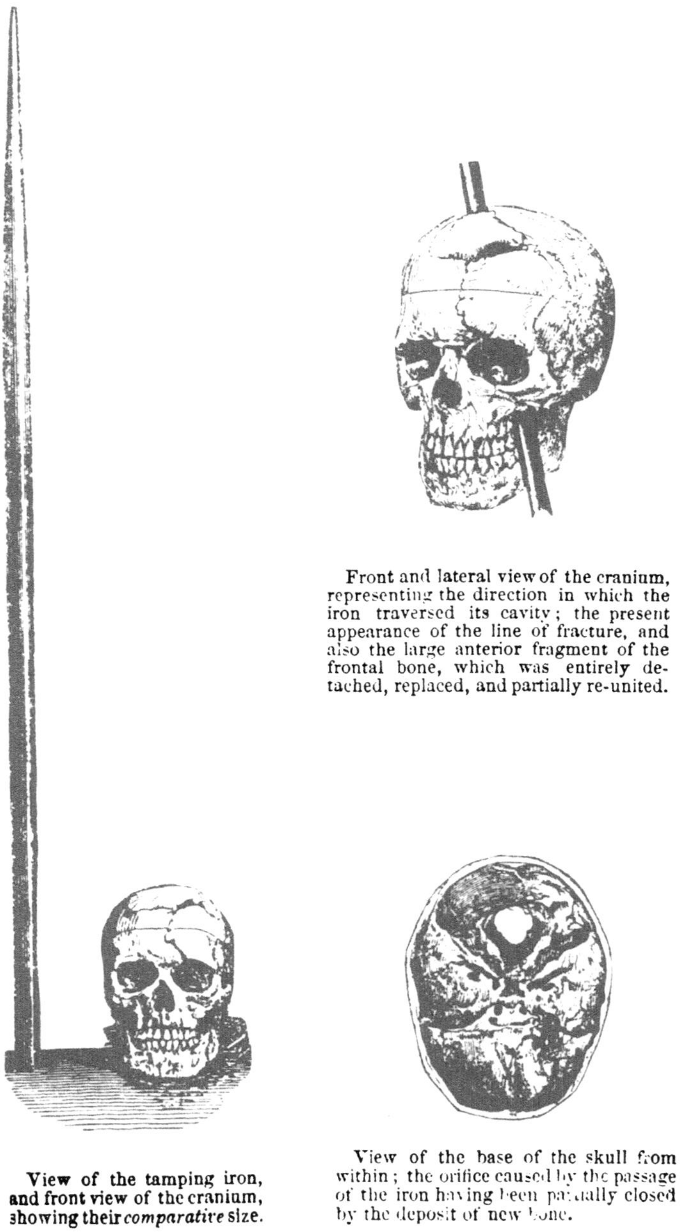

Figure 1.3 Sketch showing relation between tamping iron and Gage's skull. The iron bar was driven through Gage's left cheek and came out of the top of his head (from: Harlow, 1866–1868)

tunately no autopsy was performed, but the skull was sent to Harlow "for the benefit of science" (p. 342).

The British neurologist Sir David Ferrier (1886) was among the first to conduct comprehensive and controlled studies on the frontal lobes of non-human animals. While minimal physiological disruption was recorded, subtle psychological changes were apparent, as Ferrier noted of monkeys:

> Instead of, as before, being actively interested in their surroundings, and curiously prying into all that came within the field of their observation, they remained apathetic, or dull, or dozed off to sleep, responding only to the sensations or impressions of the moment, or varying their listlessness with restless and purposeless wanderings to and fro. While not actually deprived of intelligence, they had lost, to all appearance, the faculty of attentive and intelligent observation. (pp. 231–232)

Further, the animals became tamer and more docile following destruction of their frontal lobes, a result also reported in dogs by Goltz (1881). Goltz's experiments strongly influenced Burckhardt. Clearly, however, information regarding the functional significance of the frontal lobes was anecdotal and far from complete.

As indicated, renewed interest in psychosurgery in the 1930s was influenced by the results of contemporary experiments in animals, directed at elaborating further the function of the frontal brain areas. Carlyle Jacobsen and John F. Fulton conducted the most influential experiments. They were engaged in a programme of selectively destroying parts of the frontal cortex in chimpanzees and observing the behavioural consequences of such anatomical intrusions. Their data indicated that lesions in the prefrontal areas led to impairment of performance in a variety of tasks, including one that enforced a response delay. Briefly, in this delayed-response task a large cage was partitioned into two by an opaque screen. One of the sectors thus formed contained two food wells, each covered by a cup. The chimpanzee was put in the other half of the cage and was permitted to view, through a grille in the screen, the filling of one of the food wells. The grille was then covered, and after a specified period of time a door in the screen was opened, allowing the animal access to the other half of the cage.

Although able to enter the cage and procure the food when no delay was enforced, chimpanzees with bilateral frontal-lobe lesions were unable to cope with even the most minor delays (viz. 2 seconds).

Under the regimen of a delay between observing the well being filled and being allowed access to the wells, operated animals seemed incapable of consistently making the appropriate response. They demonstrated what is called a "delayed response deficit". It was, however, other consequences of such operations that fuelled interest in psychosurgery; in particular, the change apparent in a chimpanzee called Becky.

Prior to the operation, Becky engaged in violent temper tantrums when frustrated by such delayed-response procedures, i.e. when she made an error. Eventually Becky would not enter the experimental cage except under duress, such was her "experimental neurosis". However, following the bilateral operation, Becky's reactions to such frustration markedly changed. As Jacobsen *et al.* (1935) reported:

> ... while the subject failed repeatedly and made a far greater number of errors than it had previously, it was quite impossible to evoke even a suggestion of an "experimental neurosis". It was as if the animal had joined the "happiness cult of Elder Micheaux" and had placed its burdens on the Lord! (p. 10)

At the Second International Neurological Conference, held in London during the summer of 1935, the results of Fulton and Jacobsen's experiments were presented by Jacobsen. In the audience was the 61-year-old Professor of Neurology at the University of Lisbon, Antonio Caetano de Abreu Freire Egas Moniz. Moniz had been a member of the Portuguese parliament at the age of 29 and attended the Paris Peace Conference in 1919 as foreign minister. He became director of the new Neurological Institute at the University of Lisbon at the age of 37. His reputation spread as a result of his procedure for enabling the brain's blood vessels to be shown on X-ray, a procedure known as "cerebral angiography".

Also presented at the conference was a paper by Brickner (1936). He described the outcome of an operation conducted by Dandy which involved extirpating an individual's frontal lobes. However, it was not this paper that provoked Moniz's main interest but rather that of Fulton and Jacobsen. Fulton (1949) himself described what happened after Jacobsen had presented their results:

> Dr. Moniz arose and asked if frontal-lobe removal prevents the development of experimental neuroses in animals and eliminates frustrational behaviour why would it not be feasible to relieve anxiety states in man by surgical means? (p. 63–64)

Fulton thought that Moniz was enquiring about the complete excision of large parts of the prefrontal area in man, as they had done with chimpanzees. Walter Freeman and James Watts (1950) took up the story:

> This was too much for Fulton, but Egas Moniz marshalled his forces and finally persuaded Almeida Lima to operate upon certain patients who had proven refractory to other methods of treatment (p. xvi).

As indicated, Fulton and Jacobsen's report is conventionally regarded as providing the primary inspiration for Moniz's operations. Thus, their data are seen as crucial in the genesis of modern psychosurgery. Valenstein (1973a) referred to the "decisive influence on Moniz" (p. 390) that these data had. However, Moniz (1936a, b) does not reference any debt to Fulton and Jacobsen in his early accounts. In fact, in his reminiscence, *Mein Weg zür Leukotomie* (My road to leucotomy), Moniz (1948) set the development of his operations in quite a different context:

> It was no sudden inspiration which caused me to work out the surgical operation which I named *prefrontal leucotomy* ... after two years' deliberation, I determined to sever the connecting fibres of the neurons in question. (p. 23)

This representation was reiterated by Moniz (1956) in *How I succeeded in performing the prefrontal leucotomy*. Willett's (1960) account of the origins of psychosurgery perhaps more accurately gauged the influence of Fulton and Jacobsen's report as "merely crystallizing certain ideas along lines he had already adumbrated at the time" (p. 567). Certainly, speculations about the potential of surgery for the treatment of mental illness were "in the air" at the time. Ody (1938) claimed that he had performed psychosurgery some months before (April 1936) Moniz's early paper (June 1936) reached him. Just prior to Fulton and Jacobsen's presentation, a Dr. W. J. Mayo addressed the following remarks to a meeting of the Association of American Railroads in July 1935 (as reported in 1941 by Woltman *et al.*):

> If necessary we shall perform exploratory operations on the head at an early stage of disease and turn the light of day onto many of the pathological conditions of the brain ... Are we not in the same position in the treatment of the mentally afflicted that we were in the surgery of the abdomen, when I began fifty years ago, or as we were in the surgery of the chest? Day by day, I can see the extension of remedial means to conditions of the brain at earlier stages. (p. 200)

Further, psychiatrists in the 1930s appeared only too eager to embrace more technically impressive therapeutic innovations. The time was ripe for psychosurgery. It is no coincidence that this period in the history of psychiatry should also witness the development and rapid growth of electroconvulsive therapy.

The first operation took place on November 12, 1935. Moniz was not a neurosurgeon, but persuaded Almeida Lima to conduct the operation. Moniz and Lima (1936) reported using alcohol injections at first to destroy the white matter of the nerve fibres (rather than the grey matter of the nerve cell bodies). Later, Moniz modified this form of operation and developed leucotomy (or "leukotomy") (from the Greek " leukos" – white, and "tome" – cut; since white matter was sectioned)*.

* Leucotomy is also known as "lobotomy", especially in the United States. In the present work, however, the form *leucotomy* will be used. Similarly, many of the more specialized operations bear names ending in the suffixes "-ectomy" and "-otomy", both of which will be used here; for example, "cingul*ectomy*" or "cingul*otomy*". The suffix "-otomy" is more used in the names of certain operations, i.e. "thalamotomy".

Moniz noted that all the original twenty patients survived. Seven were considered to have recovered completely, and a further seven improved. Moniz (1956) later wrote, "We obtained cures and improvements but no failures to make us draw back" (p. 11).

The results were interpreted as being very encouraging, both by Moniz and by later supporters of psychosurgery. Moniz's activities in this area were curtailed, though, when he was shot by a leucotomized patient. The bullet lodged in his spine; Moniz retired a hemiplegic in 1944. It is unlikely that he had completed more than 100 operations. In 1949 he shared the Nobel Prize in Medicine and Physiology with Walter Hess; as the Nobel Foundation (1964) reported, "for his discovery of the therapeutic value of prefrontal leucotomy in certain psychoses" (p. 241). He died in 1955.

It fell to Walter Freeman to take over the role of "Father of Psychosurgery". Moniz's technique was modified by Freeman and Watts and was introduced into the United States in 1936. The two Americans, working at University of Georgetown, Washington, devised the "standard" technique of operating. Along with later modifications, this procedure rapidly gained popularity. Psychosurgery had truly arrived. Its arrival is illustrated by Freeman's (1971) postretirement claim that he had been "personally concerned" (p. 622) with some 3500 operations. Valenstein (1973a) estimated that some 40 000 (p. 55) of the older types of operation had been carried out in the United States. Less conservatively, Breggin (1972b) reckoned that some 50 000 patients received psychosurgical treatment in this "first wave". Tooth and Newton (1961) estimated that the figure for the United Kingdom was by 1954 some 12 000. This upsurge in interest in psychosurgery was reflected by an increase in publications on the subject (Kelly, 1975).

The First International Congress on psychosurgery took place in August 1948, in Lisbon. Walter Freeman (cf. Freeman, 1948a) was invested by Moniz as a Member of the Academy of Sciences of Lisbon. Titles and abstracts of 56 papers were received in time to be entered on the programme, but less than half of these were delivered. Various surgical techniques were described and discussed, as were the indications for various patient populations, some 8000 cases being reviewed in all.

However, this period proved to be the apex of psychosurgery. As Kelly noted, publications in this area diminished in the 1960s. There was no annual review of psychosurgery in the 1964 and subsequent editions of *Progress in Neurology and Psychiatry*, even though that journal had held such a report every year since its founding in 1946. This relative quiescence reflected a general decrease in psychosurgical activity. Frontal surgery was on the wane.

Valenstein (1973a) attributed the frantic years of psychosurgery to the need to deal efficiently with the larger number of psychiatrically disabled soldiers returning from World War II. Certainly this problem was temporary, and a subsequent decline in psychosurgery would be expected. However, it is probable that the synthesis of psychoactive chemicals, particularly the major tranquillizer chlorpromazine, in the mid-1950s, contributed substantially to the decreased incidence of surgery. Chlorpromazine offered an easier and more efficient means of managing the behaviour of highly disturbed patients. The increasing lobby critical of the seemingly imprecise methods of operation, and the adverse sequelae that were becoming more readily apparent as psychosurgery's focus of attention extended to encompass less disturbed sections of the population, possibly reinforced the winding down of psychosurgical programmes.

However, even as the decline in psychosurgery was beginning, a newer body of knowledge on brain functional organization was growing. This ultimately contributed to a surgical resurgence. As Livingston (1969), in his review entitled *The frontal lobe revisited: The case for a second look*, observed:

> In retrospect, even as lobotomy fell from grace clinical evidence consistent with earlier physiological concepts was rapidly accumulating ... On the basis of this evidence it could be postulated that the "key" to understanding the effects of frontal lobotomy lay in the elucidation of functional frontolimbic relationships – the mechanisms by which frontal lesions may alter limbic system function. (p. 92)

Here Livingston was charting a trend away from the more extensive lateral interventions of the older leucotomies towards more circumscribed lesioning of the medial and orbital frontal region. In addition, Livingston indicated the rationale underlying these newer, more restricted ventures. Unlike the lateral operations, medial and orbital surgery was considered to result specifically in changes in emotional behaviour. The intimate connection of the orbital and medial frontal areas with the limbic system was presumed to underlie such changes. Clearly, these more restricted lesions seemed more suitable to realize psychosurgery's primary aim, which was not so much to *cure* the patient's illness as to reduce the emotional impact of it.

Complementing this change in anatomical focus was a noticeable shift in the type of patient thought suitable for psychosurgery. Chronically ill, deteriorated patients who, as Valenstein (1973a) described, "have been emotionally spent for a long time" (p. 318) were clearly considered poor candidates for the newer orbital and medial procedures. Acutely ill patients, presenting a less daunting pedigree of psychopathology, were considered more suitable.

The restriction of surgery to the medial and orbital regions of the frontal cortex reflected the developing neuropsychological interest in the limbic system and its role in emotional behaviour. It undoubtedly seemed a small step from lesioning frontal regions to effect alterations in limbic system functioning to lesioning limbic system structures *per se*.

So, what Breggin (1973a) has termed the "second wave" of psychosurgery was to be mainly directed at the limbic system, a group of functionally related structures lying deep within the brain. The gradually emerging evidence that this system is intimately involved in emotional aspects of behaviour readily commended it to psychosurgeons. Its involvement in emotional behaviour was first postulated by Papez (1937):

> There is no clinical or other evidence to support this view. The new interpretation which I propose can be supported by much more data at present available in the literature, but it is evident that any such doctrine will have to stand the test of experimental and clinical experience if it is to be useful in science. Emotion is such an important function that its mechanism, whatever it is, should be placed on a structural basis. (p. 743)

However, as Maclean (1949) noted in his discussion of Papez's hypothesis, such experimental experience was readily forthcoming, for in the same year Henreich Klüver and Paul Bucy (1937) published their data on behavioural consequences of lesions of the temporal lobe on both sides of the brain of rhesus monkeys. Such a surgical procedure ablates various limbic system structures.

Five major behavioural changes emerged following the operations performed by Klüver and Bucy (1938), and the constellation of these effects became known as the "Klüver–Bucy syndrome".

(1) Psychic blindness (an inability to recognize objects by sight).

(2) Strong oral tendencies, in that all objects are examined by mouth rather than by hand.

(3) Strong tendency to attend and react to any visual stimulus – "hypermetamorphosis"

(4) Marked change in emotional behaviour, i.e. motor and vocal reactions generally associated with anger and fear are not exhibited.

(5) Increase in sexual activity.

Schreiner and Kling (1953, 1956) subsequently replicated these findings in a wide range of non-human species.

The most important finding, as far as psychosurgeons were concerned, was the attenuation of emotional behaviour. A major structure in the "circuit of emotion", as described by Papez (1937), is the *cingulate gyrus*. *Cingulectomy* (operations on the cingulate gyrus) developed from the earlier outcome of psychosurgical procedures and as a consequence of findings in animal experiments. Ward (1948), for example, reported that after ablation of the cingular gyrus (Brodman's area 24, see Chapter 2), monkeys showed no fear of man. In bolstering his argument that the cingulate gyrus was of crucial significance, he described the "unusual case of the good knight, Caspar Bonecurtius", recorded prior to 1670 by the Professor of Medicine at Basle, Felix Plater.

This knight gradually became mentally deranged over a period of two years, and his brain was examined following his death a short time later:

> At autopsy a globular tumour was found over the anterior portion of the corpus callosum which must certainly have partially destroyed the anterior portion of the cingulate gyrus. (p. 438)

Such observation on patients with tumours in these areas, together with the results of animal research, led Ward (1948) to perform bilateral anterior cingulectomy on humans. The development of cingulectomy was an important factor in the revival of psychosurgery. It is now one of the most frequently performed psychosurgical operations and is considered appropriate for a range of patients suffering from a variety of psychiatric disorders.

However, cingulectomy was not the only outcome of neuropsychological forays into the limbic system of non-human animals. The finding that wild, uncontrollable animals could be rendered tame by surgery addressed to the limbic system held other implications. As indicated previously, the work of Klüver and Bucy, as well as that of Schreiner and Kling, clearly demonstrated that limbic surgery led to a decline in emotional tone. It soon became clear that emotional docility might be produced by attention to individual structures within this system. In addition to the cingular gyrus, the amygdala readily emerged as such a structure. As Woods (1956) observed of amygdalotomized wild Baltimore rats:

> The most striking change in the behavior of these rats is that, immediately following the operation, they no longer bite the experimenter. As soon as they recover from the anaesthetic (ether) they can be handled without gloves and without fear of attack. Large (500–600 g) operated wild rats may be carried about for hours in the laboratory coat pocket without incident. (p. 369)

The implications such studies held for possible human surgical remedies were not long in receiving voice. In fact, even before this last study was published, a report by Sawa *et al.* (1954) appeared in print. This was followed closely by a series of amygdala operations conducted by Narabayashi and his associates (cf. Narabayashi and Uno, 1966).

Soon, related limbic-system components were mooted as potential surgical foci, and once again psychosurgery became a fashionable practice. In the United States, according the Valenstein's (1977) survey conducted under the auspices of the National Commission for the Protection of Human Subjects of Biomedical and Behavioral Research, just over 400 psychosurgical operations were being carried out annually at the time of the survey. A further survey carried out on their behalf revealed some 200 to 250 such operations in the United Kingdom per year: an earlier estimate given by the Royal College of Psychiatrists (1977), which was based on statistics supplied by the Department of Health and Social Security, gave figures ranging from 200 to 300*.

The Second International Congress of Psychosurgery, held in Copenhagen in 1970, heralded this revival of psychosurgery. A Third International Congress quickly followed in 1973 at Cambridge, England. The Fourth Congress was held in 1975 in Madrid. A "Renaissance of Psychosurgery", as Rylander (1973) termed it, was clearly taking place.

* The most recent figures available, however, indicate a drop in the incidence of United Kingdom operations to around 70 per annum (House of Commons (1981). *Hansard*, 8 (no. 144). 32).

2

Operative techniques

The renaissance of psychosurgery would not have been possible without three major developments: improved techniques of operation; the delineation of other areas of the brain as appropriate for surgical intervention, areas connected with and part of the limbic system; and a shift in psychosurgery's clientele to include psychiatric and behavioural "disorders" that could be classified as "illnesses" only with difficulty. It was not merely that these developments emerged at the same time that provided the new impetus for psychosurgery, although the years 1947–1951 were indeed crucial. Rather, it was the way in which they complemented each other that halted the decline in surgery and paved the way for its renewed growth.

As indicated, one of the major reasons for the decline in psychosurgery in the late 1950s and early 1960s was the disquiet about the prevalent techniques of operation. Critics characterized these procedures as imprecise and haphazard, leading to impairment of function far outweighing any possible benefits accruing from them. Consequently a great deal of time and effort was invested by psychosurgeons in trying to find more exact methods of operation. Historically, psychosurgeons have always sought to improve the technology of their business. Mention has already been made of Burckhardt's dissatisfaction with his own technique and call for better operative procedures.

Egas Moniz and Almeida Lima (1936) initially reported using injections of alcohol to destroy the subcortical nerve fibres. In the year following the publication of Moniz's monograph, Fiamberti (1937) wrote that he too had used alcohol injections in leucotomy. Another Italian, Donagio (1939), advised injections of procaine (a local anaesthetic), although he presented no case reports.

In France, Leriche (1949) reported using procaine infiltrations in his search for a method of relieving intractable pain. Although surgery for the treatment of pain lies outside the scope of this book, techniques used for its treatment will sometimes be included when they have been important in the development of psychosurgical techniques. Mandl (e.g. Mandl, 1951), working in Austria, also used procaine injections, occasionally with the addition of phenol (a powerful antiseptic) in a weak solution, to help relieve intractable pain associated with terminal cancer. In France, Abély (1952) reported using procaine injections on schizophrenics as a "non mutilante" form of psychosurgical therapy.

The development by Bucaille (1952) of a fairly precise technique of injecting procaine to relieve intractable pain can be seen as a major advance. Later, Soupault and Bucaille (1955) described their method of operation, commenting on the inaccuracy of some of the procedures used by other workers in this field.

In Argentina, Krapf and Lyonnet (1951) reported using procaine injections to predict the likely effect of permanent leucotomy. Van Wagenen and Liu (1952) also used temporary procaine block of white fibres in the frontal lobes as a means of predicting the effects of subsequent prefrontal leucotomy. Injections of procaine under pressure will, as Soupault and Bucaille observed, result in permanent lesions, whereas infiltration not under pressure produces only temporary effects. Van Wagenen and Liu reported that, in two cases out of three, temporary procaine block produced similar psychological effects to those observed following prefrontal leucotomy, and they particularly recommend procaine block in predicting relief from usual complaints of pain.

Narabayashi *et al.* (1963) reported that they had blocked or destroyed the amygdaloid nuclei by means of a mixture of oil and wax to which Lipiodol (poppy seed oil containing iodine) was added for easier identification of the area of lesion by X-ray. More unusual liquids have been injected into the brain, such as the patient's own blood by Stender (1950). No doubt other substances will be used to produce lesions by injection techniques, especially those that act more specifically at the nerve-cell level, selectively destroying certain types of cell. However, despite the development of these more sophisticated methods of injecting substances into the brain to produce limited destructive lesions, chemically mediated psychosurgery is not common. Other procedures are generally regarded as more precise. As Walder and Jaspar (1970) observed of injections:

> The disadvantage is that the injected fluid diffused readily, so that again it is impossible to predict the extent of the lesion. Efforts have been

made to control diffusion by dissolving the agent in a viscous mass. (pp. 353–354)

Indeed, early in psychosurgery's development, Moniz and Lima abandoned the use of alcohol injections and instead used an instrument called a leucotome to section white matter. This leucotome is shaped like a cannula with a knob on the top. Once the instrument was considered to be in the correct location for operation, the knob was pressed, thus pushing out a wire loop. Then the whole implement was rotated to section particular cores of brain tissue. Other leucotomes were soon developed. McGregor and Crumbie (1941) described an "improved leucotome", which had a rotating blade. McKenzie (1944) designed another leucotome, which could be inserted into the area of operation in the same manner as a cannula. By pushing the scissor-like holder upwards, a wire loop is forced out. Freeman and Watts (1942) developed a "precision leucotome", which had a blade with rounded edges calibrated in centrimetres and a movable side arm (Figure 2.1). They also used a somewhat wider blunt knife called a "radial stab incisor" to stab more deeply into the white matter. Fiamberti (1937) used a finer "needle like" leucotome for use in operating on the frontal lobes through the orbital cavity.

Freeman (1948b) designed his own form of "transorbital leucotome". Other forms of instruments have been used for the various types of psychosurgical operation; these have included spatulas, forceps, hooks, and double-

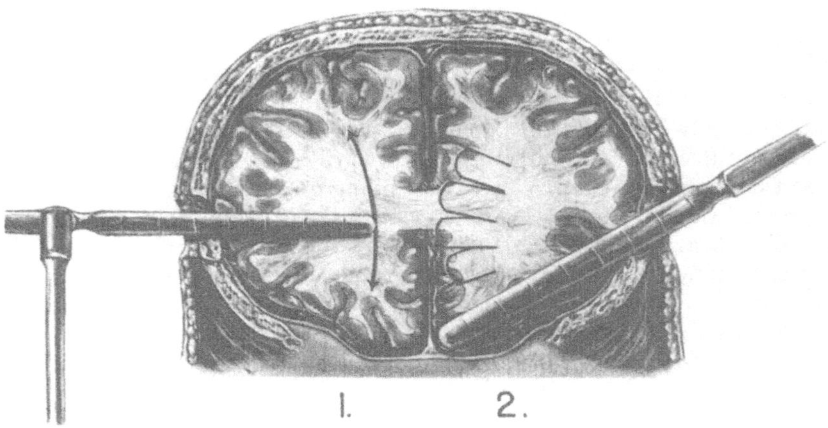

Figure 2.1 The "standard leucotomy" of Freeman and Watts. The "precision" leucotome was inserted through a burr hole in the side of the head and moved in an arc in the coronal plane. Afterwards the "radial stab incisor" was used to deepen the cuts (from: Freeman and Watts, 1950). Courtesy of Charles C. Thomas, Publishers, Springfield, Illinois

edged knives for sectioning brain tissue. McKissock (1943) viewed such developments with some scepticism:

> If one regards dispassionately the set of instruments used by almost any surgeon in the practice of his art it is indeed difficult to abstain from criticism. That they are clumsy and but ill-adapted to their work is obvious to the most uneducated eye. They compare, relatively speaking, most unfavourably with the items of the tool kit supplied with the average modern automobile. When contrasted with the delicate, but strong and beautifully designed tools of the dental surgeon they appear even more gross and unsuited for their work than at first sight. And why should this be? It is due only to us surgeons ourselves; we are as a class most unmechanically minded men, and yet we persist in inventing instruments for particular purposes each one of which we fondly imagine is better suited to achieve its end than anything that has gone before. No finer example of this tendency could be found than in the astonishing creations which have been produced in connection with prefrontal leucotomy. (p. 195)

In the operation by Moniz and Lima a hole, called a "burr hole", was made in the skull, and the leucotome was inserted through this at different angles. When the instrument was in the correct place, it was rotated so that cores of nerve fibres in the frontal lobes were sectioned.

Freeman and Watts (1942), who introduced psychosurgery into the United States, employed the Moniz technique in their first series of operations. They reported dissatisfaction with this procedure, however, and therefore modified it. Even these modifications did not yield entirely satisfactory results, and so they devised their own operative procedure. This procedure was later called the "precision" technique by Freeman and Watts (1950) and eventually consisted of three alternative operations known as the "standard", the "radical" and the "minimal" "lobotomy", depending on the extent of the lesions.

In the "standard lobotomy", described more fully by Freeman and Watts (1950), a burr hole was made on either side of the head above and behind the eye, using the coronal suture (transverse line of union across the skull between the frontal and parietal bones in the skull and often used as a reference point in psychosurgery) and the sphenoidal ridge (a wedge-shaped bone at the base of the skull) as landmarks. The hole was centred 3 cm behind the lateral wall of the orbit of the eye and 6 cm above the zygomatic arch (the cheekbone). The "precision" leucotome was inserted into the burr hole and moved in a sweeping motion so that the nerve fibres were sliced in an arc in the coronal plane, the procedure being repeated on the other side of the head. After the sweeping incisions had been made, the "radial stab incisor" was pushed into the burr hole to deepen the cuts in the white matter without damaging the larger blood vessels (see Figure 2.1).

For ease of comparison, the various psychosurgical operations, especially

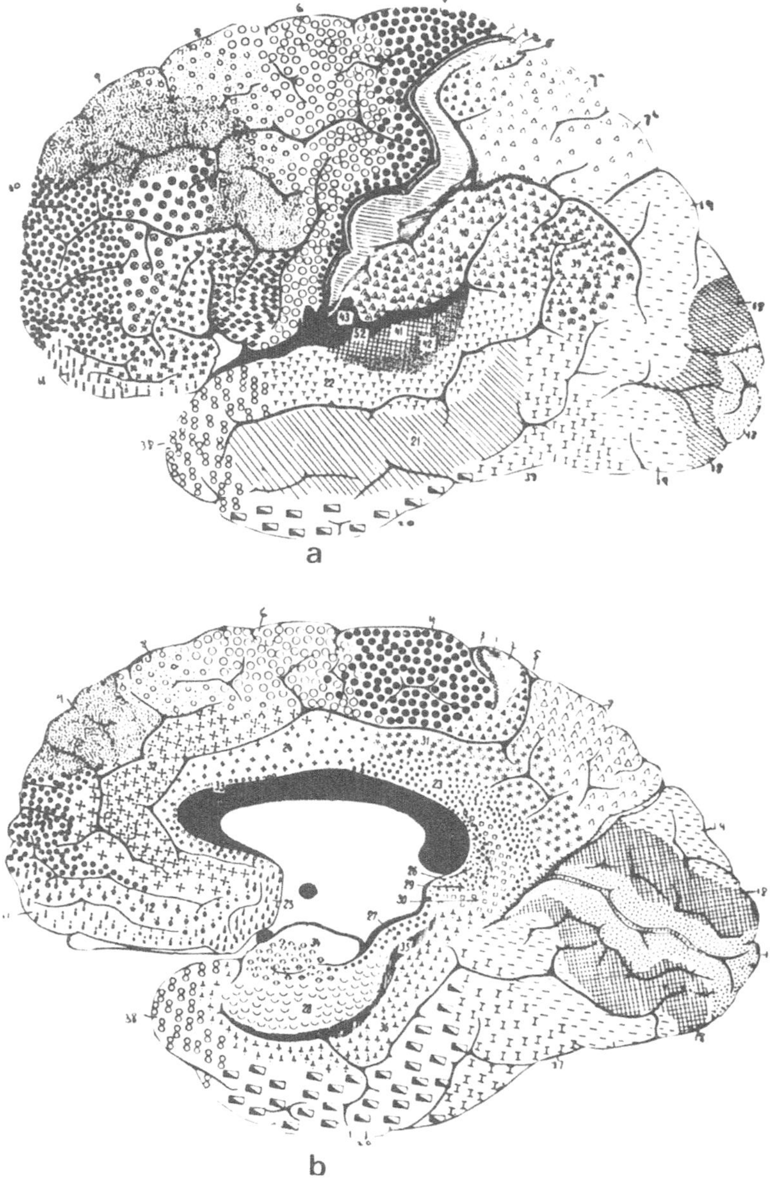

Figure 2.2 Brodmann's cytoarchitectural maps of the brain; (a) lateral and (b) medial aspects

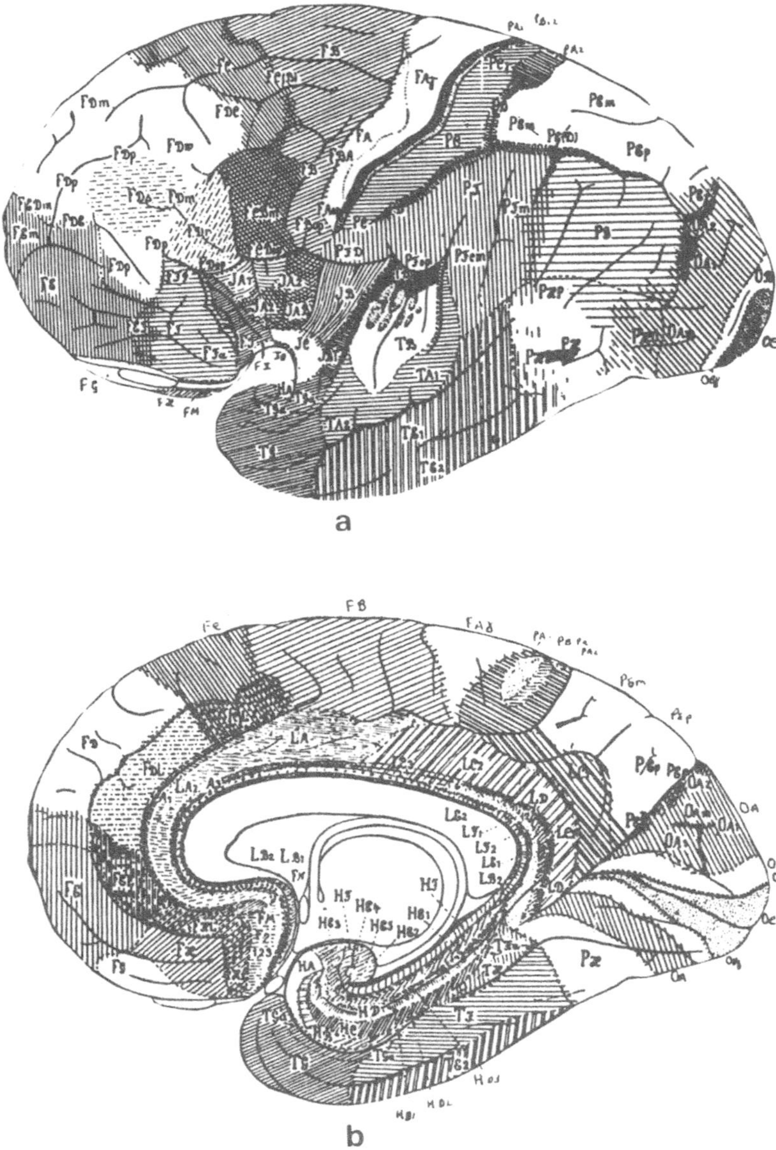

Figure 2.3 Cytoarchitectural maps of Von Economo and Koskinas; (a) lateral and (b) medial aspects

the older ones, are described in terms of the areas of Brodmann which they have as a target. Brodmann (1909) devised a system of dividing the brain into anatomical areas on the basis of the morphological variations and distributions of the nerve cell bodies of the brain (Figure 2.2). Although Von Economo and Koskinas (1925) provided a more recent division of the brain (Figure 2.3), the anatomical foci of most psychosurgical operations, especially the older ones, were described in terms of the Brodmann areas. Hence Brodmann's scheme will be adhered to in the present discussion, although by reference to the "cyto-architectural maps" ("cyto" – Greek for "cell") of Brodmann and by comparing them with those of Von Economo and

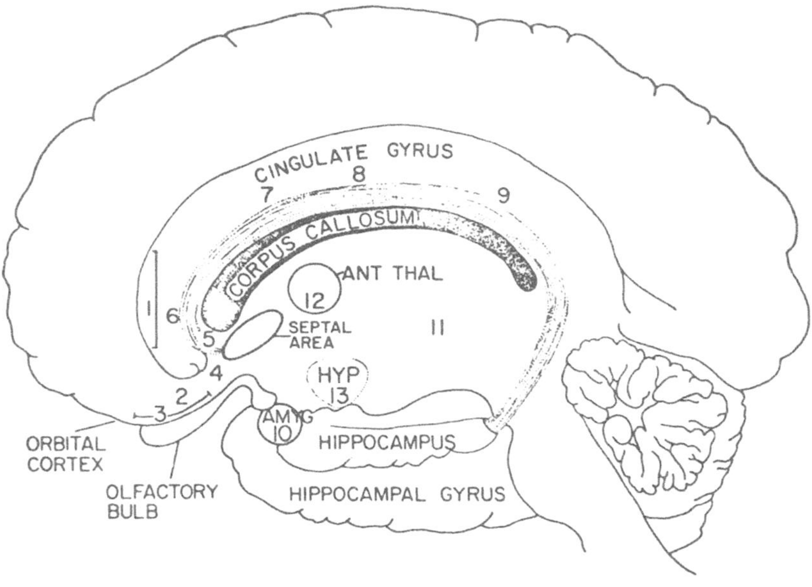

Frontal Lobe Procedures

1. Bimedial leucotomy
2. Yttrium lesions in subcortical white matter
3. Orbital undercutting
4. Basal tractotomy and substantia innominotomy
5. Anterior capsulotomy (destruction of fibers of internal capsule)
6. Mesoloviotomy (similar to rostral cingulotomy, but lesion invades genu "knee" of corpus callosum)

Cingulotomies

7. Anterior cingulotomy
8. Mid-cingulotomy
9. Posterior cingulotomy

Amygdalectomy

10. Amygdalectomy or amygdalotomy

Thalatomies

11. Dorsomedial, centromedian, parafascicular nuclei
12. Anterior thalatomy

Hypothalotomy

13. Posterior, ventromedial, and lateral hypothalamic targets

Figure 2.4 Diagram of the various psychosurgical procedures (from: Valenstein, 1977)

Koskinas, translation between the two systems is easily afforded.

Operations of various parts of the brain (Figure 2.4) can be translated into either of the two schemata. Further, reference is often made to the areas of incision in the coronal plane (that is, across the head from ear to ear) when comparing the various procedures. An incision in the coronal plane reveals grey matter (composed of nerve cell bodies) on the outside of the section, which encloses the white matter of the nerve fibres. The white matter on each side can be divided into four areas, or quadrants as they are usually called. The two quadrants of this white matter near the centre of the brain are described as being "medial" and those nearer the outside as "lateral". Two of these parts are "upper" and the others are "lower" quadrants. The system will be adopted here, although reference will occasionally be made

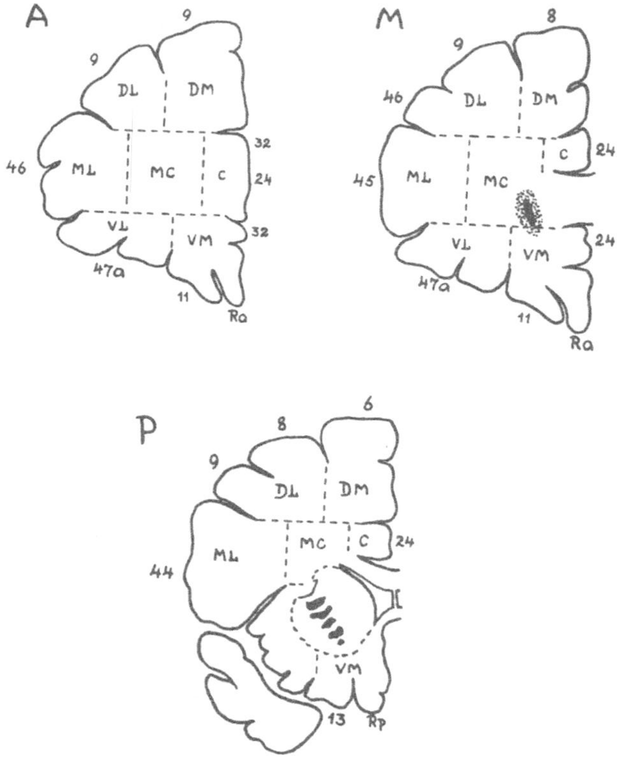

Figure 2.5 Meyer and Beck's division of coronal sections through anterior (A), middle (M) and posterior (P) planes into dorso-medial (DM), dorso-lateral (DL), mid-lateral (ML), ventro-lateral (VL), ventro-medial (VM), mid-central (MC) and cingulate (C) segments (from: Meyer and Beck, 1954). Courtesy of the publishers and Wallace and Guthrie, trustees of Wm. Ramsay Henderson Trust

to the more precise classification by Meyer and Beck (1954), who divided this coronal section into seven segments and further considered a coronal section both anterior and posterior to the standard (or middle) place of section (Figure 2.5).

As has already been noted, modifications of the standard technique were employed by Freeman and Watts. The "radical" procedure was performed in much the same way as the "standard lobotomy" except that the leucotome was inserted into the head from above and sectioning of the nerve fibres was made more posteriorly than in the standard operation. The "minimal" operation was designed to section less white matter than the "standard lobotomy". However, despite the success of the standard operation and its modifications, Freeman (1971) reported that he was still less than satisfied:

> In spite of the precision in the placement of the surgical lesions in the three grades of lobotomy, minimal, standard and radical, I became dissatisfied with the clinical end-results, and in 1946, after operations on the cadaver, applied the transorbital method described by Fiamberti. (pp. 621–622).

Fiamberti's (1937) procedure was a simpler method of operating on the frontal lobes by way of the orbital plate just above the eyes. Freeman (1948b) started using *transorbital leucotomy* (or "transorbital lobotomy" as he later described it) early in 1946, when he operated on 10 patients. He indicated that his leucotome was a better instrument than that used by Fiamberti. It was more readily driven through the bony orbital plate and more suited for the sectioning of the white matter of the frontal lobes. The operation was performed quickly and easily. The patient was generally given two to four electroconvulsive shocks within about five minutes. When the patient was unconscious, a towel was placed over the nose and mouth. The surgeon drew the eyelid away from the eyeball and inserted the leucotome, driving it through the bony cavity above the eye into the frontal lobes. If the orbital plate was too thick, a stronger instrument called an "orbiclast" was used to penetrate it. Once the leucotome was inserted to the desired depth in the frontal lobes, about 7 cm from the point of entry above the eye, the handle was moved medially and laterally so that the nerve fibres at the base of the frontal lobes were severed. The handle was then returned to its original position to determine in profile, either visually or photographically, if the desired location had been reached. The instrument was withdrawn, and pressure was applied upon the upper eyelid to control the escape of blood and cerebrospinal fluid into the orbital tissues. Sometimes, as Freeman noted (Freeman and Watts, 1950), there was "slight" discolouration of the eye due to the effusion (pouring out) of blood.

> Some of the "black eyes" are beauties, and I usually ask the family to provide the patient with sun glasses rather than explanations. Patients are encouraged to return home the day after operation. (p. 57)

Freeman regarded "transorbital lobotomy" as a relatively simple affair and described it as a minor operation; he suggested that it could be carried out by the psychiatrist. However, as Freeman (1971) indicated, Watts and he were at odds on this point of simplicity of operation:

> This method proved unacceptable to my surgical colleagues for the most part, though they were impressed by the accuracy and symmetry of the lesions. Watts and I parted company, and I proceeded on my own. (p. 622)

However, it was not just Watts who expressed concern about this type of operation. Many surgeons were doubtful regarding these "closed" or "blind" operations (so called because the practitioner operated through small burr holes in the skull and was not able to have direct vision of the area of operation). There were fears that haemorrhage from cut blood vessels could be inadvertently caused by the surgeon (even though in many such operations the aperture was washed with saline) and that such a haemorrhage might become apparent only at a belated stage. Furthermore, the surgeon could possibly section more white matter than was intended. This, it was felt, might lead to some functional impairment. Such misgivings prompted the development of alternative techniques of operation. As Watts and Murphy (1949) indicated:

> The reluctance of some neurosurgeons to perform lobotomy was partly eliminated by the open method devised by Lyerly and further developed by Poppen. However, some could not tolerate the idea of any type of cortical undercutting. They have to see what they cut, take out something, weigh it and examine it microscopically in order to feel that the operation has been done properly. Their conviction or stubbornness has led to lobotomy, gyrectomy and topectomy, which one must admit are proving a distinct contribution to the study of frontal lobe function. (p. 396)

Such an "open" procedure was no doubt more generally acceptable to neurosurgeons than the somewhat cavalier approach adopted by Freeman. Nevertheless, some surgeons continued, although reluctantly, to use the "blind" approach (McKissock, 1943).

Lyerly (1939), as indicated, was the main innovator of the "open" operation. His procedure permitted the surgeon to operate on the brain under direct vision. The operation involved making a trephine opening just back of the hairline on each side of the skull. The dura mater was then opened and part of the cerebral cortex beneath excised. A lighted speculum was inserted so that the surgeon could see and coagulate the smaller blood vessels and avoid the larger ones. Love (1943) described a modification of Lyerly's technique, a much more circumscribed procedure than the earlier extensive intrusion.

Poppen (1948) described his own "open" method of operation, and in the same year, Poppen *et al.* (1948) gave their general impressions based on the results of 470 patients subjected to this technique. Their procedure involved making two parallel incisions in the sagittal plane (that is, from the front of the skull to the back) in line with the pupil of each eye. These incisions were extended to the anterior border of the coronal suture on each side. After the scalp edges had been retracted and trephine holes in the skull made, the dura mater was opened with a semicircular incision and held back. A wedge of cortex was then excised by means of an electrosurgical suction unit, thus exposing the white tissue. The white matter was further divided by this unit. A lighted retractor was used by the surgeon to view the site of operation as well as to separate the brain tissue. A blunt speculum (a straight-line spatula) completed the leucotomy. Division in the lateral upper quadrant of the front lobes was accomplished with a curved instrument – small calibre suction tip. Once sufficient white matter was extracted, the bone buttons were replaced and the scalp incisions closed, the whole operation taking approximately one half hour.

Scarff (1948) devised a similar "open" approach, save that intervention was restricted to one side of the brain. Scarff applied this unilateral leucotomy to the relief of pain and the treatment of narcotic addiction. Throughout the history of the older forms of psychosurgery there has been continual debate as to whether unilateral leucotomy is to be preferred to bilateral leucotomy. Those in favour of the former noted that the dangers and complications observed with bilateral operations were halved with unilateral procedures. Those in favour of bilateral lesions argued that only operations on both lobes were fully effective.

An alternative method of sectioning less fibres than the standard operation was *bimedial leucotomy*. Bockoven and Greenblatt (1950) considered the latter to be a better method than the full operation and in a pilot study compared the results obtained after unilateral and bilateral leucotomy. The bimedial operation (together with the unilateral) was chosen for the Second Lobotomy Project at the Boston Psychopathic Hospital. The first project in 1943, used Poppen's bilateral open approach. In this second project, which compared the effectiveness of unilateral and bimedial leucotomy, a bilateral (full) operation was performed on a group of patients as a control. Greenblatt and Solomon (1953) described this bimedial operation in their report on the second project. This procedure, albeit bilateral, involved sectioning white matter only in the medial aspect of the Freeman and Watts' operative plane, a method later modified by Baker *et al.* (1970) using the McKenzie leucotome. Therefore, in anatomical terms, both bimedial and unilateral leucotomy involved the cutting of approximately one-half the fibres sectioned in the full bilateral (Freeman and Watts) operation (Figure 2.6).

Other modifications of the standard leucotomy restricted lesions to particularly anterior aspects of the frontal lobes. Peyton *et al.* (1948) described

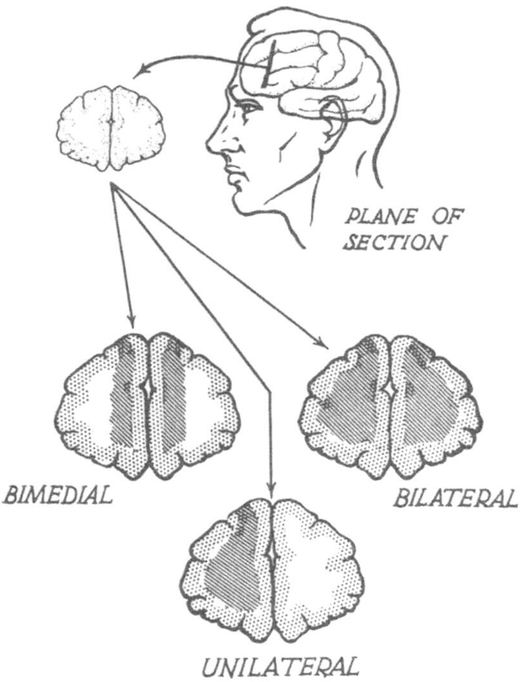

Figure 2.6 In anatomical terms bimedial and unilateral leucotomy involve the cutting of approximately one half of the fibres sectioned in the full bilateral operation of Freeman and Watts (from: Greenblatt and Solomon, 1953)

"a new form of psychosurgery" that involved removal of only the anterior part of the front lobes, a procedure similar to that proposed by Ody as early as 1938. A more anterior form of leucotomy was *topectomy*, begun in 1946 (cf. Pool, 1949). Topectomy involved bilateral removal of cortex from Brodman's regions 9 and 10. Circular areas of the frontal lobes were removed as a block, which, as Pool (1949) observed, was of prime importance.

> The cortex is removed as a block, which provides a means of estimating its extent and volume. We have weighed every specimen. We have also measured each cavity, which gives a fair idea of the volume as an added check. We think that the quantity of tissue removed is extremely important and that quantity is important in different categories of psychiatric illness. (p. 1)

No doubt it was to procedures such as this that Watts and Murphy (1949) directed their comments about some surgeons having to "see what they cut, take out something, weigh it and examine it microscopically in order to feel that the operation has been done properly".

Other modifications of the standard procedure were not based on different sites of operation (as with the above) but rather were more concerned with restricting the extent of the lesions, still using roughly the same plane of section as employed by Freeman and Watts. Jackson (1954) described his modification of the Freeman and Watts procedure. This was directed at the white matter in the lower and medial segments of the frontal lobes. Grantham (1951) likewise modified the standard operation by making lesions in the lower medial quadrant of the frontal lobes for relief of intractable pain. A few years earlier, Hofstatter *et al.* (1945) had already reported on limiting the Freeman and Watts full operation to the lower quadrants or orbital areas of the frontal lobes with some success and concluded that "The orbital areas of the frontal lobes seem to have a role in regulation of emotions" (p. 130).

It was at the First International Congress of Psychosurgery, held in Lisbon in early August 1948, that Scoville and Birdgame outlined their procedure, which was specifically aimed at the orbital areas of the frontal lobes. Scoville (1949) described his "open" method of operation, which he called "selective cortical undercutting". This procedure was aimed at three areas of the cerebral cortex: the superior surface (chiefly in areas 9 and 10 of Brodman), the orbital surface and, finally, the medial surface underlying the entire cingulate rostral gyrus both above and below the corpus callosum. Two trephine holes are drilled, either from a "superior" approach (the surgeon operating from behind the patient) or from an "inferior" approach (where he operates facing the patient), as Asenjo (1963) has described (Figure 2.7). A brain spatula is inserted into the holes, and, with the aid of a suction tip, Brodmann's areas 9 and 10 are undercut. To realize this undercutting of the orbital area, the frontal lobes are lifted so that the undersurface is exposed, allowing the medial fibres to be sectioned more easily. Finally, the whole rostral part of the cingulate gyrus above and below the corpus callosum is sectioned.

Besides Scoville's (1973) own modification of his original procedure to limit lesions to orbital undercutting, other developments were also reported. Hirose and Inugami (1958) reported to the Sixteenth Annual Meeting of the Japan Neurological Society, held in Okayama in 1957, on the introduction into Japan of orbital undercutting. Hirose (1965) later reported on "orbito-ventromedial undercutting", a modification of Scoville's procedure leaving the lateral and posterior orbital areas intact. In Britain, McKissock (1951) described an operation called "rostral leucotomy", which he noted was similar to Scoville's procedure except for being far more limited in the areas excised.

Tow and Lewin (1953) reported on a procedure that closely followed that

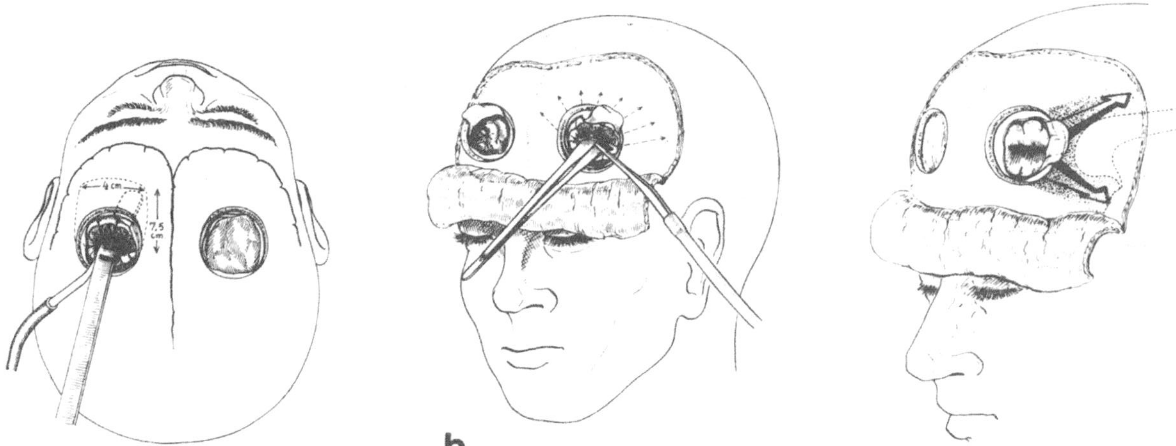

Figure 2.7 Scoville's open operation in which (a) two trephine holes are made, (b) a brain spatula is inserted and (c) Brodman's areas are undercut (from: Asenjo, 1963). Courtesy of Charles C. Thomas, Publisher, Springfield, Illinois

of Scoville, the operations being performed by Geoffrey Knight. Knight and Tredgold (1955) described this operation of restricted orbital undercutting as involving the extension of the incision in each frontal lobe for a distance of 6 cm, the last 2 cm entering the "substantia innominata" (the "unnamed substance", so called because for a long time no name was given to it) overlying Brodmann's area 13 and part of 14. Knight (1964) reported on 450 cases of operations on the orbital cortex and outlined the development of a different approach. Knight (1965) indicated that this new operation of "stereotactic tractotomy" (so called because it cut nerve tracts) concentrated on the last 2 cm of the lesion of the previous approach.

He decided to produce small lesions in this area of the substantia innominata in order to interrupt the superorbital fibres of the thalamo-frontal projection by a destructive agent that would avoid the hazards resulting from conventional cutting techniques. He used a version of McCaul's stereotactic device, an apparatus designed for a more accurate localization of areas within the brain for operation. Knight eventually inserted seeds of radioactive yttrium (^{90}Y) under X-ray control into the substantia innominata from above on both sides, corresponding to the last 2 cm of the undercutting incision. At first he used four rows of seeds but later only used three, leaving out the lateral ones. This reduction effected a more localized lesion.

Knight's use of radioactive yttrium seeds was one of a variety of techniques developed to produce small localized destructive lesions with a minimum of damage to surrounding tissue. The development of leucotomy by ultrasound (high frequency sound, generally above 20 kHz, inaudible to humans) represented one of the most technically advanced methods of producing these destructive lesions deep within the brain and was a far cry from the early mechanical and injection techniques of psychosurgery. The use of ultrasonic waves to produce lesions has many advantages over more conventional operative procedures, the main one being that damage to brain tissue resulting from the insertion of mechanical devices into the brain is avoided.

Fry *et al.* (1954) provided a description of a method of operation for primates. They clearly regarded ultrasound as a more precise technique than the then prevalent mechanical and chemical methods of producing lesions:

> The procedure described in this paper makes feasible the severing of deep fibre bundles in the central nervous system in primates or man with the following advantages over other surgical techniques: 1) no disturbance to brain tissue except in the focal region, 2) no cutting of brain tissue, 3) no disturbance to the blood vessels and 4) no opening of the dura mater. (p. 478)

In fact, it was not long before this method of producing small localized lesions was used in psychosurgery. As early as 1954, Lindstrom published an account of psychosurgery with ultrasound. Lindstrom reviewed the previous experiments using ultrasound and described his own method of operation (Figure

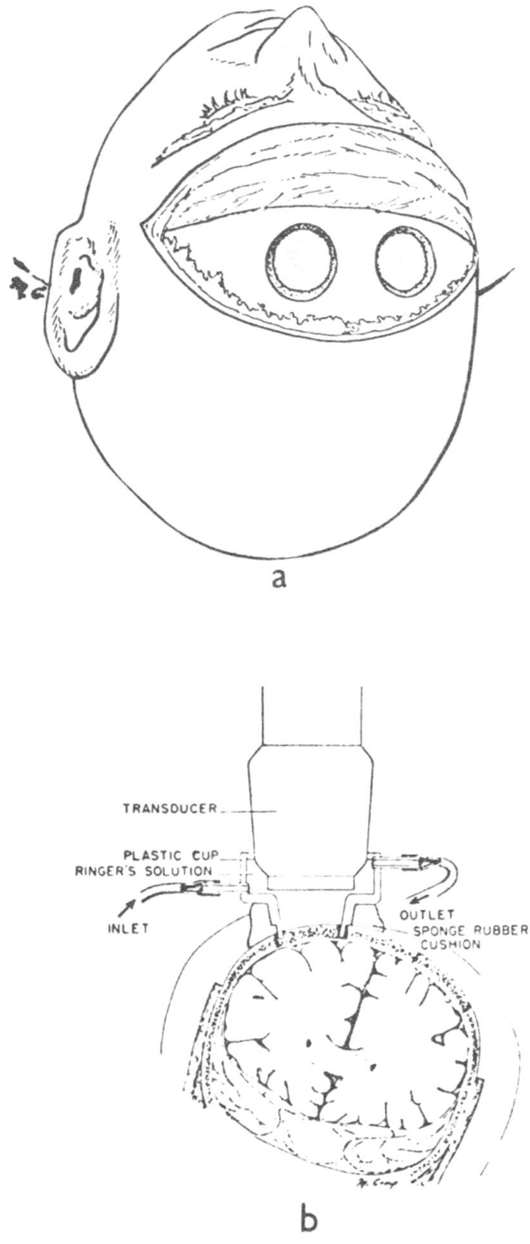

Figure 2.8 Lindstrom's method of ultrasonic operation, involving (a) the production of two trephine holes in the skull and (b) placing the ultrasonic equipment into these holes to produce deep seated and circumscribed lesions (from: Lindstrom, 1954)

2.8). With the patient under local anaesthetic, trephine holes of 1.5 inches in diameter were made in the skull. Small dural flaps were then made (contrary to the method of Fry and his associates), and a few minutes of irradiation of ultrasound was applied. In later interventions the dural flaps were omitted from the procedure. According to Lindstrom, the results were satisfactory. Further, he noted the possibility of producing *reversible* changes by ultrasound application. Fry *et al.* (1958) also noted that reversible changes could be induced by low dosages of ultrasonic irradiation and commented, "This technique of producing reversible changes offers unique opportunities for three dimensional mapping of central nervous system function" (p. 83).

At present, the use of ultrasound in psychosurgery and neurosurgery is very limited, despite these observations of its potential and Asenjo's (1963) strong advocacy that "... one hopes that this extremely interesting technique will soon be a routine surgical procedure" (p. 209). However, only Lindstrom (cf. Lindstrom, 1972) appears to have used this technique on any scale.

The development and use of operative procedures that produced temporary and reversible changes in the brain were major concerns of many psychosurgeons. Reversible changes should intimate the outcome of subsequent permanent psychosurgical interventions. One such "trial and reversible error" method of operation is cryosurgery (Richardson, 1975). Here, small localized lesions are produced by freezing discrete sections of brain tissue. Walder (1976) noted that the study of the effects of low temperatures on living animal and vegetable tissue had a long history. It could be traced to Robert Boyle's monograph on the subject in 1665 and Spallanzani's work of 1787.

An important development in the use of freezing in surgery was reported by Rowbotham *et al.* (1959). They described a cooling cannula for use in neurosurgery to produce a more localized freezing, practising first of all on excised human brains and then operating on three patients. Their cooling cannula was inserted through trephine holes to what was judged to be the centre of the tumour. Cooling lasted for half an hour, by which time a cylinder of tissue around the tip of the cannula was frozen solid. The lesion resulting from cryosurgery is typically sharply defined. Rowbotham and his associates concluded their paper with the suggestion that their procedure could be used "for certain forms of leucotomy" (p. 15).

The next major advance was reported by Cooper and Lee (1961), who described a more technically advanced brain cannula (or *cryoprobe*) using liquid nitrogen as a freezing agent to produce localized lesions. However, Morley (1976) revealed that the use of cryosurgery has declined in recent years. He indicated why:

> Most neurosurgeons today, I suspect, have no regrets at the passing of the cryoprobe. They would say that stereotactic lesions are made more conveniently and more controllably by electronically induced heat ...

> Anything the cryoprobe can do, other methods can do better – or at least as well. (p. 633)

As mentioned, heat as well as cold has been used to produce small destructive lesions in psychosurgery. These thermal lesions are made by electrocoagulation, a technique used by Grantham (1951) for the relief of intractable pain. In his procedure an electrode was inserted into the white matter, following the path of a ventricular needle (an instrument designed to enter the ventricles or cavities of the brain) under control of X-ray vision. Electric current was applied to the exposed connection of the free end of the electrode needle to produce coagulation of fibres by heat.

The use of electricity to produce lesions has a long history. Horsley and Clarke (1908) used it on animals' brains and noted that Humphrey Davy had investigated the effects of electricity on blood tissue. Bipolar electrolysis (the decomposition of cell structures by direct current as opposed to electrocoagulation using high frequency) was first used to produce localized lesions by Sellier and Verger (1898), although as Roussy (1907) observed, unipolar electrolysis had been reported in 1895 by Golsinger. They employed electrolysis to lesion parts of the thalamus of dogs. However, Walder and Jasper (1970) noted that in this technique "distant gas formation causes the lesion to assume an irregular shape, and this has so far precluded general acceptance of the method" (p. 354).

More recently, these two methods of lesioning by the use of electricity (electrocoagulation and electrolysis) were combined by Crow and his associates. Crow *et al.* (1961) described their "controlled multifocal frontal leucotomy" as a method in which gold electrodes were implanted by stereotactic means in the frontal lobes. Serial coagulations could then be made over several weeks, so that the size and location of the lesion could be varied dependent on the observed effects following each coagulation. The electrodes were removed after sufficient improvement was reported. Crow (1973) reviewed the development of his electrocoagulation technique, referring to it as "leucocoagulation". He outlined an innovation in the procedure which involved the use of a current of insufficient strength to effect a permanent lesion. Instead, it produced a temporary block in the functioning of the nerve cells. Crow observed of this method:

> Thus we have a reversible trial and error method of testing brain sites where subsequent coagulation has a predictable and beneficial effect on the patient's illness. This process we have called polarisation. (p. 371)

The use of both types of electrical destruction was noted by Wycis and Spiegel (1949) in their discussion on the neurosurgical aspects of thalamotomy. These improved techniques of performing small localized lesions, together with the development of stereotactic procedure, enabled psychosurgeons to operate on structures deep within the brain.

The development of stereotactic surgery was undoubtedly one of the most important technical advances in the history of psychosurgery. The first stereotactic apparatus for use in psychosurgery was described by Spiegel *et al.* (1947). As early as 1908, Sir Victor Horsley and R. H. Clarke had reported the development of a stereotactic apparatus for use on the brains of animals. Ranson (1934) described its use in a number of animal experiments. Although Kirschner carried out stereotactic surgery in man through the lower parts of the skull, Leksell (1974) noted that Spiegel and Wycis were the "first to have had the courage and foresight to use a stereotactic instrument for operations within the human brain". (p. 3).

The first sterotactic apparatus designed by Spiegel and his associates consisted of a frame mounted on a plaster cast of the patient's head. The cast and attached apparatus was positioned on the skull, and large windows were cut into the plaster to allow insertion of instruments into the brain as well as the taking of X-ray photographs. The ventricles of the brain were filled with air. In consequence, they stood out more clearly on the photographs, permitting the coordinates of the proposed lesions to be calculated and the place of trephination determined. Other versions have been reported by Leksell (1949), who devised a semicircular metal frame, by Escolar (1951) and by Laitinen (1971).

These instruments were used with X-rays, electroencephalograms and, of course, stereotactic atlases of the sort devised by Schaltenbrand and Bailey (1959). Coordinates were taken from the stereotactic atlases and were used to position an electrode on to a "phantom", an exact duplicate of the stereotactic machine. Under X-ray vision, these measurements were then translated on to the real machine to guide the electrode into the site of operation within the brain. Modern stereotactic surgery is now commonly used in both psychosurgery and neurosurgery and has come a long way from the somewhat crude procedures used by Spiegel and his associates in their first attempt at thalamotomy.

When describing their "Model I" stereotactic apparatus, Spiegel and his associates (1947) first detailed their thalamotomy procedure (so called because the thalamus was the focus of the operation). Thalamotomy involved the destruction of the dorsomedial thalamic nuclei in order to interrupt the thalamo-frontal connections without the deleterious side-effects of the more conventional procedures. The aim of the operation was to leave intact the association systems between the frontal lobe and other parts of the cortex; it was assumed that such a circumscribed lesion would attend only to emotional disturbance, leaving other psychological functions unaffected.

Wycis *et al.* (1950) described a modification of thalamotomy called "mesencephalothalamotomy", devised for relieving intractable pain. This operation involved lesioning the spinothalamic tract in the midbrain (that is, the long ascending pain-conducting pathways) and was based on the observations of Freeman and Watts (1946) of insensibility to pain after leucotomy. A further modification was *hypothalamotomy*, in which lesions were made in the hypothalamus. This operation, as Spiegel *et al.* (1953) reported, was usually combined with thalamotomy. Operations on the hypothalamus and the subthalamus were prompted primarily by the work of Ranson (1939), who demonstrated that lesions of the lateral parts of the hypothalamus transformed wild monkeys into tame ones. Miller and Spiegel (1940) had observed that subthalamic lesions induced transitory somnolence and diminution of reactivity in the cat. Spiegel *et al.* (1953) also reported that his group had performed lesions in the anterior thalamic nuclei (*anterior thalamotomy*), based:

> ... upon the experience that following undercutting of the cingular gyrus or sectioning of its fiber connections with the anterior nuclei in the instances of psychosis and severe psychoneurosis changes comparable to those observed after prefrontal lobotomy were noticed. (p. 387)

Mention has already been made of the importance of the work of Ward, although, Scoville (1973) claimed that it was he who provided much of the impetus for *cingulectomy*:

> In the search for selective operation ... two major schools, which I call the "orbital" and "cingulate", have developed, interrupting respectively connections from these areas to the thalamus and limbic lobe. I early introduced both approaches with my "undercutting" procedures ... and in the late 1940s I communicated my results to Eduard Busch of Denmark, Hugh Cairns at Oxford and Le Beau in Paris. (p. 30)

It was not long, though, before a number of reports were published by various members of this "cingulate school", Le Beau (1954a) claiming that his was the first published series. Le Beau (1954b) reviewed the results of his operations and outlined his techniques of anterior cingulectomy. Although cingulectomy is a bilateral operation, it was undertaken by Le Beau from a unilateral approach. A unilateral bone flap (on either the left or right side) was made in the skull, and the dura mater was reflected. The frontal lobes were withdrawn to allow a clearer view of the cingulate gyrus. This was then sectioned under X-ray vision using a *cingulotome*. More recently, Turner (1972) performed an open posterior cingulectomy instead of the usual anterior operation.

Cingulectomy and thalamotomy heralded the turning point of psychosurgery, the older types of operation focussing on the frontal lobes being displaced by surgery addressed at the limbic system. Contemporary psychosurgery is not only distinguishable by a change in anatomical interest but also by a shift in its behavioural focus. It was the finding that previously aggressive animals were "tamed" following limbic surgery that commended such operations as a method of dealing with violent and aggressive human behaviour. The recent resurgence in psychosurgery owes much to the hypothesized connection between the limbic system and agitated and aggressive behaviour.

One of the most common operations performed on persistently aggressive and violent individuals nowadays is "amygdalotomy", "amygdalectomy" or "amygdaloidectomy" – the production of lesions (usually by electro-coagulation) in the amygdala.

Williams and Freeman (1951) first reported the use of this operation in an attempt to suppress auditory hallucinations. Sawa and his associates (1954) introduced this operation into Japan. However, it was another Japanese surgeon, Narabayashi, who first performed this operation on violent patients.

Narabayashi and his colleagues (1963) described their procedure fully. A needle with concentric bipolar electrodes was inserted through burr holes in the fronto-parietal regions by stereotactic means until it reached the amygdaloid nucleus. Air encephalography was used to outline the temporal horn, above which was located the nucleus. Electrophysiological recordings and X-rays were used for the correct localization of the needle. Blocking or destruction of this structure was obtained by the injection of a mixture of oil and wax to which Lipiodol had been added.

Sano (1962) investigated other target sites for "sedative surgery". As well as *posterior–medial hypothalamotomy*, they performed *anterior cingulectomy*, *thalamotomy*, *fornicotomy* (lesioning of the fornix with a hooked knife), and *upper mesencephalic reticulotomy*.

A somewhat more common procedure for the control of aggressive behaviour is *temporal lobectomy*, so called since surgery is addressed at the temporal lobe. Obrador (1947) claimed that he was the first to carry out this form of psychosurgery. Its contemporary intricacies have been described and illustrated by Mark and Ervin (1970). Medical and neurological tests are conducted on the patient before operation. Following a decision to operate on the temporal lobe(s), a small opening is made in the scalp, the skull and the dura mater. A needle is inserted into the ventricle and radio-opaque solution injected into it so that target sites within the brain can be identified with reference to it under X-ray vision. A stereotactic apparatus is affixed to the skull at three points. Landmarks within the brain are then visualized under X-ray vision, using X-ray photographs taken with a fixed distance between the X-ray tube and X-ray cassette. With the aid of a plotting chart, measurements are taken from the X-ray films and used to place the electrode on the stereotactic apparatus within the site of operation. These measurements are translated to a "phantom" stereotactic machine as described previously. This permits the electrode to be locked on to the target before it is placed in the real stereotactic apparatus on the patient's skull. Subsequently, all moving parts of the stereotactic machine are locked into place. The electrode is then inserted into the site of operation and adjusted according to indications from electrical stimulation and from temporary temperature blocking of neural activity. Four multi-lead electrodes are planted, two in each temporal lobe. The electrodes can be left in position over several weeks and electrical stimulation carried out. Finally, stronger current is applied through the electrode to produce small localized lesions by electrocoagulation. When the desired affect has been achieved, the electrodes are withdrawn and the treatment procedure terminated.

According to Obrador (1947), the psychological aim of temporal lobectomy is "to attack the 'circuit of emotion' described by Papez" (p. 191). Mark and Ervin's notion of a limbic-centred "dyscontrol syndrome" offered a more circumscribed and specific rationale for temporal lobectomy in relation to violent behaviour. Other practitioners lesioned various parts of the limbic system in the one patient, following the hypothesis that lesioning of only one limbic structure was an insufficient interruption of the "circuit of emotion" to beneficially alter emotional behaviour. The "stereotactic limbic leucotomy" of Kelly *et al.* (1973) was one procedure involving the lesioning of various structures of the limbic system.

New forms of psychosurgery are being developed and new combinations tested. The variety of operations described in this work are many, and it must be remembered that there are many modifications of these procedures, some major and some minor. Hirose (1965) commented on the plethora of different operative procedures: "Each psychosurgeon developed the technique of his choice" (p. 1199). Robin and MacDonald (1975) added that "in short there are as many operations as neurosurgeons" (p. 46). The modern psychosurgical operation is generally a highly skilled affair; it has advanced considerably from the techniques employed by Burckhardt and seems to have answered his call for more improved techniques better suited to the new method of treatment. The question still remains, however, whether these new techniques have led to better results than those obtained by Burckhardt, thereby fulfilling the hopes expressed at the end of his report.

3

Quantitative evaluation of operative procedures

After 40 years of psychosurgery, some agreement on the matter of its efficacy might reasonably be expected. It is clear, however, that no such consensus exists. While several factors have contributed to the continuing controversy surrounding psychosurgery (many of these will be discussed in later chapters), the equivocal nature of psychosurgical data is surely of crucial importance. In the absence of adequately controlled and evaluated studies, contention is inevitable. As *The British Medical Journal* (1971) observed:

> Prefrontal leucotomy is a subject on which opinions are divergent and firmly held. The divergence is not surprising in view of the lack of knowledge. It is an astonishing fact that in the 25-year history of leucotomy, during which more than 100 000 patients must have been operated on, no prospective controlled trial has been carried out to compare its effectiveness with non-surgical treatment. (p. 595)

An editorial in the *Canadian Medical Association Journal* (1964) was even more scathing:

> ... of the 4000-odd publications concerning lobotomy to date, a ridiculously small number have paid even lip service to experimental design, adequate sampling procedures, control of the variables involved and other salutary statistical cautions. (p. 1228)

Psychosurgeons themselves are similarly given to declarations regarding the need for better designed research. However, when these pronouncements emanate from reports or studies of questionable scientific worth, they seem merely to lend artificial respectability to otherwise dubious conclusions concerning the efficacy of the particular psychosurgical procedure in question. Certainly, psychosurgeons invariably ignore their own good advice.

Thus, in spite of such statements of intent, the haphazard and poorly controlled approach persists. Uncertainty is inevitable. As the *British Medical Journal* attested:

> Where do these studies leave ue? The only impartial answer to this question must be, "In a state of uncertainty." Now the Royal College of Psychiatrists has been formed, let us hope that it will encourage the thorough investigation of these promising but unproved forms of psychiatric treatment. Perhaps the new royal college could join with the Royal College of Surgeons in arranging a prospective trial. (p. 596)

This challenge was indeed taken up by the new body. A Report of the Research Committee of the Royal College of Psychiatrists (1977) "Proposal for a prospective controlled trial" outlined the reasons in favour:

> At a time when financial considerations are of increasing importance, it is worth emphasizing the cost-benefit aspect of this study. A negative result would cause substantial saving by producing evidence that the treatment was ineffective. A positive result would, on the other hand, produce an even greater saving by extending the use of an effective treatment to many more, thereby relieving a financial burden on the patients' families and the state. (p. 177)

Indeed prospects for a controlled trial of psychosurgery in Britain seemed excellent. The Report of the Research Committee listed a number of contributing factors:

> The patients are there, the Health Service provides an appropriate setting for the selection of patients and their treatment by different methods, and the trained research personnel are available. Indeed, it is conceivable that Britain is one of the few countries in which it is possible to conduct such a trial today because all these factors are present together and political interference in clinical matters is absent. (p. 177)

However, the controlled trial was never initiated, and the present prospects, in Britain at least, seem bleak. Further, even if a properly controlled trial were started, it would be years before the full results became available. The Royal College suggested that the trial would possibly be completed within three years. However, they envisaged a follow-up of only one year. As we shall indicate later, a much more protracted follow-up would be needed to properly assess the long-term effects.

Alternative methods of large-scale assessment have been tried. A survey would certainly appear to be a less contentious means of evaluating psychosurgery. This would involve writing to the various centres where psychosurgery is carried out and obtaining from the surgeons the results of their operations. Valenstein (1977) recently reported the results of one such survey on the efficacy of neurosurgery for pain performed in the United States. It is likely that a similar procedure for psychosurgery could be carried out in the United Kingdom. If good indications for psychosurgery were obtained, then this information could no doubt be used in support of a renewed application for a controlled trial.

This survey method has been used twice before in the United Kingdom. The Board of Control: England and Wales (1947) reported the results of one such survey. This was primarily the work of the Board's Medical Commissioner, Dr. Isobel Wilson, and its Statistical Officer, Mr. E. H. Warland. The survey was based upon questionnaires sent to all hospitals in England and Wales that had conducted psychosurgery up to the end of 1944. Returns from one hospital and two "licensed houses" were not included in the reports. The results from two Scottish hospitals were added to the survey. In all, 1000 cases were reviewed. Some years later a second survey was carried out by Tooth and Newton (1961). This covered all those patients who underwent a single operation during the years 1942–1954 and can therefore be seen as a follow-up to the earlier survey. Results were presented for 10 365 patients.

Although a nationwide survey provides useful clues about the efficiency of psychosurgery on a large number of patients, advantages of a large sample have to be offset by the disadvantages arising from loss of important detailed information. A questionnaire can be a tedious instrument to devise, complete and analyse. In consequence, questionnaires are invariably brief and the questions posed limited by practical constraints. Tooth and Newton (1961) explained:

> In planning the survey, it was recognised that the information hospitals could reasonably be expected to supply would be limited to facts and observations that would normally be recorded in the case notes of the patients concerned. In addition to this basic information hospitals were asked to supply an up-to-date clinical grading of patients who were in hospital at the time of the survey and of those discharged patients who had been examined within six months prior to completing the questionnaire. Very few hospitals were able to arrange a special follow-up for the purpose of the survey and a comparatively large group of patients who had left hospital were not graded. (p. 2)

The difficulty in obtaining full information on all the patients undergoing psychosurgery is a problem that can jeopardize the validity of the survey's findings. Non-return of questionnaires remains a serious hazard in any survey work. It is difficult, if not impossible, to estimate whether the sample of questionnaires returned is a fair and unbiased representation of the total population. Similar difficulties arise with regard to those patients who cannot be traced.

More serious and specific criticisms, however, relate to the use of such techniques in the evaluation of psychosurgery. Assessment of results of the operation is done by extracting information from the case notes. The impressions of patients' conditions before and after psychosurgery contained in case notes, being subjective in nature, hardly constitute a vigorous and objective evaluation of psychosurgery. The lack of comparability of reports from different hospitals is a serious complication of such survey work. Although the same diagnostic categories and terms of improvement may be employed, there is no guarantee that all hospitals will employ them in the same way. Comparisons between patients subjected to psychosurgery and those receiving no operation is difficult. Comparison with other therapies and assessment of any possible placebo effects are virtually impossible. In summary, therefore, the survey method of evaluating psychosurgery is simply a collation of uncontrolled case reports. Indeed, because of the problems detailed above, this technique of assessing psychosurgical procedures is probably less reliable than any single uncontrolled study. In the Preface to the report by Tooth and Newton (1961), G. E. Godber, the Chief Medical Officer of the Ministry of Health, noted the limitations of the survey:

> The results cannot afford a measure of the value of leucotomy, nor are they intended to be used as a basis of comparison with other methods of treatment particularly by the new drugs now available. They do, however, convey a general idea of what has happened to those patients suffering from different forms of mental derangement who had a leucotomy operation in the period covered by the survey.

In desperation, other methods of evaluation have been called for by various authorities. An editorial in the *Year Book of Neurology and Neurosurgery* (1976) declared:

> The whole situation cries out for analysis of results of psychosurgery; if an impartial panel cannot be chosen (since all have prejudices), at least one of equal numbers of advocates or opponents could be brought together. (p. 482)

One attempt was made to do this. The Massachussetts Task Force on Psychosurgery, headed by Stone (1975), was an attempt to reconcile the divergent views of its members, drawn from various bands of the spectrum of the psychosurgery controversy. Indeed, a report was produced; the almost impossible task of pooling the different opinions had apparently been achieved. However, inspection of the Massachussetts document reveals two reports, not one; a majority report and a minority one. The majority report was supported by those not practically involved in psychosurgery, while the minority one mainly attracted signatures of neurosurgeons and psychiatrists. Clearly, the task of reconciling the seemingly irreconcilable had not been wholly successful.

Another method of evaluation was chosen by the National Commission. Apart from two special projects commissioned by this body, Eliott Valenstein (1977) was invited to undertake an evaluation of published accounts of psychosurgery. Valenstein's assessment focused on published reports in English from 1971 to 1976. Some 153 papers that presented data on psychosurgery were collated; of these, the 26 articles presenting data from the United States were closely reviewed.

There have been similar evaluations of psychosurgery in the past. However, such reviews have often been very cursory in nature. Frequently, the whole of the published literature of psychosurgery is summarized in a couple of pages and an authoritative (if not authoritarian) assertion of efficacy derived. Further, some reviewers have selected only a very modest sample of reports as illustrative of the general field. Different reviewers have chosen different samples as representative. Finally, there has been frequently little attempt to differentiate between various psychosurgical procedures or different patient populations.

The main criticism of past reviews of psychosurgery is that they lack systematic and critical analysis. Problems raised by the comparability of diagnosis and diagnostic criteria between different periods of time, countries and psychiatrists are rarely, if ever, considered. Matters relating to experimental design and control are invariably neglected. A sort of "scientific egalitarianism" pervades these reviews; poorly controlled and designed studies with modest follow-ups are afforded the same weight as studies that have attempted to control some of the possible confounding variables and have engaged in lengthy follow-ups. Clearly, one carefully controlled study is substantially more informative than a host of uncontrolled efforts characterized by bias, slapdash evaluative methods, naive assumptions about "improvement" and the lack of long-term follow-up.

Unfortunately, as we indicated earlier, most psychosurgical studies fall into the latter category. Anecdotal testimonies of dramatic cure, bizarre assessment procedures (e.g. pre- and postoperative photographs), unsophisticated and casual methods of follow-up (e.g. the receipt of Christmas cards from the patient) and "amateur" statistics (e.g. sometimes the number of patients displayed in tables exceeds the total number of cases presented in the report, and occasionally patients mysteriously vanish from statistics halfway through a report) are far from atypical. While these examples are culled from the early clump of studies on psychosurgery, there is little to suggest that contemporary studies have substantially transcended such dubious methodological practices.

Valenstein (1977) judged the scientific status of English-language reports published 1970–1976, contained in his review. One of six categories of scientific merit was assigned to each of the "data articles" reviewed. These categories were based on a 96-point rating scale, which was developed by May and Van Putten (1974) to assess the scientific status of reports on the results of various therapies in the treatment of schizophrenia. They commented that their scale was constructed to assess "design or relevance":

> ... i.e. the degree of confidence with which the findings of a particular study can be applied to the treatment of schizophrenia, based on the reported design, execution and analysis of results. (p. 375)

Factors included in the rating scale were, use of control groups, independent evaluators of treatment effect, length of follow-up, appropriate statistical analysis of results, use of objective tests and degree of contamination by non-surgical variables (e.g. improved hospital care and attention). The category containing studies with the highest scientific merit (i.e. D.R. I and II) would include reports with adequately matched controls, objective tests, independent assessors and long-term follow-up. The lowest category would include anecdotal case reports.

Valenstein's analysis indicated that over 90% of all articles published on psychosurgery (1970–1976) were placed in categories four to six, about half being allocated to the lowest category of all. Category four, we are told:

> ... would be given only to articles of low scientific value. It is unlikely, for example, that an animal study with such a low rating would be accepted for publication by the editors of a respected experimental journal. (p. 60)

It is crucial for reviewers to temper their evaluation according to the strengths of the study. However, many reviewers of psychosurgery uncritically accept the results presented in such poorly designed studies. They reproduce the "recovery and improvement rates" reported therein and make no attempt to assess the worth of these findings. A common tactic is to average the percentage of patients reported improved across the studies sampled for review. This simple-minded "head counting" approach characterizes much of the evaluation of psychosurgery. Factors such as the status of the assessors of the treatment, relapse rates, contamination of results by non-surgical variables and placebo effects are all ignored.

The only way, therefore, to carry out a proper evaluation is to present both a *quantitative* and *qualitative* analysis of the psychosurgery literature. In the *quantitative* analysis, a simple, intuitive "head counting" inspection is undertaken. To this must be grafted a *qualitative* assessment. This frequently omitted part of the evaluation is crucial.

The rest of this chapter will be devoted to the *quantitative* evaluation of psychosurgical studies, with regard first to overall results and second to different patient populations and different psychosurgical procedures. Of special interest here is the comparison of the old and new wave procedures. A detailed and critical *qualitative* analysis will develop over the course of the next four chapters.

At the outset it must be noted that the task facing any evaluator of psychosurgery from the published literature is a daunting one. Given the vast number of reports, some sort of selection must take place. Obviously, selection readily permits bias. It could be claimed that reports sampled for review were chosen to fit in with preconceived notions regarding efficacy, rather than to project a truly representative sample. To avoid such criticism the criteria used to select reports for evaluation should be detailed.

The aim of the present review is to evaluate the relative efficacy of various operative procedures of both the old and new "waves" of psychosurgery, as well as to examine the indications for various patient populations. Papers reporting results related to these will, therefore, be reviewed. In some cases, however, there are numerous reports on the efficacy of a particular psychosurgical procedure (e.g. the "standard" operation) in the treatment of a specific psychiatric disorder (e.g. schizophrenia). As a general principle, therefore, only large-scale studies or those most frequently cited in the literature will be reviewed in the present chapter. In particular, greater attention will be directed towards procedures of the "second wave". The so-called "controlled" studies will be critically analysed in Chapter 4. Studies reporting adverse operative sequelae will be reviewed in Chapter 5. Other studies with particular points of interest will be considered in all five chapters addressed to the critical evaluation of psychosurgery's empirical status.

The most suitable format for a general review of psychosurgery is the presentation of results in tables. Hence, only studies whose results are amenable to presentation in this form will be reviewed in this chapter. Comparison between studies, operative procedures and patient populations can, therefore, be easily made by the reader. In the first series of tables, summaries of results will be presented for different operative procedures. Later tables will depict results according to psychiatric disorder.

One problem encountered is that a series of papers may give data on the same patients. This is particularly true in the case of reports charting the experiences of certain psychosurgeons over several years (the various papers of Freeman and Knight provide examples of these). In the tables, therefore, data from successive reports on the same patients will be presented only once, usually from the most recent account. In some instances, a paper may claim to be reviewing the effects of psychosurgery on a certain number of patients but provides a detailed analysis of only a sample of operatees. In such cases, the actual number fully assessed will be presented in the tables, and the total operative sample from which this number was drawn will be given in parentheses below this figure. Reasons for the smaller sample will be given in the "Remarks" column.

The diagnostic categories given in the tables are essentially those used in the original paper. For the sake of space, however, in those cases in which more than one diagnostic label is applied, only the primary diagnosis will be given. Similarly, in lists of psychiatric diagnoses given in the tables, those diagnostic labels which have been assigned to only a very few cases will be excluded and the patients assigned to the "others" category.

A major difficulty in tabulating the results of psychosurgical procedures is that different criteria have been used to assess the outcome of operations. The two major methods of evaluation have been "discharge rates" and "improvement rates." The former was a more common system of expressing results of psychosurgery in the "first wave" and consisted of calculating, as a percentage of the total number of operatees, all those patients who were discharged following surgery.

Improvement rates are presently the more common method of expressing postoperative outcome. Here, patients are generally assigned to one of a number of categories of "improvement" and the percentage of patients in each category calculated. The number of categories of "improvement" varies considerably from paper to paper. Sometimes only a rudimentary assessment is made, and therefore outcome measures consist solely of "percentage of patients improved", "success" or "good results"; gradations of improvement are not included. For the purpose of the present tables, four categories will be employed: "marked improvement", "some improvement", "no improvement" and "worse".

Grade 1: Marked Improvement. Patient has either completely recovered or markedly improved; is on little or no medication; occasionally or never consults psychiatrists; generally functions at 75–100% of ability.

Grade 2: Some Improvement. Patient has shown some improvement; takes medication regularly; consults psychiatrists regularly; generally functions at 25–75% of ability.

Grade 3: No Improvement. Patient's condition is not (or only very minimally or temporarily) improved; is under constant psychiatric care; generally functions at below 25% of ability.

Grade 4: Worse. Patient's psychiatric disorder has worsened or general condition has deteriorated due to advance operative sequelae; includes patients whose deaths can in some way be attributable to operation and also suicides.

Obviously, such categories are somewhat arbitrary. They do not represent objective divisions along a continuum of outcome of psychosurgery. They are only intended as a guide to outcome for comparison between studies and a basis for further later critical analysis. The first category would include patients for whom psychosurgery could be considered a success. The second consists of only partial successes, while the third contains essentially failures. The final category includes all those patients for whom psychosurgery has had a detrimental effect on their condition.

Naturally, exact matching of original categories and the present divisions cannot always be adequately made. In some cases certain attributes that characterize one category in the original report might be included in the description of another division in the present scheme. The general principle that will operate in classification is, therefore, that the initial attribute listed for each category in the present systems is considered critical and will essentially determine a patient's status. In addition, changes may be made to original classifications where supplementary information concerning the patient's postoperative adjustment suggests that this is appropriate.

For those studies that give more than four categories, the results will be translated into the present system by combining some of the original categories. Indications of the original categories and how they have been translated into the present system will be detailed in the column following that presenting results. Where the original studies employ less categories than in the present review (e.g. an "improved" category that does not differentiate between "much" and "some" improvement), the general result will be noted in the main body of the table at the midpoint between the pertinent divisions.

Obviously, many problems arise when summarizing in tabular form information contained in papers. Such difficulties will be indicated in the "remarks" section for each individual report. Indeed, any factors of special note will be detailed in this column.

Tables 3.1–3.13 present a summary of the data given in over 50 papers reporting results of the major psychosurgical procedures. In each table the results of several studies examining roughly the same operation are displayed. Procedures might then be quantitatively compared. It should be noted here that "prefrontal" in the tables refers mainly to the standard operation and its minor modifications. Comparison can also be made of the efficacy of a particular procedure for a variety of disorders.

From these data, the overall "improvement rates" for the studies have been arranged in three further tables. In the first of these (Table 3.14), results of essentially "first wave" procedures (prefrontal, transorbital, bimedial, orbital and rostral) can be compared. In the second (Table 3.15) are arranged studies reporting operations of the "mid-period" (stereotactic tractotomy and cingulectomy). Finally, results of the more circumscribed procedures deemed to be characteristic of the "second wave" (thalamotomy, hypothalamotomy, amygdalectomy, multi-target limbic leucotomy, capsulotomy and mesoloviotomy) are presented for comparison in the third of these tables (Table 3.16).

From these results, an average rate of improvement can be calculated for each operative procedure. The total number of patients in each of the categories of improvement are expressed as a percentage of the total number of operatees subjected to that operation. Table 3.17 presents a rank order of efficacy of the major psychosurgical procedures with the associated "marked improvement" percentage. Given the weakness of psychosurgical data and their susceptibility to bias, coupled with the drastic nature of the intervention, only category 1 allocations can reasonably be submitted as successful outcomes. As can be seen from the table, capsulotomy (devised to lesion fibres connecting the frontal lobes and the thalamus in the internal capsule) would appear to yield the most favourable results on the basis of this quantitative "head counting" technique. It must be noted, however, that very few individuals have been subjected to it, and the range of patients undergoing this procedure has to date been extremely limited. The high status accorded to cingulectomy would appear to be based on a somewhat firmer foundation, given the plethora of studies that have employed it. Rostral leucotomy and thalamotomy would appear to be the poorest psychosurgical procedures in terms of efficacy. The results for amygdalectomy are also comparatively poor, being only slightly better than those for the largely discredited standard or prefrontal operation. These observations on the relative efficacy of cingulectomy and amygdalectomy are also supported by Valenstein's (1977) findings from his survey of some of the American psychosurgical studies.

Table 3.17 also presents the rank order of efficacy of psychosurgery in the treatment of various disorders. Patients diagnosed as "sexual deviants" would appear to be most indicated for psychosurgery, although as before, it must be noted that only a few such patients have undergone hypothalamic psychosurgery. Further, the theoretical indications for this procedure are poor (cf. Chapter 8), and it is unlikely that its effects are specific (cf. Chapters 7 and 9). As many other commentators suggest, obsessional neurosis would appear to be indicated for psychosurgery, whereas schizophrenia does not appear to be greatly helped by psychosurgical procedures. Similarly, aggression/hyperkinesis seems poorly indicated.

Finally, Table 3.18 presents a comparison of operations for various disorders. Cingulectomy would appear to be indicated over other procedures for most disorders, except perhaps for depression and schizophrenia. For the former, the orbital procedures would appear to offer greater benefit, whereas for schizophrenia, mesoloviotomy (lesion of the rostral part of the "genu," i.e. the knee of the corpus callosum) seems to yield surprisingly good results, although this finding is based on only one study in which only 17 schizophrenics underwent surgery.

Thus, using the "head counting" technique, it would appear that certain psychosurgical procedures are efficacious in the treatment of certain psychiatric disorders. Many other reviewers of psychosurgery, although their studies were based on less data, have come to the same conclusion. However, any evaluation of psychosurgery cannot rely solely on "improvement rate". This quantitative approach leaves unanswered many important questions. What problems are encountered when comparing the various psychosurgical studies? How long was the improvement maintained? What would have happened to the patient if no treatment had been applied? To what extent can "improvement rates" be linked specifically to the surgical lesion, rather than to improved postoperative care and attention, or to the expectancy of therapeutic benefit by the patient or others? Are unspecific effects, i.e. adverse operative sequelae, likely to outweigh possible benefits? These and other crucial questions will be carefully examined in the next four chapters.

Table 3.1 Results of various studies of the operation of prefrontal leucotomy

Study	*Date*	*Samp. no.*	*Diagnoses*	*M. imp* *1*	*S. imp.* *2*	*No imp.* *3*	*Worse* *4*	*Original categories*	*Remarks*
Rao and Govindaswamy	1944	25	25 Schizophrenics	28	24	40	8	1 = "recovered" 2 = "improved" 3 = "no change" 4 = "deteriorated" (p. 218)	
Board of Control	1947	1000	599 Schizophrenia	16[1]	46[1]	32	6[2]	1 = "recovered"	[1] Includes some patients who had relapsed
			250 Manic-depressive	45[1]	33[1]	13	9[2]	2 = "improved"	[2] Includes patients who had died (many of them as a result of the operation)
			29 Obsessional neurosis	59[1]	31[1]	3	7[2]	3 = "no change"	
			5 Other neurosis	40	40	-	20	4 = "worse"	
			25 Delusional insanity	20	48	24	8[2]	(p. 7)	
			92 Others	16[1]	49[1]	25	10[2]		
			1000 Total	25[1]	43[1]	25	7[2]		
Freeman and Watts	1950	596[1]	328 Schizophrenias	35	38	27		1 = "good"	[1] Excluding "pain" patients
			147 Involutional psychoses	60	24	14		2 = "fair"	[2] Including operative deaths
			121 Obsessive and psychoneuroses	57	28	15		3 and 4 = "poor" (p. 508)	
			596 Total	45	33	22			
Hohman *et al.*	1951	254 234[1]	171 Schizophrenia	6	59	33	2	1 = "recovered"	[1] Insufficient details given of postoperative condition for other 20 patients
			55 Affective disorders	29	49	20	2	2 = "better"	
			8 Obsessive–compulsive disorders	100	-	-	-	3 = "same" 4 = "worse" (p. 531)	
			234 Total	14	55	29	2		

Moore	1952	71	66[1]	50 Schizophrenia	46	30	24		1 = "recovered" and "much improved"	[1] 4 patients died (2 as a result of the operation) and 1 was untraced
				8 Affective psychosis	75	25	–		2 = "improved"	
				7 Obsessional neurosis	71	–	29		3 and 4 = "unchanged" (p. 126)	
				1 Anorexia nervosa	100	–	–			
				66 Total	53	26	21			
Tooth and Newton	1961	11127	9284[1]	6146 Schizophrenic	30	33	32	5[2]	1 = D1 "total recovery", D2 "social recovery", D3 + H1 "greatly improved"	[1] Excludes 462 patients who had more than one operation; 300 patients for whom the questionnaires were incomplete, 1081 patients whose deaths were not attributable to operation
				2139 Affective	63	19	11	7[2]	2 = D4 "family invalid", H2 "social improvement", H5 "family burden", H3 "social defect"	[2] Includes patients who had died due to the operation
				999 Other	59	26	8	7[2]	3 = H4 "no change"	
				9284 Total	41	28	25	6[2]	4 = H5 "worse" and "dead" (pp. 8–9)	

Table 3.2 Results of various studies of the operation of transorbital leucotomy

Study	*Date*	*Samp. no.*		*Diagnoses*	*M. imp.* *1*	*S. imp.* *2*	*No imp.* *3*	*Worse* *4*	*Original categories*	*Remarks*
Jones and Shanklin	1950	74	52[1]	39 Schizophrenia	41	15	44		1 = "Good"	[1] These were patients followed up from 1 to 2 years
				7 Manic-depressive psychosis	72	14	14		2 = "Fair"	
				6 Other	67	33	–		3 and 4 = "Poor" (pp. 124–126)	
				52 Total	48	17	35			
Freeman and Watts	1950	262	252[1]	150 Schizophrenias	33	26	41[2]		1 = "Good"	[1] 10 "pain" patients excluded [2] includes operative deaths
				68 Involutional psychoses	44	28	28[2]		2 = "Fair"	
				34 Obsessive psychoneuroses	65	24	11		3 and 4 = "Poor" (p. 512)	
				252 Total	40	26	34[2]			
Wilson *et al.*	1953		400	267 Schizophrenia	49	23	26	2	1 = "Out of hospital" and "Good"	
				48 Psychosis with mental deficiency	48	21	29	2	2 = "Fair"	
				20 Psychosis with epilepsy	25	35	35	5	3 = "Unimproved"	
				20 Manic-depressive psychosis	65	20	15	–	4 = "Operative deaths" (p. 881)	
				17 Psychopathic personality	35	35	30	–		
				28 Other	54	21	21	4		
				400 Total	48	24	26	2		

Table 3.3 Results of various studies of the operation of bimedial leucotomy

Study	*Date*	*Samp. no.*		*Diagnoses*	*M. imp.* *1*	*S. imp.* *2*	*No imp.* *3*	*Worse* *4*	*Original Categories*	*Remarks*
Fleming and Baker	1972	44	42[1]	23 Psychoneurosis	44	39	17		1 = "excellent"	[1] 2 patients unavailable for assessment
				12 Schizophrenia	25	25	50		2 = "satisfactory"	
				6 Personality disorder	50	50	–		3 + 4 = "unsatisfactory"	
				1 Involutional melancholia	100	–	–		(pp. 326–327)	
				42 Total	38	38	24			
Bernstein *et al.*	1975		43	27 Obsessive compulsive	81	4	11	4	1 = "+3"; and "+4"; "symptom free"	
				10 Schizophrenic	50	10	10	30	2 = "+2"; "fair improvement"	
				5 Hypochondriac	100	–	–	–	3 = "0" and "+1"; "no" or "minimal symptomatic improvement"	
				1 Manic-depressive	100	–	–	–	(Also calculated on the basis of a similar rating scale of adverse sequelae)	
				43 Total	77	5	11	7	(p. 1043)	

Table 3.4 Results of various studies of the operation of orbital leucotomy

Study	*Date*	*Samp. no.*	*Diagnoses*	*M. imp.* *1*	*S. imp.* *2*	*No imp.* *3*	*Worse* *4*	*Original categories*	*Remarks*
Tow and Lewin	1953	20	10 Schizophrenia	20	60[1]	20		1 = "Recovered" 2 = "Improved" 3 = "No change" or "Improved slightly" (p. 646)	[1] Includes 3 patients who relapsed and 1 who had suddenly died [2] Includes 1 patient who had relapsed [3] Includes patients who had died
			4 Agitated depression	50	50[2]				
			2 Manic depressive psychosis	50	50				
			2 Chronic anxiety state	50	–	50			
			2 Others	50	50				
			20 Total	35	40[3]	25			
Ström-Olsen and Northfield	1955	27	15 Schizophrenia	33[1]	34	33		1 = "Recovered" 2 = "Improved" 3 = "Unchanged" and "Slightly improved" (p. 986)	[1] Includes patients considered sufficiently improved to be discharged [2] 1 patient died as a result of operation
			4 Chronic anxiety	75	25				
			8 Other	25	63		12[2]		
			27 Total	37	41	18	4[2]		
Knight and Tredgold	1955	59 52[1]	12 Schizophrenic state	42	42	8	8	1 = A; "markedly improved" 2 = B; "some improvement" 3 = C; "unchanged" 4 = D; "somewhat worse" and E; "markedly worse" (p. 983)	[1] 4 patients untraced and a further 3 excluded because they had undergone previous psychosurgery
			11 Obsessional state	18	55	27			
			11 Anxiety state	73	18	9			
			10 Reactive depression	50	50				
			5 Hysteria	20	40	40			
			2 Endogenous depression	100	–				
			1 Psychopathic personality	–	100	–	–		
			52 Total	44	40	14	2		
Sykes and Tredgold[1]	1964	350 207[2]	64 Reactive depression	67	24	9		1 = I; "completely relieved" and II; "Improved, no treatment required." 2 = III; "Improved but still requiring treatment" 3 = IV; "unchanged" 4 = IV; "worse" (p. 610)	[1] Includes some patients reviewed in previous reports [2] The rest of the patients were not fully assessed
			32 Recurrent depression	69	19	12			
			16 Involutional depression	62	25	13			
			28 Anxiety state	39	46	11	4		
			24 Obsessional	29	46	25			
			14 Schizophrenic	29	36	35			
			29 "Others" and "Mixed"	21	52	27			
			207 Total	50	35	14	1		

Table 3.5 Results of various studies of the operation of rostral leucotomy

Study	*Date*	*Samp. no.*	*Diagnoses*	*M. imp. 1*	*S. imp. 2*	*No imp. 3*	*Worse 4*	*Original categories*	*Remarks*
McKissock	1951	160 84[1]	?	23	56	19	2[2]	1 = "Greatly improved" 2 = "Moderately improved" and "slightly improved" 3 = "No improvement" 4 = "Died" (p. 93)	[1] 76 patients were not followed up [2] Patients died
Pippard	1955a	240 220[1]	33 Tension states	33	30	37		1 = "good" 2 = "fair" 3 and 4 = "poor" (p. 762)	[1] 13 patients were untraced and 7 had unilateral leucotomies and were therefore excluded from detailed analysis [2] Includes 1 operative death [3] Includes 4 operative deaths
			26 Obsessional states	46	15	39			
			23 Psychopathic personality	22	9	69			
			14 Hypochondriasis	21	7	72[2]			
			32 Schizophrenia and paranoid illness	12	16	72[2]			
			26 Single depressions	58	15	27			
			26 Recurrent, mainly endogenous, depression	38	27	35			
			15 Recurrent, more reactive depression	67	13	20			
			4 Manic and depressive attacks		25	75[2]			
			21 Mental illness in reaction to or in association with organic disease	42	10	48			
			220 Total	36	17	47[3]			

Table 3.6 Results of various studies of the operation of stereotaxic tractotomy

Study	Date	Samp. no.		Diagnoses	M. imp. 1	S. imp. 2	No imp. 3	Worse 4	Original categories	Remarks
Ström-Olsen and Carlisle	1971	210	150[1]	75 Depression	56	24	20	–	1 = { I; "Completely recovered" II; "Improved – no treatment required" }	[1] All series A patients who had adequate follow-up
				46 Anxiety state	41	24	35	–	2 = III; "Improved but still needing treatment"	
				20 Obsessional neurosis	50	15	30	5	3 = IV; "Changed"	
				5 Schizophrenia	–	40	60	–	4 = "Worse"	
				4 Other	50	25	25	–	(p. 142)	
				150 Total	49	23	27	1		
Göktepe *et al.*	1975	208[1]	134[2]	78 Depression	68	20	12	–	1 = I; "Recovered" and II; "Well"	[1] Report on next series of patients from Ström-Olsen and Carlisle
				24 Anxiety	62	21	17	–	2 = III; "Improved"	[2] Only 134 patients were available for full assessment
				18 Obsessional neurosis	50	33	17	–	3 = IV; "Unchanged"	
				4 Schizophrenia	–	50	50	–	4 = V; "Worse"	
				10 Other	10	40	50	–	(p. 275)	
				134 Total	58	25	17	–		

Table 3.7 Results of various studies of the operation of cingulectomy

Study	*Date*	*Samp. no.*		*Diagnoses*	*M. imp.* *1*	*S. imp.* *2*	*No imp.* *3*	*Worse* *4*	*Original categories*	*Remarks*
Whitty *et al.*	1952	29	24[1]	10 Schizophrenia	–	10	90	–	1 = "cured" or "much improved"	[1] Includes only patients observed from 1½–3 yrs. after operation
				4 Obsessional neurosis	75	25	–	–	2 = "improvement" and "slightly improved"	
				10 Others	10	20	70	–	3 = "unchanged" (pp. 477–478)	
				24 Total	17	17	66	–		
Le Beau	1954b	50	30[1]	11 Mental retardation and agitation	73[2]		27		1 = "good results" i.e. "complete or nearly complete cure" (p. 270)	[1] 2 children had died, 14 epileptics have been excluded, another 4 patients were not accounted for, unless they were cases in which postoperative sequelae were reported
				9 Depressive states	33[3]		67			[2] There were 3 out of 4 with obsessional neurosis
				6 Excited states	33		67			[3] There were 2 out of 3 cases with hysteria
				4 Psychoses with violence	75		25			
				30 Total	43		57			
Tow and Armstrong	1954		17	10 Schizophrenics	–	10[1]	90	–	No categories given	[1] 1 patient showing continued improvement at follow up
				7 Others	–	–	90	10[3]		[2] 10 other patients showed some improvement but relapsed
				17 Total	–	6[1]	88[2]	6[3]		[3] Postoperative death
Sano	1962		14	14 Agitated Idiocy	50		50		1 and 2 = "effective" 3 and 4 = "not effective" (p. 119)	
Brown and Lighthill	1968		110	37 Obsessive–compulsive					1 = 1; "well" and 2; "greatly improved"	[1] It is not possible to give improvement rates for each diagnostic category, since no information was applied in the original report
				31 Affective disorders					2 = 3; "improved" and 4; "slightly improved"	
				24 Anxiety–tension states					3 = 5; "unimproved"	
				10 Anxiety hysteria					4 = 6; "worse" (p. 516)	
				4 Involutional psychoses						
				4 Others						
				110 Total	87[1]	7	5	1		

Table 3.7 (continued)

Study	*Date*	*Samp. no.*		*Diagnoses*	*M. imp. 1*	*S. imp. 2*	*No imp. 3*	*Worse 4*	*Original categories*	*Remarks*
Paillas *et al.*	1971		20[1]	20 Obsessional neurosis	45[2]	30	25		1 = "spectacular improvement" 2 = "improvement" 3 = "no improvement" (p. 918)	[1] 5 of these cases underwent prefrontal leucotomy [2] Although 12 cases were described as spectacular improvement, 3 of these had relapsed and have been included in the "some improvement" category
Gaches *et al.*	1972	351	20[1]	20 Obsessive syndromes	80	10	10		1 = III; "complete recovery" and II; "considerable improvement" 2 = I; "slight improvement" 3 = 0 "no improvement" (p. 233)	[1] These patients were selected on the basis of diagnosis; another 11 patients with the same diagnosis were excluded
Laitinen and Vilkki	1972		20	10 Schizophrenic anxiety 10 Others 20 Total	70 20 45	30 60 45	 20 10		1 = "Good" 2 = "Fair" 3 and 4 "Poor" (p. 246)	
Mingrino and Schergna	1972		10	10[1] Aggressiveness	20	30	50		1 = "Good" 2 = "Fair" 3 and 4 = "Poor" (p. 260)	[1] Patients were also epileptic and all but 1 were mentally retarded
Richardson	1972		12	12 "Severe disability secondary to emotional illness" (p. 1223)	84	8	-	8	1 = excellent 2 = good 4 = "frontal lobe syndrome" (p. 1222)	
Balasubramaniam *et al.*	1973a	34	28	11 Pethidine addiction 11 Morphine addiction 6 Alcohol addiction 28 Total	91 73 67 79		9 27 33 21		1 = "Successes" 2 = "Failure": "Even if the patient takes one tablet or injection in the postoperative period, the result is considered a failure" (p. 64)	

Meyer *et al.*	1973	75	68[1]	26 Schizophrenia	42	42	16		1 = +3; "well"	[1] The other 7 cases were not evaluated
				22 Depression	50	41	9		and +2; "marked improvement"	
				12 Alcoholism	42	17	8	33	2 = +1; "moderate improvement"	
				3 Obsessive compulsive	67	33			and −1; "slight improvement"	
				5 Others	20	80	–	–	3 = −2; "none"	
									4 = −3; "worse"	
				68 Total	44	40	10	6	(p. 47)	
Ballantine *et al.*	1977	238	149[1]	149 "mood disturbance" (p. 335)	49	38	13		1 = 5; "well" and 4; "markedly improved" 2 = 3; "moderately improved" and 2; "slightly improved" 3 = 1; "no improvement" 4 = 0; "worse" (p. 335)	[1] 34 "pain" patients are excluded, a further 15 patients had died and no reason was given for the exclusion of the other 40 patients
Martin *et al.*	1977	68	67[1]	29 Schizophrenia	45	48	7		1 = "excellent"	[1] 1 patient diagnosed as suffering from intractable pain has been excluded from the presentation
				27 Neurotic depression	41	37	22	–	2 = "moderate" and "slight"	
				4 Psychotic depression	75		25	–	3 = "none"	
				6 Alcoholic	100		–	–	(p. 384)	
				1 Emotionally unstable personality	100		–	–		
				67 Total	51	37	12	–		
Bailey *et al.*	1977		200[1]	88 Manic depressive	98	2	–	–	1 = { "++++": "very marked improvement"; "+++": "remission of all symptoms"; "++": "well, marked improvement" }	Postoperative suicides (2%) of operative deaths (0.5%) but were not included in a "worse" category
				40 Schizo-affective	88	10	2	–		
				36 Anxiety-phobic	97	3	–	–		
				36 Obsessive/antisocial-compulsive	83	14	3	–		
				200 Total	93	6	1	–	2 = { "+": a significant relief of symptoms but the patient still requires continuing medication and supportive treatment" }	
									3 = "−" "no improvement" (p. 230)	

Table 3.8 Results of various studies of the operation of thalamotomy

Study	*Date*	*Samp. no.*	*Diagnoses*	*M. imp.* *1*	*S. imp.* *2*	*No imp.* *3*	*Worse* *4*	*Original categories*	*Remarks*
Spiegel *et al.*	1953	61 51[1]	37 Schizophrenia	27	30	43	–	1 = A; "returned home" and B; "able to return home"	[1] 2 operative deaths and the "first three cases were not included because only rather small lesions had been produced" (p. 386)
			5 Anxiety neurosis	80	20	–	–	2 = C; "hospitalized but are relieved of some of their symptoms"	[2] Does not include 2 operative deaths
			4 Affective reaction types	25	25	50		3 = D; "patients who are not improved"	[3] Includes temporary improvement
			3 Obsessive-compulsive neurosis	–	33	67	–	4 = "Worse" (p. 386)	
			2 Paranoid state		–	100	–		
			51[2] Total	29	28	43	–		
Andy and Jurko	1972	30	30 "hyperresponsive syndrome" "aggression," "hyperkinesia" and "pathoaffect"	20	47	33	–	1 = "good" 2 = "fair" 3 = "poor" (p. 128)	

Table 3.9 Results of various studies of the operation of hypothalamotomy

Study	*Date*	*Samp. no.*	*Diagnoses*	*M. imp.* *1*	*S. imp.* *2*	*No imp.* *3*	*Worse* *4*	*Original categories*	*Remarks*
Schvarcz *et al.*	1972	1	11 "Severe hetero- and/or autoaggressiveness" (p. 357)	64	27	9	–	1 = "Marked improvement" 2 = "Improvement" 3 = "Failure" (p. 358)	
Sano *et al.*	1972	53 43[1]	43 "Violent, aggressive or restless" (p. 66)	30	65	5	–	1 = "Excellent results" 2 = "Good results" 3 = "Unchanged" (p. 66)	[1] "Followed up 2–8 years" (1 operative death not included)
Müller *et al.*	1973	22	20[1] "Sexual deviants" 2 Others	75 –	15 100	5 –	5[2] –	1 = "Good" 2 = "Fair" 3 = "Poor" (p. 121)	[1] Mainly "homosexual deviations" [2] 1 patient died 6 days after operation
			22 Total (p. 113)	68	22	5	5[2]		
Balasubramaniam *et al.*	1971	8	8 "Patients who are restless or exhibit destructive tendencies" (p. 227)	37	50	13	–	1 = A; "Where there is no need of any drug" and B; "Very much docile and given to occasional outbursts only" 2 = C; "Manageable when given drugs though not leading a useful life" 3 = D; "Transient improvement but relapsed" and E; "No change" 4 = F; "Died" (p. 229)	
Balasubramaniam *et al.*	1973b	21[1]	21 "Hyperkinetic behaviour disorders" (p. 138)	81 (1 + 2)		19 (3 + 4)		1 = "17 of 21 cases had become quiet and manageable and could be considered to have had good results" (p. 141)	[1] May include patients of earlier paper

Table 3.9 (continued)

Study	*Date*	*Samp. no.*	*Diagnoses*	*M. imp.* 1	*S. imp.* 2	*No imp.* 3	*Worse* 4	*Original categories*	*Remarks*
Dieckmann and Hassler	1975	6	6 "Sexual deviations" (p. 179)	83	17			1 = "Good" 2 = "Fair" (p. 183)	
Dieckmann and Hassler	1977	4	4 "Sexual violence" (p. 451)	100				1 = "Marked reduction of their sex drive" (p. 460)	
Schvarcz	1977	33	33 "Strong history of aggressive violent behavior" (p. 433)	80 (M. imp. and S. imp. combined)		20 (No imp. and Worse combined)		102 = "Satisfactory overall results were obtained in 80 per cent" (p. 433)	
Nádvornik *et al.*	1977	10	10 "Hedonic manifestations in chronic alcoholism and paedophilia" (p. 440)	60	30		10[1]	1 = "Normal life" or cessation of "deviation" 2 = "Improvement" (p. 446)	[1] Adverse sequelae of operation
Rubio *et al.*	1977	31 24[1]	24 "Oligophrenia erethica" (or "agitated idiocy") (p. 439)	71	13	8	8	1 = "excellent" 2 = "good" 3 = "unchanged" 4 = "dead" (p. 441)	[1] "Only 24 patients had an adequate follow-up of diverse causes" (p. 439)

Table 3.10 Results of various studies of the operation of amygdalectomy

Study	*Date*	*Samp. no.*	*Diagnoses*	*M. imp.* *1*	*S. imp.* *2*	*No imp.* *3*	*Worse* *4*	*Original categories*	*Remarks*
Narabayashi and Uno	1966	40	40 "Behavior disorders" (p. 168)	45	33	22	–	1 = A; "dramatic and marked improvement" 2 = B; "Fairly improved" and C; "Slightly improved" 3 = D; "Not changed" (p. 169)	[1] 20 cases were excluded because "the family of which sent no answer at all and the cases, answers about which by the family were considered rather unreliable" (p. 168)
Balasubramaniam *et al.*	1970	115	115 "Hyperkinetic and behavior disorders" (p. 18)	38	37	17	8	1 = A; "No need of any drugs" and B; "Very docile and given to occasional outbursts only" 2 = C; "Manageable when given drugs though not leading a useful life" and D; "Transient improvement" 3 = E; "No change" 4 = F; "Died" (p. 21)	
Vaernet and Madsen	1970	12[1]	12 "Psychotics with aggressive behaviour" (p. 858)	67[2]	25	8		1 = "No aggression" and "marked improvement" (p. 862)	[1] 3 patients underwent a further basofrontal tractotomy [2] Includes 4 out of 5 schizophrenics
Kiloh *et al.*	1974	18	18 "Aggressive behaviour of an incapacitating degree" (p. 430)	22	28[1]	50		1 = "Marked improvement" 2 = "Slight improvement" 3 = "No change" (p. 440)	[1] Authors noted for 2 patients "slight improvement but not attributed to operations" (p. 440)

Table 3.11 Results of various studies of the operation of limbic leucotomy

Study	*Date*	*Samp. no.*	*Diagnoses*	*M. imp.* *1*	*S. imp.* *2*	*No imp.* *3*	*Worse* *4*	*Original categories*	*Remarks*
Mitchell-Heggs *et al.*	1977	120 66[1]	27 Obsessional neurosis	66	22	4	8	1 = I; "symptom free"	[1] First 66 patients who had been followed up for a mean period of 16 months
			15 Chronic anxiety	27	40	20	13	and II; "much improved"	
			9 Depression	56	22	22	-	2 = III; "improved"	
			7 Schizophrenia	57	29	14		3 = IV; "unchanged"	
			8 Other	25	13	25	37	4 = V; "worse"	
			-					(pp. 369–370)	
			66 Total	50	26	14	10		

Table 3.12 Results of various studies of the operation of capsulotomy

Study	*Date*	*Samp. no.*	*Diagnoses*	*M. imp.* *1*	*S. imp.* *2*	*No imp.* *3*	*Worse* *4*	*Original categories*	*Remarks*
López Ibor and López-Ibor Aliño	1977	75 57[1]	57 Obsessive neuroses	74	17	9		1 = I; "Full recovery" II; "Leads a normal life, but obsession may persist" 2 = III; "Slight improvement" 3 = IV; "No improvement" 4 = V; "Worse" (p. 153)	[1] Results of 18 "other diagnoses" not given
Bingley *et al.*	1977	35	35 Obsessive compulsive neurosis	71	29			1 = A; "free from symptoms" and B; "much improved" 2 = C; "slightly improved" 3 = D; "unchanged" or "worse" (pp. 293–294)	

Table 3.13 Results of various studies of the operation of mesoloviotomy

Study	*Date*	*Samp. no.*	*Diagnoses*	*M. imp.* *1*	*S. imp.* *2*	*No imp.* *3*	*Worse* *4*	*Original categories*	*Remarks*
Laitinen and Vilkki	1973a	38	17 Schizophrenia	82	12	6		1 = I; "Symptom free"	
			10 Anxiety neurosis	50	30	20		and II; "Much improved"	
			5 Affective psychosis	20	40	40		2 = III; "Improved"	
			6 Others	33	17	50		3 = IV; "Not improved"	
			—					4 = IV; "Worse"	
			38 Total	58	21	21	-	(p. 78)	

Table 3.14 Summary of outcome of "first-wave" procedures

Study	*Date*	*Operation*	*No.*	*W.* 4	*No imp.* 3	*S. imp.* 2	*M. imp.* 1
Rao and Govindaswamy	1944	Prefrontal	25	8	40	24	28
Board of Control	1947	Prefrontal	1000	7	25	43	25
Freeman and Watts	1950	Prefrontal	596		22	33	45
Hohman *et al.*	1951	Prefrontal	234	2	29	55	14
Moore	1952	Prefrontal	66		21	26	53
Tooth and Newton	1961	Prefrontal	9284	6	25	28	41
Jones and Shanklin	1950	Transorbital	52		35	17	48
Freeman and Watts	1950	Transorbital	252		34	26	40
Wilson *et al.*	1953	Transorbital	400	2	26	24	48
Fleming and Baker	1972	Bimedial	42		17	39	44
Bernstein *et al.*	1975	Bimedial	43	7	11	5	77
Tow and Lewin	1953	Orbital	20	–	25	40	35
Ström-Olsen and Northfield	1955	Orbital	27	4	18	41	37
Knight and Tredgold	1955	Orbital	52	2	14	40	44
Sykes and Tredgold	1964	Orbital	207	1	14	35	50
McKissock	1951	Rostral	84	2	19	56	23
Pippard	1955a	Rostral	220		47	17	36

Table 3.15 Summary of outcome of "mid-period" procedures

Study	*Date*	*Operation*	*No.*	*W.* 4	*No imp.* 3	*S. imp.* 2	*M. imp.* 1
Ström-Olsen and Carlisle	1971	Tractotomy	150	1	27	23	49
Göktepe *et al.*	1975	Tractotomy	134	–	17	25	58
Whitty *et al.*	1952	Cingulectomy	24	–	66	17	17
Le Beau	1954b	Cingulectomy	30		57		43
Tow and Armstrong	1954	Cingulectomy	17	6	88	6	–
Sano	1962	Cingulectomy	14		50	50	
Brown and Lighthill	1968	Cingulectomy	110	1	5	7	87
Paillas *et al.*	1971	Cingulectomy	20	–	25	30	45
Gaches *et al.*	1972	Cingulectomy	20	–	10	10	80
Laitinen and Vilkki	1972	Cingulectomy	20	–	10	45	45
Mingrino and Schergna	1972	Cingulectomy	10	–	50	30	20
Richardson	1972	Cingulectomy	12	8	–	8	84
Balasubramaniam *et al.*	1973a	Cingulectomy	28		21		79
Meyer *et al.*	1973	Cingulectomy	68	6	10	40	44
Ballantine *et al.*	1977	Cingulectomy	149	–	13	38	49
Martin *et al.*	1977	Cingulectomy	67	–	12	37	51
Bailey *et al.*	1977	Cingulectomy	200	–	1	6	93

Table 3.16 Summary of outcome of "second-wave" procedures

Study	*Date*	*Operation*	*No.*	*W.* *4*	*No imp.* *3*	*S. imp.* *2*	*M. imp.* *1*
Spiegel *et al.*	1953	Thalamotomy	51	–	43	28	29
Andy and Jurko	1972	Thalamotomy	30	–	33	47	20
Schvarcz *et al.*	1972	Hypothalamotomy	11	–	9	27	64
Sano *et al.*	1972	Hypothalamotomy	43	–	5	65	30
Müller *et al.*	1973	Hypothalamotomy	22	5	5	22	68
Balasubramaniam *et al.*	1971	Hypothalamotomy	8	–	13	50	37
Balasubramaniam *et al.*	1973b	Hypothalamotomy	21	19		81	
Dieckmann and Hassler	1975	Hypothalamotomy	6	–		17	83
Dieckmann and Hassler	1977	Hypothalamotomy	4	–		–	100
Schvarcz	1977	Hypothalamotomy	33	20		80	
Nádvornik *et al.*	1977	Hypothalamotomy	10	10	–	30	60
Rubio *et al.*	1977	Hypothalamotomy	24	8	8	13	71
Narabayashi and Uno	1966	Amygdalectomy	40	–	22	33	45
Balasubramaniam *et al.*	1970	Amygdalectomy	115	8	17	37	38
Vaernet and Madsen	1970	Amygdalectomy	12	–	8	25	67
Kiloh *et al.*	1974	Amygdalectomy	18		50	28	22
Mitchell-Heggs *et al.*	1977	Limbic	66	10	14	26	50
López Ibor and López-Ibor Aliño	1977	Capsulotomy	57	–	9	17	74
Bingley *et al.*	1977	Capsulotomy	35	–	–	29	71
Laitinen and Vilkki	1973a	Mesoloviotomy	38	–	21	21	58

Table 3.17 Efficacy of psychosurgical procedures – percentage of operatees showing marked improvement, i.e. category 1

Operation	%	*Disorder*	%
Capsulotomy	73	Sexual "deviation"	72
Cingulectomy	66	Obsessional neurosis	62
Bimedial	58	Manic-depression	59
Mesoloviotomy	58	Depression	57
Hypothalamotomy	55	Anxiety/tension	51
Tractotomy	53	Aggression/hyperkinesis ("behaviour disorders")	43
Limbic	50		
Orbital	47	Schizophrenia	30
Transorbital	45		
Amygdalectomy	40		
Prefrontal	39		
Rostral	32		
Thalamotomy	25		

Table 3.18 Comparison of various psychosurgical procedures in the treatment of certain disorders percentages of patients judged to have shown "marked improvement" following operation

	Thalamotomy	*Rostral*	*Prefrontal*	*Amygdalectomy*	*Transorbital*	*Orbital*	*Limbic*	*Tractotomy*	*Hypothalamotomy*	*Mesoloviotomy*	*Bimedial*	*Cingulectomy*	*Capsulotomy*
Sexual "deviation"	–	–	–	–	–	–	–	–	72	–	–	–	–
Obsessional neurosis	0	46	61	–	65	23	66	50	–	–	81	72	73
Manic-depression	–	0	45	–	67	50	–	–		–	100	98	–
Depression	–	40	59	–	44	66	56	62	–	–	–	45	–
Anxiety/tension	80	33	25	–	–	51	27	49	–	50	–	94	–
Aggression/hyperkinesis ("behaviour disorders")	20	–	–	40	–	–	–	–	58	–	20	–	–
Schizophrenia	27	12	29	–	43	31	57	0	–	82	36	36	

4

Patient populations undergoing psychosurgery

A close examination of which types of patients, if any, benefit from psychosurgery is a crucial first step in any critical assessment. However, at the outset it should be emphasized that many inconsistencies in diagnosis are encountered in reports from different periods of time, different countries and different psychiatrists; there can even be inconsistencies within the same reports. Such diagnostic variations constitute a major "stumbling block" in the evaluation of psychosurgery. Conflicting opinions regarding prognosis constitute another related difficulty. The implications of problems with diagnosis and prognosis will be carefully reviewed in the present chapter. In particular, their bearing on the popular contemporary assertion that operations of the "second wave" offer better treatment prospects than the older procedures will be critically examined.

It is only in the comparatively recent history of psychiatry that diagnostic considerations have been considered important. Given the purely custodial nature of institutions for the insane in the past, it is hardly surprising that little attention was paid to carefully differentiating between psychiatric disorders for the purposes of therapy. Most patients were treated in the same manner, regardless of condition.

The variety of psychiatric treatments available has clearly increased in recent years. It has consequently become essential to distinguish reliably between different psychiatric conditions if therapy and condition are to be fruitfully matched. Conversely, the adequate division of psychiatric disturbances into distinct classes of disorders has furthered the search for specifically tailored therapies. The intimate and reciprocal interaction between treatment development and diagnostic refinement can be clearly seen. Psychiatric diagnosis is no longer unnecessary; in contemporary mainstream psychiatry, it is regarded as fundamental. Kendell (1975) explained:

> Without diagnosis or some comparable method of classification, ... without a criterion for distinguishing between sickness and health, and between one sort of sickness and another, there could never be any rational planning of psychiatric services. Indeed all scientific communication would be impossible and our professional journals would be restricted to individual case reports, anecdotes and statements of opinion. (pp. 6–7)

Without a classification system of some sort, then, systematic treatment evaluation is impossible. Further, the reliability of the diagnostic scheme is crucial; sensible comparison and evaluation requires reliable and consistent diagnostic practices.

However, very few accounts of psychosurgery have tackled the problem of diagnostic reliability. Rather, it has been assumed that patient populations attracting the same diagnostic label in reports from different periods of time, from different countries and from different psychiatrists are analogous. Thus, it is supposed, for example, that a patient currently diagnosed as schizophrenic would have received the same diagnosis in the "first wave." Let us examine the validity of such assumptions.

In comparing diagnoses of patients from different periods of time, three possible sources of variation should be considered: the introduction of different classification systems in psychiatry; changes in the concepts of various disorders, such that some disorders embrace symptoms now which previously were not included as part of that disorder; and a deliberate shift in psychiatric disorders deemed appropriate for psychosurgery.

As Kendell (1975) has detailed, there has been a succession of revisions of the *International Classification of Diseases* (known as *ICD*) in recent years. Such changes can make comparison between psychosurgery reports from different eras extremely difficult. For example, there are notable differences between the American versions of *ICD-6* and *ICD-8* (cf. Spitzer and Wilson, 1968). With the adoption of a new system, certain patients could well receive a different diagnostic label from the one they would have attracted under a previous regime.

The problem of diagnostic consistency is compounded further by the reluctance of some psychiatrists to amend their diagnoses in accordance with a new classification. Kendell (1973), comparing diagnoses made before and after the introduction of *ICD-8*, noted that the new system had made very little difference to many English psychiatrists. In the proceedings of the

Fourth International Congress of Psychosurgery, years after the introduction of *ICD-8*, only Hirose (1977) and Mitchell-Heggs *et al.* (1977) furnished the international codings.

Apart from the problem presented by the introduction of successive international classifications, there are indications that, even under the regime of the same classification system, marked changes in diagnostic concepts and practices have occurred. Such temporal fluctuations in psychiatric diagnosis have long been recognized. The studies of Masserman and Carmichael (1938) and Hunt *et al.* (1953) have demonstrated inconsistencies in psychiatric diagnoses over time. Their results have led Zubin (1967) to conclude that "the consistency over time of diagnosis is for the most part low" (p. 386).

The introduction of new methods of treatment can lead to quite dramatic changes in the pattern of psychiatric diagnosis. For example, a change in the diagnosis of neurotic conditions over a 15-year period was reported at the Maudsley Hospital in London by Hare (1974). It was noted that there was an increase in the proportion of neurotic cases diagnosed as depression with the introduction of drugs for depressive states. A subsequent increase in the proportion of diagnoses of phobia paralleled the introduction of behaviour therapy.

Finally, comparison between temporally displaced psychiatric studies is furthered hampered in the case of psychosurgery by a change in the choice of disorders considered appropriate for treatment. Today's patients are generally less chronically disturbed and have a better prognosis without treatment than those operated on during the "first wave" of psychosurgery (cf. Valenstein, 1977). The present selectivity has undoubtedly been occasioned by "first wave" experiences. It is a point made by Post and Schurr (1977) in their account of the changes in patient populations deemed suitable for surgery at their neurosurgical unit in London. In Japan, Hirose (1973) detailed a similar shift.

In general, the data from Britain reveal a marked decline in the proportion of schizophrenic patients receiving psychosurgery (Table 4.1). The first figure in the Table is derived from all patients subjected to psychosurgery prior to 1944 in England and Wales (Board of Control, 1947). Tooth and Newton's (1961) study covers all single operations from 1942 to 1954 in England and Wales. The final figure in the table is based upon Valenstein's (1977) analysis of the total number of psychosurgery patients in each diagnostic

Table 4.1 Comparison of the percentages of schizophrenics in the UK who underwent psychosurgery from its inception until 1976

Study	Board of Control (1947)	Tooth and Newton (1961)	Post and Schurr (1977)		Valenstein (1977)
Period	-1944	1942–1954	1953–1958 :	1969–1974	1970–1976
Percentage of all operatees diagnosed as schizophrenic	60	64	7	0	3

category reported for the United Kingdom in the years 1971–1976. According to Valenstein's analysis, "depression" (42%), "obsessive–compulsive neurosis" (22%), "fear and anxiety" (19%) and "epilepsy with psychotic disorders" (8%) would apppear to be the preferred targets for psychosurgery.

In addition to these inconsistencies over time, striking geographic variations in diagnostic practices can be detected. A number of reports, in particular those by Lewis (1946), Shepherd (1957), Roth (1959), Kramer (1969) and Zubin (1969) make explicit mention of possible differences in diagnostic practices between countries, especially between the United States and the United Kingdom.

The *United States–United Kingdom* (US–UK) *Diagnostic Project*, described by Zubin (1969), closely examined the comparable diagnostic procedures of American and British psychiatrists. Marked differences between the two countries in diagnostic practice were reported (e.g. Gurland *et al.*, 1970; Cooper *et al.*, 1972), despite the fact that both countries had adopted the same classification system (*ICD-8*) and the same glossary (the British one). The major finding was that the diagnosis of schizophrenia was made more often by American psychiatrists than by their British counterparts. It appeared that the concept of schizophrenia differed substantially between the two countries. In their monograph on this project, Cooper and his associates concluded:

> ... the New York concept of schizophrenia is much broader than that used in London and embraces many patients who would be regarded by British psychiatrists as suffering from depressive illnesses, neurotic illnesses or personality disorders, and nearly all those who would be regarded as suffering from mania. (p. 139)

The implications of geographical inconsistencies in diagnosis are compounded further in the case of psychosurgery by variations in the diagnostic categories that attract surgery in different countries. Valenstein's (1977) analysis reveals clear differences between Britain and the United States in this respect. In contrast to the current British preferences, listed earlier, the main American targets are "depression" (38%), "schizophrenia and other psychoses" (21%), "obsessive–compulsive disorders" (10%) and "aggression" (9%).

Thus, psychosurgery is still frequently employed with patients diagnosed as "schizophrenic" in the United States, although the current proportion is considerably less than that apparent in the "first wave" of surgery. This difference is in all probability bound up with the more widespread use of the schizophrenic diagnosis in the United States. Included in the American "schizophrenic" population are likely to be patients who would not have attracted this diagnostic label in the United Kingdom. An important implication of geographical inconsistencies in diagnosis becomes apparent.

Psychosurgeons in the United States have always regarded schizophrenia as an indication for psychosurgery to a much greater extent than their British counterparts. Their preferences undoubtedly reflect their different experiences with the disorder. The data cited in Chapter 3 attest to the conflicting indications for psychosurgery on schizophrenic patients. One variable that underlies the conflict is country of study; the more favourable results generally arise from the United States. It is possible that divergent diagnostic practices regarding schizophrenia underlie the differences in results. The relatively broad and inclusive concept of schizophrenia held in the United States may serve to include patients with more favourable prognoses (irrespective of treatment) than those encompassed by the more circumscribed British diagnostic concept. Thus, better outcomes primarily reflect the inclusion of patients with better chances of recovery anyway.

Finally, even psychiatrists from the same country and at the same time cannot always reliably agree on diagnosis. In the 1930s and 1940s, a series of reports (e.g. Doering and Raymond, 1934; Masserman and Carmichael, 1938; Gordon, 1946; Ash, 1949) drew attention to the problems of the reliability of psychiatric diagnosis. More recently, Spitzer and Fleiss (1974) reviewed much of the previous data, applying a statistic called *Cohen's Kappa* to compensate for chance agreement. Their analysis reveals that the reliability of psychiatric diagnosis is far from perfect and has not notably improved over the years. Spitzer and Wilson (1975) commented:

> Most of the studies involved diagnosticians of similar background and training, a factor that one would expect to contribute to good reliability. In addition, in some of the studies, special efforts were made to have the participant diagnosticians come to some agreement regarding diagnostic principles before beginning the study. One can only assume, therefore, that agreement between average diagnosticians of different orientations and backgrounds, as they work in routine clinical settings, is even poorer. (p. 22)

Clearly, such unreliability has implications for evaluations of the effectiveness of any treatment intervention. Hetherington *et al.* (1972) illustrated the problems with regard to the psychosurgical treatment of schizophrenia. They noted that two papers, one by Sykes and Tredgold (1964) and the other by Baker *et al.* (1970), reported unsatisfactory results in apparent contrast to the report of Miller (1967). Hetherington and coworkers accounted for this discrepancy in terms of diagnostic variation:

> Conversation with Miller revealed that the discrepancy was probably due to the interpretation of the meaning of schizophrenia. Miller and his colleagues actually studied what would now be referred to as schizo-affectives. (p. 333)

This example essentially confirms our earlier analysis. It also serves to underscore the contention that diagnostic variation is an extremely important consideration in the evaluation of psychosurgery.

There are several reasons for doubting that, even within a single psychosurgery report, patients bearing the same label are, in fact, really homogeneous with respect to disorder. For example, many reports contain information on patients who have been assigned diagnostic labels at different periods of time. Further, the diagnoses presented in a single report may have been derived from several psychiatrists. As Turner (1972) has pointed out, patients come to the psychosurgeon from a variety of sources.

In summary, therefore, comparison between reports from different periods of time, from different countries or between different psychiatrists should be made with extreme caution. Even within the same report, homogeneity cannot be taken for granted. Such considerations have important implications for the evaluation of psychosurgery. They strongly advise against the uncritical acceptance of reports of the efficacy of psychosurgical procedures. Much of the disagreement over the suitability of various psychiatric conditions (especially schizophrenia) for psychosurgery can, in part, be accounted for in terms of inconsistencies in diagnosis. Further, as we illustrated earlier, inaccurate diagnoses can artificially inflate apparent rates of success. This occurs when patients with a favourable prognosis (irrespective of treatment) are assigned a diagnostic label denoting a condition with an unfavourable prognosis. The positive American results for psychosurgery with schizophrenia undoubtedly reflect artefacts of this sort.

Clearly, success rates with psychosurgery for a given patient group can be sensibly evaluated only relative to recovery rates without treatments for that group (even this ignores the placebo effects of the treatment milieu, an influence that will be considered later). How does psychosurgery fare in comparisons of this sort? How do the newer operations fare relative to the older procedure? It is to these questions that we shall address much of the remainder of this chapter.

The first point to emphasize is that patients do indeed recover from a variety of psychiatric disorders without any specific therapeutic intervention. Further, it is clear that certain patient characteristics have an important bearing on the likelihood of improvement without therapy. Diagnosis would seem to be the most important of these characteristics.

The forecasting of the course and outcome of a disorder and the choice of treatment for it are two aspects of what Zubin (1967) referred to as the "predictive validity" of psychiatric diagnosis. Different diagnostic categories imply different treatments and different prognoses with and without treatment. It is, however, virtually impossible to obtain "pure" baselines for rates of improvement, i.e. recovery rates in the absence of specific therapeutic interventions, since, at present, most patients who receive a diagnosis also receive some specified treatment. Practical and ethical considerations militate against the withholding of treatment in order to observe the course and outcome of psychiatric disorders. Other methods have, however, been devised.

One method of providing "pure" baselines is to adopt data from the past, i.e. before administration of specific therapies became routine. This procedure was used by Staudt and Zubin (1957) in their investigation of early physical methods of treatment in psychiatry (including psychosurgery). Staudt and Zubin (1957) concluded:

> Generally speaking, most of these studies indicate about a 30–40% improvement rate maintained at follow-up by these so called spontaneous remissions or by those who had non-specific treatment. (p. 176)

Staudt and Zubin (1957) plotted the percentage of schizophrenics (given non-specific treatment) recovered, much improved and improved at follow-up intervals up to five years after admission to hospital. These figures were based upon the studies reviewed earlier. Comparison can then be made with the outcome of the psychosurgical studies they reviewed (Figure 4.1). The untreated curve shows a fairly even course during the 5-year period.

For psychosurgery, however, the course is much more variable. At two

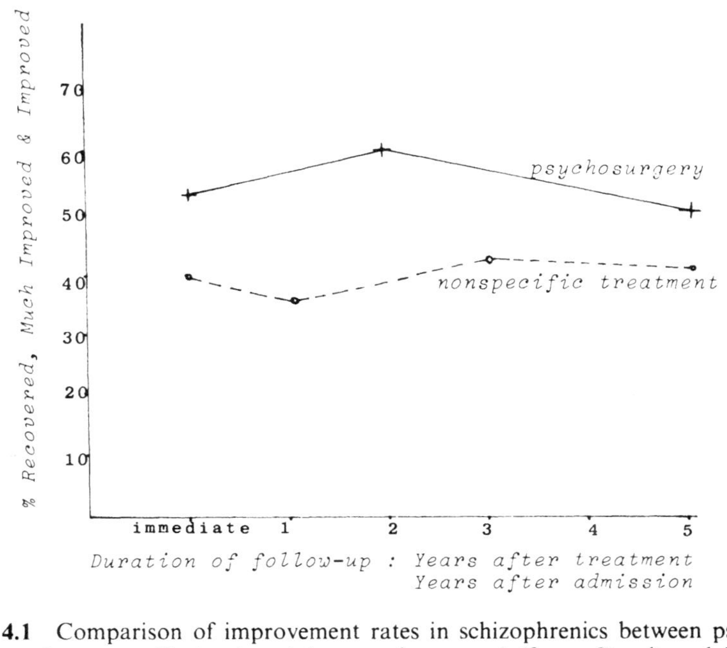

Figure 4.1 Comparison of improvement rates in schizophrenics between psychosurgery and non-specific treatment (pre-psychosurgery) (from: Staudt and Zubin, 1957). Copyright (1957) by the American Psychological Association; Reprinted by permission

years the outcome was better than immediately after the operation. This is often referred to as "delayed operation response." After five years, the outcome was poorer than immediately after the operation. While the psychosurgery patients demonstrated better immediate outcome (between 50 and 60%) than did the untreated group, they suffered substantial relapse over time, so that by the end of five years, aggregate outcome had approached the non-specific rate of 40%. Although similar findings were reported for the other somatotherapies or organic therapies reviewed, Staudt and Zubin claimed that these other therapies at least saved life. This advantage was not claimed for psychosurgery (Figure 4.2).

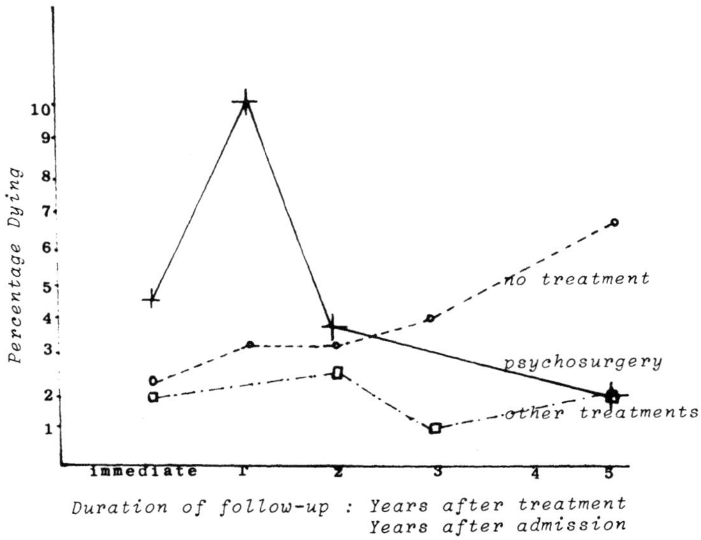

Figure 4.2 Comparison of incidence of deaths among schizophrenics between psychosurgery, no treatment and other treatments (from: Staudt and Zubin, 1957). Copyright (1957) by the American Psychological Association; Reprinted by permission

There are, however, difficulties with baseline data from the pre-psychosurgery era. Staudt and Zubin elaborated:

> These data ought not to be used as standards or baselines since, as we have seen, they were derived from total hospital populations. Moreover, diagnostic criteria have changed and probably the character of the patient population has changed, too, as a consequence of mental health education, interest in psychiatry, and increased use of specific therapies in private practice as well as in hospitals. (p. 187)

It would, therefore, appear unwise to adopt uncritically data from the past for the purpose of control. Nevertheless, such patients have frequently comprised the control groups against which organic therapies have been compared. However, it should be appreciated that any biases in such control data favour the treatment to be compared, since the developments cited above clearly imply a trend towards better untreated prognosis over the years.

Several studies have employed no-treatment controls selected from the contemporaries of the patients to be treated. Staudt and Zubin reviewed a "representable" number of such studies. Generally, there appeared to be a greater improvement in the treatment group compared to the untreated controls (except in the case of Metrazol therapy). However, only one study of psychosurgery is included in this review. This is a study by Friedman *et al.* (1951), which reported dramatic differences in improvement rates between control and treatment groups in favour of psychosurgery. On follow-up at two years, 3% of the 100 controls showed substantial improvement, whereas the comparable figure for the leucotomized patients was 57.8%. However, caution is warranted. The outcome after two years for the control group is extremely poor compared to that observed for the non-specific treatment subjects in Figure 4.1 and the control groups reviewed by Staudt and Zubin. These authors drew attention to the problems of such control groups. They

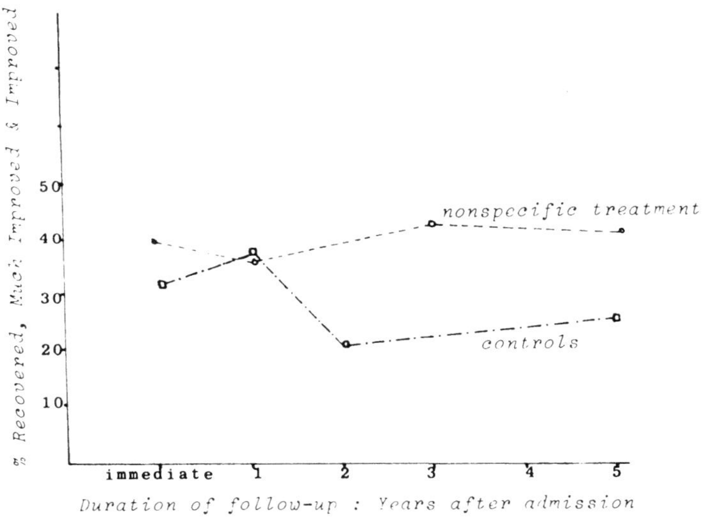

Figure 4.3 Comparison of outcome between schizophrenics given non-specific treatment (pre-psychosurgery) and those used as controls in somatotherapy studies (from: Staudt and Zubin, 1957). Copyright (1957) by the American Psychological Association; Reprinted by permission

noted that, on the whole, the prognosis for the control groups of this period was much worse than that for the non-specific treatment groups of the pre-shock or pre-psychosurgery area (Figure 4.3):

> One reason may be that in the shock era only poorer patients, that is, those with unfavourable prognosis, were available as controls, other patients being given the benefit of the specific treatments. There is also a second possibility, namely, that chronic deteriorated cases may have been selected as controls. (p. 183)

The psychosurgery literature reveals few studies that have even attempted to compare the outcome of leucotomized patients with that of contemporary untreated controls. Staudt and Zubin (1957) included only one such psychosurgery study in their review of the somatotherapies. Nevertheless, their criticism that pretreatment prognoses of treated patients were generally more favourable than those of their controls can be well documented in the case of psychosurgery. As is revealed by the following review of such "controlled" studies by psychosurgery, matching psychosurgery candidates and controls on the basis of prognosis has in most projects been rudimentary and generally biased in favour of the treatment group.

An early study that attempted to compare operatees with untreated controls was that undertaken by Penrose (1944). This was a survey of the effects of a number of organic therapies in Ontario hospitals. Penrose compared the number of operatees remaining in hospital with that of a similar group of patients, matched with the treated group for age and duration of illness. At follow-up, approximately two years posttreatment, six patients remained on the hospital books, compared to an expected 16.87. However, caution should be exercised with respect to this finding. Penrose's survey of patients treated by shock therapy indicated differential improvement rates in favour of the treatment between treated patients and their controls at two-year follow-up. By the end of five years, however, there was no great difference in discharge rates. This result essentially confirms the findings of Staudt and Zubin (1957) with respect to the outcome of shock therapy. It should serve to illustrate the dangers of assuming that immediate or two-year differences in discharge rates between operatees and controls will be maintained at longer follow-up (cf. Figure 4.1).

Worthing *et al.* (1951) used a similar method of comparison to evaluate the results of leucotomy. They observed of their 600 cases (mainly schizophrenics) subjected to the Lyerly modification of the "standard" technique:

> ... the number out of the hospital tends to stabilize at about 35% of the total operated cases. This figure is not reached until about 2 years after operation and there is indication that it does not fall off during the third and even fourth post operative year (group 1–100); thus, the result appears to be stable. (p. 328)

However, inspection of their data does reveal that the number of patients out of hospital at four-year follow-up for the first group of patients (1–100) had indeed dropped, albeit slightly (38 to 36). From some patients in this group, follow-up was only three years, since they underwent operation at a later date than the first patients. The last date of operation for this group was April 6, 1948, and follow-up for the whole group took place on April 21, 1951. It is possible, therefore, that by the end of a full five-year follow-up for all patients, relapse rates would reduce the improvement rate of the operatees towards that of the controls.

A frequently cited study that compared an operated group to a contemporary untreated group was the first Columbia–Greystone Project, designed to study the effects of topectomy. A group of 24 operatees was matched to the same number of controls. The first group received psychosurgery, while the second underwent a "sham" operation. Four months afterwards, 20 of the operatees were recommended for parole by an independent board, while only four of the controls received such a recommendation. However, due to a number of reasons, only 16 of the operatees were in fact released. At the end of 30 months, seven of these 16 were still out of hospital and had never returned. A further three had been readmitted but were out of hospital at follow-up. The four controls had not returned to the hospital.

These results, as reported by Landis *et al.* (1950), reveal that the difference between the discharge rates for the two groups at the 30 month follow-up is less marked than at 4 months and is not statistically significant. It must be noted that only a few months after the original leucotomy, two of the operatees and six controls underwent psychosurgery; therefore, strict comparison between the two groups at the longer follow-up period was rendered impossible. Further, although the two groups were supposedly matched, the authors' own account casts some doubts on the validity of the matching procedure. Landis *et al.* (1950) explained:

> The decision as to which of each pair should be operated was made by the medical and surgical specialists on the basis of which of the two was the best "risk" for operation. (p. 127)

Despite May's (1974) assertion to the contrary, such a procedure would appear to bias the results *in favour* of the operated group. That the control group had a poorer pretreatment prognosis was suggested by Hoch *et al.* (1956) and is confirmed by a closer inspection of the data presented by Mettler (1949).

First, the two groups were not comparable with respect to disorder. Of the 24 operatees, 17 received diagnoses other than schizophrenia, while all but two of the controls were diagnosed as schizophrenic (more hebephrenics were in this latter group as well). The effects of such inadequate matching of diagnoses with different associated untreated prognoses has already been detailed. Another crucial variable upon which the two groups were inadequately matched with respect to prognosis was length of institutionalization. The average period of hospitalization was greater for the controls (67 months) than for the operatees (51 months). Of the controls, only three patients had been institutionalized for two years or less, compared to eight of the operatees. Of the eight, *six* were adjudged to have demonstrated "lasting improvement" (p. 315) after leucotomy.

That six of the operatees who had periods of hospitalization shorter than two years demonstrated lasting improvement, out of a total of nine patients assigned to the "lasting improvement" category (p. 315) suggest that postoperative course was influenced markedly by preoperative status. Given the better status of the operatees, i.e. more patients in the operated group had institutional stays of less than two years duration, the results accordingly are likely to be biased in favour of psychosurgery.

This study has been examined in some detail, since it is frequently cited as one of the most carefully controlled and systematically planned psychosurgery projects. That such major methodological defects flaw this supposedly well-designed study should indicate the status of the rest of the so-called "controlled" studies.

The second Columbia–Greystone Project (the "Rocklands Investigation"), designed to study the effects of various forms of surgical intervention (including transorbital leucotomy) in the treatment of mental disorder, found no significant difference between discharge rates for the controls (one out of six patients) and for the operatees (two out of 25 patients), despite the controls having poor prognoses (Mettler, 1952).

The Connecticut Lobotomy Cooperative Study, mentioned by Staudt and Zubin (1957), investigated the effects of the Lyerly or "open" operative procedure, mainly on schizophrenics. An operated group (254 patients) was compared with a control group of 100 patients who had been originally selected for surgery. However, since family permission had not been granted, no operation was performed on the control patients. Friedman *et al.* (1951) compared the outcomes for the two groups. At the follow-up of two years, 3% of the 100 controls showed much improvement whereas the comparable figure for the leucotomized patients was 57.8%. Only 2% of the control group were discharged from hospital, compared to 37% of the operatees.

As Staudt and Zubin (1957) observed, the outcome of the controls would appear to be markedly worse than that of the non-specific treatment group of the previous era (compare Figures 4.1 and 4.3). Further, there were some important differences between the operatees and their controls. For example, the control group contained more women than men (80% compared to 59%), more patients over the age of 50 (30% compared to 13%), more patients with a longer duration of illness (39% over 12 years of illness compared to 25%) and more patients with a longer duration of hospitalization (88% over two years compared to 76%).

Further inspection of the Friedman *et al.* report indicates that 48% of control group patients had been in hospital for over eight years, as opposed to only 24% of the leucotomized group. Close examination of the graph presented by Friedman *et al.* reveals that degree of improvement is, in fact, inversely related to length of pretreatment hospitalization. Eight years seems to be an important cutoff point here. If the operated group had comprised more long-stay patients, it is likely that the recovery rate observed following leucotomy would not have deviated substantially from that depicted for the non-specific treatment patients in Figure 4.1.

Another study that used a similar style of control group was the West Virginia Lobotomy Project. In this study, Freeman *et al.* (1954) reported on the clinical effects of transorbital leucotomy on 228 operatees. A control group of 200 unoperated patients comprised those candidates for surgery whose relatives had refused permission for operation. At one year follow-up, 85 of the 224 survivors of psychosurgery were out of hospital, compared to only five of the controls. Although the percentage of patients discharged after leucotomy is not large (37%), nevertheless it represents a considerable improvement over the untreated group.

However, detailed results were only presented at one year follow-up. Evidence was presented that relapses had already taken place by the time the paper was written. A longer period of observation would be needed to ensure that the difference between discharge rates would be maintained over a number of years.

A major problem with this study is that no evidence of matching was presented. Whether the controls were indeed comparable to the operatees in terms of prognoses cannot be ascertained. Although it was stated that the two groups had both been selected for psychosurgery, this does not imply that they were indeed comparable. That the relatives of the controls refused permission could indicate a poorer prognosis for the control group.

Interest of the relatives in the project was considered to be a major factor affecting discharge rates of leucotomized patients, as these authors observed.

> Experience has shown that the chance of getting a patient home after lobotomy is about doubled if the relatives can be persuaded to adopt responsibility for the patient within two weeks after operation. (p. 941)

Further, inspection of the method of discharge reveals that the two groups were not treated analogously.

> About a week after one of the operative sessions a large group of relatives was invited to meet at the hospital to learn about transorbital lobotomy. The superintendent discussed for them the function of the hospital in caring for the patients, and one of us (W.F.) described the nature of the operation and the responsibilities of the families in caring for the patients after release. About 20 patients already operated on were sitting with their relatives in the auditorium, so that relatives of patients yet

> to be operated on had a chance to see the immediate results of transorbital lobotomy. This meeting resulted in so many patients being released that similar meetings were held on later occasions. (p. 941)

Clearly, this procedure substantially favours discharge for the operated group.

A further study employing this sort of control group was reported by Medina *et al.* (1954). Twenty-five operatees were matched with a similar number of controls (mainly consisting of patients whose relatives had refused permission for operation) on nine criteria: race, age, sex, preoperative diagnosis, period of hospitalization, age at time of hospitalization, years of formal education, marital status and occupational level. Each group contained 19 schizophrenics and six affective psychoses. Severity of individual psychosis was judged by social behaviour and impairment of affect. A further 18 operatees for whom no adequate controls could be found were also subjected to investigation.

Only one control was placed in the *marked improvement category*, whereas ten of the original operatees were assigned this rating and one was assessed as completely recovered. Of the whole operated group (43 in all), 13 were placed in the former category and seven in the latter. Of these 20, 25% were reported as reaching their "peak of adjustment" within one year of operation and 60% within five years. A further 40% continued to improve up to eight-year follow-up. Such belated improvement would no doubt be interpreted as being due to "delayed operative response." Unfortunately, relapses were also noted in the same period. As these authors observed of five of the combined group of 20 operatees achieving the two highest categories:

> 5 have shown signs of regressing to a lower adjustment level within the last few years. 2 of these 5 were patients for whom complete recoveries had been reported in a report published within a year after operation. (p. 28)

Thus, although improvement can appear fairly immediately, as revealed by the Petersen and Buchstein (1942) report, relapses can occur after a considerable period of time and are only observed at long-term follow-up. Most of the studies reported here would not have picked up such relapses. This study, with its "delayed operative responses" and relapses, demonstrates the need for long-term comparison with untreated controls. It must be noted that this is one of the only controlled studies in which improvement rates are used to compare the two groups. The better assessment of "intra-hospital improvement" for the operatees may not be independent of the knowledge that these patients had undergone psychosurgery or that the operation made these patients easier to manage without necessarily greatly improving their psychiatric condition. (Only one operatee was sufficiently improved to be out of hospital at 12-year follow-up.) Finally, very few of these controlled studies have employed independent evaluators.

The Veterans Administration Lobotomy Research Project (Jenkins *et al.*, 1954) was designed to investigate the effects mainly of standard leucotomies. Operatees were matched to controls. However, according to the authors, allocation to surgery was made "on a therapeutic basis" (p. 85). Those with more severe symptoms were apparently allocated to the treatment group. Comparison of 60 schizophrenic "rigidly matched pairs" in terms of number and severity of symptoms reveals that 30 operatees were categorized as "definitely improved," while only 14 control patients achieved this status. On a measure of "normality," eight of the operatees were assigned to the "definitely improved" category, compared with five of the controls. These authors concluded that "although both groups tend to show improvement, the operated one still shows more tendency to improvement than do control cases. This difference is reliable at the 0.01 level of confidence" (p. 85).

These results should, however, be seen in the context of a follow-up of a very short duration. Only a year earlier, the first 30 patients were evaluated at *three-month* follow-up by Jenkins and Holsopple (1953).

The later report by Ball *et al.* (1959) included the patients reviewed in earlier studies by Jenkins *et al.* In the later paper, Ball *et al.* compared 185 controls with 188 leucotomees, supposedly comparable with respect to age, diagnosis and duration of illness. Most of the leucotomees had undergone the standard (Poppen modification) form of operation. The rest underwent bimedial, undercutting and transorbital leucotomies. Discharge rates were lower for the transorbital leucotomees than for the controls over five-year follow-up. The undercutting patients showed slightly greater improvement than controls. Significantly better discharge rates were reported for both the standard and bimedial groups of patients than for the controls at four-year follow-up. Unfortunately, confounding of results occurred thereafter due to the administration of certain drugs (mainly chlorpromazine), so that some two thirds of the patients at the time of five-year follow-up were on some form of antipsychotic medication.

Apart from this latter factor, a number of methodological defects flaw this study. First, the two groups were not strictly comparable with respect to diagnoses: more schizophrenics were included in the control group. Second, it would appear that the operatees had poorer preoperative prognoses than controls. Further, the rater knew whether or not the patient had been leucotomized. Finally, Ball *et al.* (1959) and Jenkins and Holsopple (1953) reported difficulty in keeping postoperative treatment similar for both leucotomees and controls.

A study by Powell (1955) employed a similar control group and was designed to study the effects of transorbital leucotomy. Most of the operatees were schizophrenics (59 of 71), some of whom had had more than one operation. Significantly more *controls* were discharged than operatees.

However, as Robin and MacDonald (1975) have observed, it would appear that the pretreatment prognoses of the operatees were worse than for the controls, which could account for differences in improvement rates.

Scherer and associates compared 22 leucotomees (Lyerly modification of the "standard" operation) with a similar number of controls, all fairly well equated for age, education, length of hospitalization, diagnostic classification and degree of cooperation (Scherer *et al.*, 1957). Although the leucotomees were better at some tests than the controls, Scherer *et al.* (1957) nevertheless concluded:

> Quantitative analysis of the lobotomized patients' behavior and examination of psychiatrists' progress notes suggest that in some respects the operated group is not doing as well clinically as the nonoperated group. (p. 298)

At five-year follow-up, seven leucotomees were discharged, compared to four controls; the difference was not statistically significant.

In a large-scale study, Barahal (1958) reported on some 1095 leucotomees (mainly schizophrenics), who were compared with 606 controls. The controls were described as patients

> . . . who were recommended for prefrontal lobotomy but for whom operative permits could not be obtained. This was used as a control series, as in every respect other than the operation itself these patients were considerably comparable to the operation series. (p. 656)

Only 2% of controls, compared to 21% of leucotomees, were discharged at five- to ten-year follow-up. Unfortunately, no matching criteria were given and, as Zubin (1958) observed of the selection of controls:

> Whether Dr. Barahal's unlobotomized patients constitute an adequate control group is questionable. It is likely that the reasons for rejecting an operation are not independent of psychiatric status, or of the family's attitude toward the return of the patient, or of the eventual outcome. (p. 685)

Three retrospective studies were reported by Robin (1958a, b; 1959). In the first of these, 198 controls (derived from the same hospital records) were matched to 198 operatees for chronicity, age on admission, sex and "under treatment at the same time" (to compensate, no doubt, for non-specific treatment affects). Robin (1958a) concluded that at ten-year follow-up leucotomy did not appear to improve the chances of discharge from hospital, accelerate discharge, reduce chances of readmission, delay readmission, reduce numbers of readmission, reduce total period of admission, improve hospital behaviour as judged at ward level, or significantly increase the death rate.

Similarly, at ten-year follow-up, no significant differences between discharge rates for 91 leucotomized schizophrenics and for controls (mainly schizophrenics) were reported by Robin (1959). May (1974) criticized these studies and suggested that the leucotomees had poorer preoperative prognoses than controls. He also pointed out the matching of diagnosis was inadequate, since the control group comprised fewer schizophrenics.

Similarly, May suggested that the leucotomized group of 60 schizophrenics reported by Robin (1958b) were more disturbed than their 60 schizophrenic controls. Sixty pairs of patients were matched on the basis of sex, age of admission and length of admission as well as a large number of factors, including total length of previous hospital admission(s), civil state (single, married, etc.), stability of occupational record, family history of mental illness and suicide, school progress, heterosexual attainment (friendships, an engagement, etc.), personality profile, age and acuteness of onset of first symptoms, number of remissions in the illness and previous treatment history.

Robin concluded:

> The general results show leucotomy to offer no advantage in the treatment of schizophrenia. A large number of discharges in the leucotomy group is counter-balanced by a larger number of readmissions. The total period in Runwell after operation and in all mental institutions is comparable in the treated and untreated groups. (p. 128)

This finding supports Staudt and Zubin's (1957) observation (see Figure 4.1) that although operatees show better initial improvement than controls, nevertheless, due to a high relapse at the end of five years, improvement rates for both are comparable.

Comparing 132 leucotomized schizophrenics with 71 schizophrenic controls, Witton and Ellsworth (1962) reported discharge rates at two and a half years after operation or selection for operation, after two and a half years of drug treatment and after a further two and a half years "unclassified treatment" in which both groups were treated similarly. After the latter period, no group differences were apparent; approximately one quarter of patients in both groups had been released.

One of the most widely cited controlled studies of psychosurgery is that carried out by McKenzie and Kaczanowski (1964). In an attempt to assess the clinical efficacy of the "standard" type of operation, these authors retrospectively matched 183 operatees to 183 controls. Operations had been carried out between the years 1955 and 1957. Length of hospitalization was reported as being comparable between the two groups, as were chronicity, sex, diagnosis and age. The control group contained 58 patients who would have been considered for surgery but permission for operation was refused by relatives. They reported that there was no significant difference in rate of hospital discharge between the two groups, despite "some methodological bias in favour of the operated group" (p. 1195). The sample was an heterogeneous group of patients who were investigated in respect to intermittency and chronicity of illness. The authors noted that "leucotomy, *if* successful in intermittently ill subjects, is likely to be rather stabilizing" (p. 1195, italic in original).

The last controlled study to be reviewed here that focused on the effects of psychosurgery in the treatment of schizophrenia was by Nicholas (1967). Leucotomized patients (mean postoperative period was 11 years) who had been admitted to a special rehabilitation unit were compared to all non-leucotomized patients. No significant difference between the two groups is apparent from the data presented.

Very few studies have compared the effects of leucotomy on other diagnostic categories in the context of controlled studies. One attempt to assess the efficacy of modified leucotomy in the treatment of severe agoraphobia was reported in a retrospective study by Marks *et al.* (1966). Of their 22 patients, nine (Series B) underwent bimedial leucotomy, while all but two of the remainder (Series A) had the Jackson modification of the standard operation described in Chapter 2. These were matched with controls on the basis of sex, age at treatment, symptom type and duration, and age at onset of illness. Sixteen controls were found to be suitable on these criteria following a search in the hospital records.

Both groups were judged to be comparable in the severity of their agoraphobia and general anxiety. Ratings (a five-point rating scale was used) were made on a variety of measures. These ratings were made on extracts of case records taken just before operation, three months after it and at one-, three- and five-year follow-up. For the controls, the equivalent data for assessment was date of discharge from the institution of admission. Marks *et al.* (1966) concluded:

> Leucotomy patients did significantly better than controls with respect to phobias and general anxiety; depression remained mild; work adjustment improved markedly. Maximum improvement of general anxiety occurred within the first three months, whereas phobias continued to improve after the first year. (p. 768) In longstanding cases of severe agoraphobia with prominent anxiety, modified leucotomy produced more useful sustained improvement than other forms of treatment. (p. 769)

However, inspection of their summary graphs reveals that the differences between the operated and control groups were slight, especially for the phobic patients receiving bimedial operations. For general anxiety, maximum change occurred in Series A patients at three months, but then a relapse was noted towards the three-year follow-up. Similarly, improvement for the bimedial leucotomy group (Series B) appeared greatest at three months and subsequently declined such that at three years their mean improvement rating was indistinguishable from that reported for the control group. For depression, no real differences were observed. The control patients, if anything, seemed to have improved slightly more than both series of operatees at five-year follow-up. Considering readmissions, the rates for control and treatment seemed comparable.

Two earlier studies had examined psychosurgery in the context of obsessive–compulsive disorders. Ingram (1961) reported that 39% of 46 non-leucotomized patients had improved at follow-up, compared to 56% (i.e. 10) of 18 leucotomees. Matching was, however, poor, and follow-up was variable. Further, as Robin and MacDonald (1975) have pointed out, the difference between the two groups at follow-up was not statistically reliable. Similarly, Pollitt's (1960) study also failed to find significant differences between leucotomized and control groups of obsessionals.

In a more recent study, Tan *et al.* (1971) examined the effectiveness of bimedial leucotomy in the treatment of patients diagnosed as suffering from obsessive–compulsive neurosis. Comparison was made between 23 leucotomized patients and 13 controls. The two groups were matched on symptom severity, type and duration, as well as on age. The major difference between the two groups was the longer symptom duration of the operatees compared with the controls (15 years compared to 8 years). Ratings were made on several measures (obsessions and compulsions, anxiety, depression, work and social activities). These ratings were made on extracts of case notes immediately before leucotomy and then three months after, followed by ratings at one-, three- and five-year follow-up. The point of comparison for the controls was the date of discharge from the index admission. These authors concluded of their results:

> Leucotomy patients did significantly better than controls with respect to obsessions and general anxiety. Obsessions were reduced from a severe to a moderate degree of handicap. Work adjustment improved. Personality changes after operation were mild and not related to outcome. Maximum improvement of obsessions and general anxiety occurred within the first three months. Improvement for both was maintained over 5 years follow-up. The present study, using carefully matched controls, suggests that modified leucotomy is a useful treatment in highly selected patients with long-standing severe obsessions and anxiety. (p. 163)

An inspection of the graphs provided with this study reveals that average differences between the two groups on all four measures are clinically marginal; on the order of one point on a five-point rating scale. On three of the scales, the leucotomized group averaged a score of about two whereas the controls averaged about three. At the outset, both groups achieved roughly the same score on the measure of anxiety. At three months, the leucotomized group's rating had improved more than that of the controls. However, by the five-year follow-up, the two groups attracted largely similar scores.

A further point for consideration is that six of the leucotomized patients had to undergo a further operation. Of these, the authors noted that some time after the operation one committed suicide, while a second had a major epileptic seizure. Another two patients who received only one operation died. A further patient complained of impotence, while another "was cautioned by the police for making improper advances to young girls" (p. 161). Still another suffered two episodes of psychotic depression (ameliorated by ECT). The authors noted that eight of the leucotomized patients developed severe or moderate leucotomy effects. No similar effects were reported for the control group, although two control patients had manifested a total of four suicide attempts by follow-up. These informal data certainly mitigate the claim that the operations dramatically improved *overall* prognosis for the operated group compared to the controls.

As this review has revealed, all these controlled studies are characterized by serious methodological flaws. One of the most serious defects is that operatees were not often adequately matched with their controls on important variables. All too often the pretreatment prognosis of the control group was far worse than that of the operated group. Better postoperative care and attention for the leucotomees as well as non-independent assessment of outcome bias the results in favour of the treatment group. Length of follow-up has usually been short, and therefore long-term differences between treatment and control groups cannot be studied. Finally, possible "placebo" effects of the operation have been generally ignored.

Given the disparities in methodology, exact comparison between these studies is difficult. However, considered together, they do little to commend earlier psychosurgical procedures over no treatment at all. The optimistic claims for psychosurgery would not seem to be grounded on a substantive and firm data base. Differential improvement rates are either non-existent, marginal, evaporate with longer follow-up, or are greatly undermined by procedural flaws. It must be conceded, however, that the operations described in these studies were conducted during the "first wave" of psychosurgery. Perhaps, it has been argued, the newer procedures offer greater comfort.

Although it is a widely held belief that contemporary psychosurgical procedures are more effective than the older forms of operation, no formal tests (i.e. prospective controlled trials) have been cited to demonstrate this. Instead, the newer procedures are attributed greater efficacy on the basis of the improvement rates they engender relative to those previously reported with the older operations.

These are good grounds for challenging the validity of this sort of comparison. It assumes that the respective patient populations are indeed comparable. However, as we indicated previously, diagnostic practices have changed considerably in the intervening years. There are also considerable grounds for suspecting that the pretreatment prognoses of contemporary psychosurgery candidates are far better than those of their "first wave" counterparts. Three areas of evidence point in this direction.

First of all, there are several reports that attest to a general improvement in prognoses for most psychiatric disorders over the years (cf. Staudt and Zubin, 1957). The prospect for untreated patients was noted to have improved, even over the duration of the "first wave" of psychosurgery, in both the United States and in Britain (cf. Bond, 1954; Harris and Norris, 1954). More recently, both Wing (1966) and Hare (1974) related a further improvement in the prognosis of schizophrenia; Hare commented that "schizophrenia is becoming a milder disease from causes unassociated with the provision of psychiatric care and treatment" (p. 287).

Another factor contributing to an improved pretreatment prognosis in contemporary psychosurgery candidates has been the diminishing pool of patients available for operation. As the popularity of earlier psychosurgical procedures increased, more and more patients were treated by surgery. Thus, increasingly, candidates had to be drawn from less chronic and less disturbed sectors of the patient population, since most of the others not deemed "operative risks" had already undergone psychosurgery. The newer procedures, then, by default had to tackle patients with a better prognosis.

Finally, there is evidence of a conscious selection of patients in contemporary psychosurgery to ensure candidates with better pretreatment prognoses than the "first wave" operatees. Many early reports argued that it was the less disturbed patients, with briefer histories of hospitalization and illness, who responded better to psychosurgery. For example, the control study of Freeman *et al.* (1954) on the effects of transorbital leucotomy cited above found that the shorter the period of prior hospitalization, the better the chance of discharge following surgery; the schizophrenics in their sample demonstrated better results when operated upon within the first two years of hospitalization. Results of this sort have undoubtedly influenced current selection practices.

Present preferences are revealed in several contemporary accounts. Freeman (1971), for example, stated:

> ... it seems evident that frontal lobotomy is more successful in early cases of schizophrenia. In the chronic cases it has limited value. In a dangerous disease such as schizophrenia it may prove safer to operate than to wait. (p. 624)

Brown (1973), commenting on the use of multiple limbic targets for schizophrenia, made much the same point.

Thus, contemporary psychosurgery is in the main practised on patients with a better pretreatment prognosis than that characteristic of early surgical candidates. This shift clearly confers a substantial advantage on the newer procedures. Any gains in efficacy may simply reflect the fact that present psychosurgical candidates have better prospects, irrespective of treatment.

From our previous discussion, we might speculate that psychosurgery's successes have always been among those patients with good pretreatment prognosis, i.e. patients with better than average prospects of improvement without specific treatment. Oltman and Friedman (1961) were certainly convinced of this:

> . . . Prefrontal lobotomy, like all other known modes of therapy in schizophrenia, achieves its optimal aims in patients whose illness is associated with very favourable prognostic criteria. (p. 71)

In the light of their early experiences, many psychosurgeons constructed profiles on "pen-pictures" of "ideal" and "poor" candidates for surgery. For example, Greenblatt *et al.* (1950) presented the following description of the "ideal" leucotomy candidate:

> The patient most likely to improve with lobotomy has achieved a measure of maturity before illness (married, children, college graduate), has shown at some time a tendency to attacks with improvement (previous attacks of mental disease), has an anatomically intact brain (free of brain damage), has a good prepsychotic adjustment (good community, family and work adjustment; sociable, lacking irritability), has evidence of considerable external stress (major precipitating factors in illness), and develops the psychosis acutely (one month or less). The duration of illness and hospitalisation is relatively short (illness less than four years, hospitalisation less than two years). ... (p. 294)

The "poor" candidate, in contrast, was characterized as follows:

> The profile of the individual who is most likely to fail with lobotomy indicates a lesser level of personality development preoperatively (high school or some college, student or unskilled laborer); this patient shows signs of brain damage, has had little external stress accompanying onset of illness. The psychosis is insidious in onset, of long duration (illness and hospitalization ten years or more) and the patient has not had the benefit of any somatic treatment. (p. 294)

Freeman and Watts (1950) also listed prognostic indicators for psychosurgery:

> Sex: Proportionately more women than men are able to leave institutions, probably because of the greater protection afforded them in the home.
> Race: Eleven out of thirteen negro females have been greatly benefited by operation, which is a higher proportion than for white females....
> Education: College-trained people show better results than grade-school products....
> Occupation: In contrast to educational achievement, the simpler occupations witness a greater resumption of useful activity....
> Religion: Jewish people show a higher rate of success than others. This

> probably hinges upon the greater family solidarity manifested by these people. (p. 515)

Jackson and Jaco (1954) similarly presented profiles of the patients most and least likely to benefit from transorbital leucotomy. Factors significantly related to postoperative improvement were as follows:

> 1. Sex: female. 2. Color: Negro. 3. Diagnosis: involutional or schizophrenic, mixed or paranoid types. 4. Duration of illness: less than 2 years. 5. Duration of hospitalization: less than 1 year. 6. Previous treatment: less than 10 EST's. 7. Marital status: married. 8. Education: 11–12 years. 9. Occupation: service occupations. 10. Church affiliation: Protestant–Baptist or Methodist. 11. Venereal history: positive. 12. Readmission status: present. (p. 357)

Patients least likely to improve were characterized as follows:

> 1. Sex: male. 2. Color: white. 3. Diagnosis: psychosis with mental deficiency, psychosis with convulsive disorders, or psychosis with meningeoncephalitis. 4. Duration of illness: 10 or more years. 5. Duration of hospitalization: 2 or more years. 6. Previous treatment: 15 or more ICT's, or over 70 EST's. 7. Marital status: single. 8. Education: illiterate or 6 years. 9. Occupation: agriculture. 10. Church affiliation: Catholic, nor none. 11. Venereal history: negative. 12. Readmission status: none. (p. 357)

Viewed overall, these profiles of "ideal" and "poor" psychosurgical candidates are quite illuminating. Presumably, on the basis of Jackson and Jaco's profiles, any surgeon contemplating transorbital leucotomy should seek out female syphilitic, married, black Baptists and avoid white Catholic bachelors with no history of venereal disease! Clearly, many of these supposed indicators are correlated with postoperative outcome only inasmuch as they reflect the operation of more fundamental factors. For example, Freeman and Watts' (1950) observation that Jewish and female operatees are more liable to get discharged undoubtedly reflects the environmental circumstances particular to these patients, a point that the researchers readily concede.

More importantly, it should be noted that many of the prognostic indicators listed for psychosurgery correspond closely with the determinants of prognosis *without treatment*, i.e. the profiles of "ideal" and "poor" candidates for psychosurgery match the characteristics considered to be favourable and unfavourable prognostic indicators irrespective of treatment. Rees (1978) listed the general indicators of prognosis in schizophrenic disorders:

> *Favourable Indicators*
> 1. An acute onset of illness. 2. Precipitation by environmental or physical factors. 3. Well-adjusted, stable previous personality. 4. The presence of true affective components in the illness. 5. A pyknic (eurymorphic)

> physique. 6. A history of previous attacks from which the patient had made a complete recovery.
> *Unfavourable Indicators*
> 1. Long duration of illness, over two years. 2. A gradual onset. 3. An unstable, ill-adjusted previous personality. 4. An early age of onset. 5. Marked leptomorphic physique. 6. Absence of clear precipitating factors. (p. 179)

They are clearly similar to the descriptions of "ideal" and "poor" psychosurgical candidates presented earlier.

The studies of Lorr and his associates (cf. Lorr *et al.*, 1955) add further weight to our argument here. Examining the characteristics that predicted outcome in leucotomees and control patients, they observed that the factors related to improvement following leucotomy correspond exactly to the prognostic indicators in the control patients. Lorr *et al.* concluded

> These findings strongly suggest that although lobotomy results in the improvement of many patients with chronic schizophrenia, the nature of the process of improvement in schizophrenia following lobotomy does not differ greatly from that which may occur without lobotomy. (p. 43)

The suspicion that the success or failure of psychosurgery hinges on candidates' prospects for improvement irrespective of treatment necessarily weakens the case that psychosurgery is an effective treatment.

The assertions in these profiles that blacks, Jews and women constitute good surgical candidates (cf. Freeman and Watts, 1950; Jackson and Jaco, 1954) undoubtedly underlie the criticism that psychosurgical interventions have been directed disproportionately at these groups. Let us briefly examine the pertinent demographic data.

There is certainly evidence that more women than men have undergone psychosurgery. In the United Kingdom, the Board of Control's (1947) report indicated that of 1000 operatees, some 65% were female; Tooth and Newton's (1961) later survey showed that of 10 365 operatees, nearly 60% were women. Valenstein (1977) conducted a sex ratio analysis of all the US articles on psychosurgery published after 1970, noting that some 56% of psychosurgery patients were female.

However, a greater proportion of female operatees does not necessarily reflect a "sexist" bias in the selection of candidates. Reitman (1948), for example, observed that the ratio of women to men in the Netherne Hospital, England, was approximately 2:1, which "was found to be closely followed in the operation figures" (p. 86). Valenstein (1977) reported that the sex ratio observed by him was not significantly different from that of the sample from which operatees would be drawn and therefore did not "support the belief that females are being preferentially selected for psychosurgery" (p. 89). The sex ratio of about three women to two male operatees observed in the United

Kingdom closely mirrors the makeup of the general psychiatric population (Department of Health and Social Security, 1977). Thus, it is in the general area of psychiatric diagnosis and intervention that we should look first for bias, rather than in psychosurgical practices *per se*. However, the demographic data give psychosurgeons no cause for complacency; the selection practices attending psychosurgery clearly perpetuate the already existing imbalances in the sexual composition of psychiatric clientele (see also Chapter 11).

It is virtually impossible to examine selection bias on the basis of culture or race, since most psychosurgery reports present no relevant data. According to Valenstein's (1977) review of the literature and his correspondence with neurosurgeons, no overall bias of this sort occurs. Nevertheless, suggestions that certain minority groups constitute ideal candidates for psychosurgery, coupled with Mark *et al.*'s (1967) remarks about black rioters in the United States (see Chapter 11), cannot have lessened fears about psychosurgery's possible use as an instrument of oppression.

In conclusion, determining which patient populations, if any, benefit from the various psychosurgical procedures has proved a difficult business. Variations in diagnostic criteria and conceptions of mental illness both between and within studies ensure this. Inconsistencies in diagnostic practices are compounded further by temporal and geographic shifts in the diagnostic categories deemed suitable for surgery. Our analysis does suggest strongly, though, that the reasonably favourable American experience with schizophrenic patients, not borne out by British results, is an artefact of the American predilection for diagnosing schizophrenia and the consequent inclusion under that rubric of patients with much better pretreatment prospects than those generally associated with schizophrenia.

In addition, it would seem that the outcome of psychosurgery generally hinges on the pretreatment prognosis of its clientele. A gradual improvement over the years in the pretreatment prognosis of psychiatric patients, coupled with a shift of focus within psychosurgery from chronic to more acutely disturbed individuals, confers an undoubted advantage on contemporary procedures; better results would be expected irrespective of the efficacy of the newer operations. Finally, our analysis of the so-called controlled studies casts serious doubt on whether psychosurgery, or at least the "first wave" procedures, offered real benefit to any patient category. While the newer procedures have yet to receive any sort of controlled investigation, there is little reason to suspect that they would fare any better than their earlier counterparts in an evaluation of this sort.

5

Adverse sequelae

By itself, the improvement rate associated with a particular psychosurgical procedure is clearly an insufficient index of efficacy. Any possible benefits must be weighed against potential adverse operative sequelae. Such untoward side effects must be expected given the complex functional integration of diverse brain areas and the fact that psychosurgery interrupts histologically normal brain tissue. It should never be assumed *a priori* that the effects of the operation will be specific, modifying only circumscribed patterns of undesirable behaviour and leaving unaffected other psychological functions. Indeed, one of the most persistent criticisms of psychosurgery has been that the effects of operations are, in fact, more diffuse, leading to a fairly general dampening of function; i.e. alterations in target symptoms or behaviours occur embedded in a complex constellation of behavioural changes.

The elaboration of possible side effects undoubtedly contributed to the decline in popularity of earlier operations and provided some of the impetus for the development of more restrained procedures, which, because of their more circumscribed character, would supposedly engender more specific behavioural effects.

At present, there would, in fact, appear to be some consensus that the adverse sequelae of newer psychosurgical procedures are less severe and less frequent than those associated with operations of the "first wave". However, some critics of contemporary psychosurgery maintain that what benefits accrue from these procedures are still bought at the expense of a general blunting of function.

Evaluation is difficult; it is rarely the case that proper systematic investigation of adverse sequelae is conducted. Further, analyses of side effects are generally reported separately from the data on clinical efficacy. Accounts detailing rates of improvement usually devote themselves only to the most superficial analysis of operative side effects. For example, Tables 5.1, 5.2 and 5.3 present data on adverse operative sequelae from the studies reviewed in Chapter 3. Generally, data will be presented here on the same number of patients subjected to more detailed analysis in the earlier tables (Tables 3.1–3.13) presented in Chapter 3 (i.e. figures presented in the "No" column of those tables). Similarly, the percentage of patients reported as having deteriorated as a result of their operation will be the same here as in the previous tables. These figures are included here since deterioration in general clinical

Table 5.1 Comparison of adverse operative sequelae from "first-wave" procedures

	Study	*Date*	*No.*	*Worse*	*Dead*	*Surgical/ neurological complications*	*Seizures*	*Incontinence*	*Weight*	*Person/soc./ behavioural disorders*	*Memory*	*Cognitive/ abstract impairment*
Prefrontal	Rao and Govindaswamy	1944	25	8*	0	?	–	12	✓	✓	–	–
	Board of Control	1947	1000	1	3	–	3	–	–	1	–	–
	Freeman and Watts	1950	623	1	2	?	12	✓	✓	✓	✓	✓
	Hohman *et al.*	1951	254	2	1[1]	–	6	✓	–	✓	–	–
	Moore	1952	71	?	3	–	7	✓	–	–	–	–
Transorbital	Tooth and Newton	1961	9284	2	4	–	1	–	–	–	–	–
	Jones and Shanklin	1950	52	?	0	0	0	0	0	0	0	0
	Freeman and Watts	1950	252	1[2]	1[2]	1[2]	?	?	?	18	?	?
	Wilson *et al.*	1953	400	2	2	✓	–	?	–	–	–	–
Bimedial	Fleming and Baker	1972	42	?	0[3]	2	3[3]	1	✓	✓	–	?
	Bernstein *et al.*	1975	43	7	0	7	21	–	40	✓	–	–
Orbital	Tow and Lewin	1953	20	0	0	–	10	25	50	10	✓	?
	Ström-Olsen and Northfield	1955	27	4	4	–	4	✓	–	✓	✓	0
	Knight and Tredgold	1955	52	2	1[4]	–	–	✓	–	?	10	✓
	Sykes and Tredgold	1964	207	1	2[5]	3[5]	18[6]	–	–	60	7	✓
Rostral	McKissock	1951	84	2	2	✓	–	✓	–	–	–	–
	Pippard	1955a	220	?	1[7]	13	7	10	–	8	–	–

* All figures in main body of table are percentages.
[1] of 367 patients
[2] of 400 patients
[3] of 70 patients
[4] of 175 patients
[5] of 350 patients
[6] of 177 patients
[7] of 240 patients

condition must, obviously, be regarded as a major adverse sequela. Occasionally, especially when dealing with percentage of patients dying as a result of surgery, figures are given based on the total number subjected to operation (usually the figure included under the "Sample" column of the tables in Chapter 3). In such cases, the figure on which the percentage was based will be given in the "Notes" column.

Instances where the original report asserts that no patient suffered a particular complication will also be recorded in Tables 5.1, 5.2 and 5.3. Where some patients are known to have experienced some particular adverse sequelae but the style of the report precludes the calculation of the percentage, a check in the appropriate column will be used to record such effects. Finally, in those instances where there is a query as to the percentage of patients who suffered a particular complication (or that any experienced it at all), a question mark will be entered in the relevant column.

An inspection of the tables readily reveals that for many reports there are dashes in several columns; that is, no indication was given of whether a particular complication was suffered by any of the operatees. In most cases, therefore, it is difficult to estimate the percentage of patients showing a

Table 5.2 Comparison of adverse operative sequelae from "mid-period" procedures

	Study	*Date*	*No.*	*Worse*	*Dead*	*Surgical/ neurological complications*	*Seizures*	*Incontinence*	*Weight*	*Person/soc./ behavioural disorders*	*Memory*	*Cognitive/ abstract impairment*
Tractotomy	Ström-Olsen and Carlisle	1971	150	1*	0	√	1	0	9	14	–	?
	Göktepe *et al.*	1975	134	0	1	–	2	–	–	7	–	–
Cingulectomy	Whitty *et al.*	1952	24	0	3[1]	3[1]	10[1]	31[1]	–	√	√	–
	Le Beau	1954b	30	?	4[2]	8[2]	–	–	–	?	–	0
	Tow and Armstrong	1954	17	6	6	6	18	24	–	√	–	–
	Sano	1962	14	?	0	–	–	–	–	–	–	–
	Brown and Lighthill	1968	110	1	0	1	√	33	–	–	√	0
	Paillas *et al.*	1971	20	0	0	–	0	–	–	–	√	–
	Gaches *et al.*	1972	20	0	10[3]	–	√	75	–	√	–	0
	Laitinen and Vílkki	1972	20	0	0	√	–	75	–	√	0	√
	Mingrino and Schergna	1972	10	?	–	–	–	–	–	–	√	0
	Richardson	1972	12	8	0	8	–	√	–	√	–	–
	Balasubramaniam *et al.*	1973	28	?	0	–	–	–	–	–	–	–
	Meyer *et al.*	1973	68	6	0	4[4]	1	–	–	–	–	√
	Ballantine *et al.*	1977	149	0	0	–	√	–	–	–	√	0
	Martin *et al.*	1977	67	0	0	6[5]	0	–	–	–	–	0
	Bailey *et al.*	1977	200	0	1	1	–	–	3	√	–	0[6]

* All figures in main body of table are percentages.
[1] of 29 patients
[2] of 50 patients
[3] of 31 patients
[4] of 75 patients
[5] of 68 patients
[6] of 94 patients

Table 5.3 Comparison of adverse operative sequelae from "second-wave" procedures

	Study	*Date*	*No.*	*Worse*	*Dead*	*Surgical/ neurological complications*	*Seizures*	*Incontinence*	*Weight*	*Person/soc./ behavioural disorders*	*Memory*	*Cognitive/ abstract impairment*
Thalamotomy	Spiegel *et al.*	1953	51	0*	–	–	–	–	–	√	√	√
	Andy and Jurko	1972	30	0	3	–	–	–	–	–	–	–
Hypothalamotomy	Schvarcz *et al.*	1972	11	0	–	–	–	–	–	–	–	0
	Sano *et al.*	1972	43	0	2	–	–	–	√	–	–	0
	Müller *et al.*	1973	22	5	5	5	–	–	5	√	–	–
	Balasubramaniam *et al.*	1971	8	8	0	13	–	–	√	–	–	–
	Balasubramaniam	1973b	21	?	0	10	–	–	–	–	–	–
	Dieckmann and Hassler	1975	6	0	0	–	–	–	√	√	–	–
	Dieckmann and Hassler	1977	4	0	0	–	–	–	50	–	–	–
	Schvarcz	1977	33	?	0	√	–	3	–	–	–	0
	Nádvornik *et al.*	1977	10	10	0	√	–	–	20	–	0	0
	Rubio *et al.*	1977	24	8	4	38	–	–	–	–	–	–
Amygdalectomy	Narabayashi and Uno	1966	40	0	–	–	–	–	–	–	–	–
	Balasubramaniam *et al.*	1973b	115	8	?	–	–	–	0	–	0	0
	Vaernet and Madsen	1970	12	0	–	–	–	–	–	–	–	–
	Kiloh *et al.*	1974	18	0	0	6	31[1]	–	–	–	–	0
Limbic	Mitchell-Heggs *et al.*	1977	66	10	0	2	0	√	0	√	√	0
Capsulotomy	López Ibor and López-Ibor Aliño	1977	57	0	0	–	–	–	–	–	–	0
	Bingley *et al.*	1977	35	0	0	2	0	–	√	–	–	0
Mesoloviotomy	Laitinen and Vilkki	1973a	38	0	–	2[2]	–	–	–	–	0[3]	0[4]

* All figures in main body of table are percentages.
[1] of 13 non-epileptic patients
[2] of 46 patients
[3] of 24 patients
[4] of 20 patients

particular undesirable side effect. With so many omissions it is obviously difficult to estimate the rate at which adverse side effects occur in psychosurgery. Table 5.4 is an attempt to provide a summary of adverse operative sequelae for various psychosurgical procedures.

Clearly, while such tables are a useful summary of the adverse sequelae

Table 5.4 Summary of adverse operative sequelae for various psychosurgical procedures

Operation	*No. of studies*	*No.*	*Worse*	*Dead*	*Surgical/ neurological complications*	*Seizures*	*Incontinence*	*Weight*	*Person/soc./ behavioural disorders*	*Memory*	*Cognitive/ abstract impairment*
Prefrontal	6	11257	(11257)[1] 2	(11410) 4	(648) √	(11272) 2	(973) √	(648) √	(1942) √	(663) √	(663) √
Transorbital	3	704	(800) 2	(852) 2	√	(52) 0	(52) 0	(52) 0	(304) 15	(52) 0	(52) 0
Bimedial	2	85	(43) 7	0	5	(113) 10	(42) 1	√	(42) √	–	–
Orbital	4	306	1	(419) 2	(330) 3	(224) 16	(47) √	(20) √	(254) √	(286) √	(99) √
Rostral	2	304	(84) 2	(224) 1	√	(220) 7	(220) 10	–	(220) 8	–	–
Tractotomy	2	284	1	1	(150) √	3	(150) 0	(150) 9	– 11	–	(150) ?
Cingulectomy	15	789	(707) 1	(825) 1	(561) 3	(201) 3	(198) 32	(224) √	(261) √	(169) √	(500) 0
Thalamotomy	2	81	0			–	–	–	–	–	–
Hypothalamotomy	10	182	(128) 2	(171) 2	(75) 18	–	(4) 75	(36) 14	(43) 0	(33) 0	(10) 0
Amygdalectomy	4	185	5	(133) 0	(18) 6	(13) 31	–	(115) 0	–	(115) 0	–
Limbic	1	66	10	0	2	0	√	0	√	√	0
Capsulotomy	2	92	0	0	(35) 2	(35) 0	–	(35) √	–	– 0	–
Mesoloviotomy	1	38	– 0	–	(46) 2	–	–	–	–	(24) 0	(20) 0

[1] Numbers in parentheses refer to the total number of patients upon which each percentage figure was based

reported by many studies, they represent a necessarily incomplete picture of undesirable postoperative changes. They offer merely a sketchy and undoubtedly conservative impression of the adverse sequelae associated with various psychosurgical procedures. It is only with the addition of supplementary information from separate investigations of undesirable side effects that something approaching a true picture of the hazards associated with psychosurgery can be constructed. Let us now examine in more detail what these two sources of information reveal about the various operative procedures.

For prefrontal leucotomy, the percentage of patients reported to have deteriorated varies somewhat (Table 5.1), with an average deterioration rate of about 2% (Table 5.4). In most cases, the notable exceptions being Board of Control (1947) and Freeman and Watts (1950), few details are given about these deteriorated cases.

Obviously, death constitutes the most serious side effect associated with any psychosurgical procedure. It has been claimed that the older forms of operation were particularly liable in this respect; the average operative death rate for prefrontal leucotomy would appear to be in the region of 4% (see Tables 5.1 and 5.4). As to the cause of death, few studies present adequate postmortem data, although, as Partridge (1950) has suggested, the most frequent cause of surgical mortality would appear to be cerebral haemorrhage (cf. Board of Control, 1947; Macklay, 1953; Moore, 1952). Other fairly common causes of death would appear to be cerebral abscess (Board of Control, 1947; Macklay, 1953) and respiratory complications (Board of Control, 1947; Hohman *et al.*, 1951; Macklay, 1953; Partridge, 1950).

The most likely and serious of the non-fatal hazards of the older forms of psychosurgery would once again appear to have been haemorrhage (Rao and Govindaswamy, 1944; Partridge, 1950; Robin and MacDonald, 1975). Freeman and Watts (1950) reported that it occurred in about 4% of their cases and occasionally was associated with paralysis (Freeman, 1953, p. 489). Oedema and trophic disturbances have also been noted (Freeman and Watts, 1950; Halpern, 1947; Reitman, 1946; Ziegler and Osgood, 1945). However, these neurological sequelae have been apparent only after more extensive examination (Reitman, 1946).

One of the most common and potentially serious complications of surgery is postoperative seizure (Freeman and Watts, 1950). Most of the reports of prefrontal leucotomy do provide data on the incidence of seizures following surgery. Its incidence appears to vary, with an average reported rate of about 2% (Table 5.4). A few studies have scanned the general electrical activity of the brain after surgery by means of electroencephalography (EEG) in order, among other things, to predict postoperative seizures; EEG data have, however, proved inconclusive in this regard and generally disappointing (Cohn, 1945; Stevens and Mosovich, 1947; Freeman and Watts, 1950).

Incontinence, especially of urine, has occasionally been reported to follow prefrontal leucotomy. After death and epilepsy, Partridge (1950) described it as "the next most troublesome complication" (p. 28). Few reports, however, give any indication of its frequency or severity. However, most researchers suggest that it is only temporary (Freeman and Watts, 1950; Hohman *et al.*, 1951; Moore, 1952; Rao and Govindaswamy, 1944). Frequency and urgency of micturition would indeed appear to be markedly increased (at least temporarily), but faecal incontinence less so (Freeman and Watts, 1950; Partridge, 1950).

Weight gains have also been noted after prefrontal leucotomy. Partridge (1950) claimed that these were observed in approximately 90% of the 300 cases he investigated, although there are suggestions that it can be attributed to an increased appetite (Freeman and Watts, 1950; Partridge, 1950; Rao and Govindaswamy, 1944). With regard to gastrointestinal activity following prefrontal leucotomy, the situation is far from clear (cf. Carmody, 1950; Pirovano, 1952). Reitman (1947) and Reed (1948) both reported at least temporary increase in gastric acidity in the postoperative phase. Vargha *et al.* (1951), however, reported a diminution of acidity following prefrontal leucotomy.

Cardiovascular system responses following prefrontal leucotomy have also been investigated. Freeman and Watts (1950) reported temporary lowering of blood pressure. Other reported changes include elevation of temperature, variation of blood pressure and bradycardia (Peterson and Buchstein, 1942; Kolb, 1949; Kalinowsky and Hoch, 1952).

Insensitivity to pain following prefrontal leucotomy has been noted by many authorities (e.g. Otenasek, 1948; Scarff, 1948; Freeman and Watts, 1950; Pötzl, 1950). It does not appear, however, that the pain threshold or perception of pain itself is altered (Chapman *et al.*, 1950).

The adverse operative sequelae that have come under most scrutiny have been those which have been categorized as "personality," "social" or "behavioural" disorders. The range of those which have been reported following prefrontal leucotomy is extensive. Occasionally, some inertia, apathy, lethargy or indifference is noted in the period immediately after surgery (Kolb, 1949; Freeman and Watts, 1950; Landis, 1951). Sometimes this diminution in activity may persist for a while (Partridge, 1950). The inertia phase may be followed by an increase in activity leading to restlessness (Frankl and Mayer-Gross, 1947; Kolb, 1949; Freeman and Watts, 1950). Occasionally the two conditions alternate (Hutton *et al.*, 1941). It is, however, the euphoria with a tendency to joke and pun (*Witzelsucht*), carelessness and lack of restraint or disinhibition that have most frequently attracted attention. Such behaviour has often been subsumed under the label "frontal-lobe syndrome," which, according to Freeman (1953), "... is compounded of indolence, carelessness, rudeness, profanity, and 'the loud laugh that speaks the vacant mind'" (p. 490).

Freeman observed that it occurred in about 9% of the 600 survivors of prefrontal leucotomy. Harlow's (1866–1868) description of the changes in Phineas Gage brought about by the accident to the frontal lobes, detailed in Chapter 1, is similar to the many accounts of the postleucotomy patient (Kolb, 1949; Partridge, 1950; Freeman and Watts, 1950; Hoch, 1951; Kalinowsky and Hoch, 1952; Walsh, 1978).

Lack of spontaneity or initiative has also been reported after prefrontal leucotomy (Rao and Govindaswamy, 1944; Board of Control, 1947; Partridge, 1950; Freeman and Watts, 1950; Hoch, 1951). If, as Freeman and Watts (1950) claimed, "the problem in psychosurgery is to cut sufficient pathways in the frontal lobes to reduce the affective charge of the psychosis or neurosis to a point where the ideas no longer disable the patient" (p. 75), then it is hardly surprising that the emotional aspects of the leucotomee's life are altered by the surgery. Many authorities also attest to the reduction of the so-called "morbid emotional state" (Hutton *et al.*, 1941; Walker, 1944; Kolb, 1949; Partridge, 1950; Hoch, 1951; Landis, 1951; Sargant, 1951; Kalinowsky and Hoch, 1952; Brennan *et al.*, 1955).

Adverse emotional changes following prefrontal leucotomy have also been noted (Hoch, 1951; Shevitz, 1976). The most characteristic of these are the changes dubbed "affective incontinence" by Rylander (1939). The term denotes a tendency of prefrontal leucotomy patients to react with exaggerated emotional displays, whether it be tears or laughter, to somewhat trivial events. At the same time they may react with seemingly calm indifference to genuinely distressful happenings. These emotional disturbances are characterized by their short duration and lack of depth of real feeling. Indeed, the analogy has been drawn (cf. Harlow, 1866–1868) between the behaviour of the patient following frontal lobe disruption and that of the child (cf. "surgically induced childhood," – Freeman and Watts, 1950, p. 188). Obstinacy, stubbornness, temper tantrums, playfulness, lack of restraint of manner, speech and morals, as well as lack of thought for consequences have all been described as typical of the prefrontal leucotomee. While such behaviour may cause embarrassment to relatives and in some cases may be extremely antisocial (cf. Board of Control, 1947; Freeman, 1953), the patient is frequently unperturbed by his/her actions. Kolb (1949), following Rylander, proposed that "the fixed personality traits of the individual appear to be exaggerated by damage to the frontal lobes" (p. 127).

Increases in sexual desire or activity have been claimed by some researchers to follow prefrontal leucotomy (Levine and Alpert, 1951; Castelletti, 1951), although no real change in sexual behaviour has been reported by others (Walker, 1944; Pomeroy, 1956; Zlotlow and Paganini, 1959). Freeman (1973) recorded a socially disruptive increase in libido in female patients following prefrontal leucotomy, although he contended that in some cases increments in sexual activity represented a return to normality (cf. Partridge, 1950).

Although impairment of memory does not appear to be a particular hazard of prefrontal leucotomy, there are indications that a percentage of patients exhibit some form of confusion, disorientation and amnesia after surgery (Freeman and Watts, 1950). A particularly interesting phenomenon reported by some authorities is the denial of operation (Frank, 1946; Freeman and Watts, 1950; Hutton *et al.*, 1941). Paganini and Zlotlow (1960) investigated this denial and concluded that it was not "a neurological phenomenon, due to the damaged brain of the patient" (p. 266) but rather reflected "an extension, continuation of further manifestation of the basic mechanism of denial used by the patient in his severe mental illness" (p. 266).

With regard to deficits in the cognitive or abstract sphere, there are indications that general intelligence might have suffered in some leucotomees (Rao and Govindaswamy, 1944; Board of Control, 1947). On formal testing with standard psychometric and psychological tests, which are purported to test general intelligence, a number of studies have reported no essential impairment (cf. Worchel and Lylerly, 1941; McGregor and Crumbie, 1941; Fleming, 1942; Freeman and Watts, 1942; Strom-Olsen *et al.*, 1943; Porteus and Kepner, 1944; Frank, 1946; Crown, 1951; Medina *et al.*, 1954). A few reports have indicated otherwise (Rylander, 1947; Yacorzynski *et al.*, 1948; Malmo, 1948; Petrie, 1949; Rosvold and Mishkin, 1950).

However, even among those studies which have reported no essential change in "general intelligence," a finer-grain analysis of the operatees' performance, especially on some subtests, has indicated subtle deficits. These have been investigated more systematically by means of specially designed tests. As Walsh (1978) has noted, three major areas of impairment have been identified:

1. lessened ability to formulate an adequate plan for the solution of a problem;
2. lessened ability to utilize information from their errors to modify subsequent action;
3. some inflexibility in conceptual behaviour. (p. 148)

Evidence of difficulties in planning following frontal lobe surgery comes from studies using the Porteus Maze Test. A large number of studies attest to deficits in Porteus Maze performance (cf. Porteus and Kepner, 1944; Greenblatt *et al.*, 1947; Malmo, 1948; Petrie, 1952; Crown, 1951; Landis, 1951; Smith, 1960).

The second area of cognitive impairment concerns the patient's inability to profit from mistakes, i.e. errors are repeated even when the patient has had the error explicitly pointed out. Using formal psychometric procedures together with more informal observation of performance on other tasks, a number of investigators have reported perseveration after prefrontal leucotomy (Rosvold and Mishkin, 1950; Poppen *et al.*, 1965; Drewe, 1974, 1975).

The final cognitive deficit noted after prefrontal leucotomy is impairment of abstract thought (Freeman and Watts, 1942, 1950; Kisker, 1944; Goldstein,

1949; Halstead *et al.*, 1946). This deficit has been described as "concreteness" – the patient becomes fixed on the here and now, restricted to the literal. According to Halstead *et al.* (1946), this deficit reflects an impairment of "biologic intelligence," which is defined as "usable intelligence, i.e., his capacity for adaptive behaviour" (p. 218).

Together with the "standard" form of operation, transorbital leucotomy would appear to be the most common psychosurgical procedure of the first wave. Its popularity seems surprising given the reservations voiced by many surgeons. While the percentage of patients reported to have deteriorated after operation appears to be equal for both procedures as revealed by Table 5.4 (2% for each), operative mortality would appear to be considerably lower with the newer operation. Freeman (1953) noted, however, that death resulting specifically from cerebral haemorrhage was a greater hazard with the newer procedure, and even if not fatal, such haemorrhaging could at least lead to transient paralysis (Freeman, 1953; Wilson *et al.*, 1953). Furthermore, misdirected incisions and the breaking of leucotomes during operation were also more common (Freeman, 1953).

As can be seen from Table 5.1 postoperative seizures are not reported to be a particular complications with transorbital leucotomy; their incidence as reported by Freeman (1953), almost 2%, is considerably lower than for the earlier procedure (over 25% in that series). Similarly, both incontinence and obesity would appear to be less prevalent (Freeman, 1953; Wilson *et al.*, 1953).

The occurrence of adverse personality, social and behavioural side effects after transorbital leucotomy has received relatively scant attention. Freeman (1953) admitted that six patients out of 1200 survivors of transorbital leucotomy suffered the "frontal lobe syndrome," considerably less than that observed in the 600 leucotomees. Further, these six may have suffered from "non-fatal haemorrhage into both frontal lobes" (p. 490).

The operation of bimedial leucotomy would appear, according to Table 5.1 to result in some 7% of operatees being substantially worse after surgery. Although no patients were reported to have died in either of the two reports of bimedial leucotomy, one patient seems to have died as an indirect result of operation in the series reported by Bernstein *et al.* (1975). Further, some 44% of operatees displayed signs of "organic brain syndrome." Although there would appear to be inconsistencies in the data of Bernstein *et al.*, the postoperative convulsive seizure rate seems to be about 20%. Incontinence would not seem to have been a particular complication (Baker *et al.*, 1970; Bernstein *et al.*, 1975), and while weight gains were reported by Baker *et al.*, no frequency data were presented. Bernstein *et al.* observed that obesity was a complication in some 17 (40%) of their cases.

As to personality changes, Bernstein *et al.* noted a fair amount of variability. Baker *et al.* observed "occasional undue changes in moral code, anger, sexuality or interpersonal relationships" (p. 40) and declared that "one hesitates to interfere with moral codes, with patterns of anger and sexuality and with the interpersonal balance in families" (p. 41). Since these changes were rather dramatic in some cases, the hesitancy shown by Baker *et al.* can be readily understood.

Unfortunately, in neither series was information presented regarding memory or cognitive or abstract impairment, although "deficits in drive, recent memory and intellectual functioning" (p. 1043) were included in the description of "organic brain syndrome" given by Bernstein *et al.* (1975).

The percentage of patients reported to have deteriorated following orbital leucotomy would appear to be half that cited for prefrontal leucotomy (Table 5.4). Altogether the overall mortality rate associated with the orbital operation would appear to be approximately 1%. Knight (1964) reported that six patients had died out of 463 cases up to the end of 1962. Scoville and Bettis (1977) reported the death rate to be some 4% (of 109 cases). Death resulted mainly from seizure, clot, cancer or coronary.

One patient reported by Ström-Olsen and Northfield (1955) exhibited hyperpyrexia (extremely high temperatures) and remained in a comatose state for 48 hours. Three patients completely lost their sense of smell after the operation, possibly "through injury to the olfactory-bulb, tract or cortex" (p. 987) in two of these cases. The incidence of seizures after orbital undercutting (16%) would appear to be considerably higher than that following prefrontal leucotomy (2%) (see Table 5.4).

Although precise figures are unavailable, it has been asserted that the incidence of incontinence after orbital undercutting is lower than that for the older operations (Knight and Tredgold, 1955; Ström-Olsen and Northfield, 1955; Sykes and Tredgold, 1964; Tow and Lewin, 1953). The only report of noticeable weight gains after orbital undercutting is that of Tow and Lewin (1953).

With respect to behavioural complications, it has been submitted that relative to the standard operation, orbital undercutting attracts similar but less severe side effects (Knight and Tredgold, 1955; Scoville and Bettis, 1977; Ström-Olsen and Northfield, 1955; Sykes and Tredgold, 1964).

Memory disturbances after orbital undercutting have received scant attention. Both Knight and Tredgold (1955) and Sykes and Tredgold (1964) reported impairment (10% of leucotomees for the former and 7% for the latter). Both Tow and Lewin (1953) and Ström-Olsen and Northfield (1955) reported no signs of intellectual impairment.

The technique of rostral leucotomy has never achieved anything like the status of orbital undercutting as an alternative to the standard operation. Overall, about 2% of patients appear to have deteriorated after rostral leucotomy. It is impossible to determine exactly how many patients deteriorated in the sample investigated by Pippard (1955a), since these patients were merely included in the "poor" category of results.

Of the 100 rostral leucotomies described by McKissock (1951), two died as a result of surgery, although no indications were given of the actual cause of death in either case. McKissock reported that both deaths were in the "open" series of operations (63 patients). There were no deaths in the blind rostral leucotomy series (37 patients), although Pippard reported a further death in the blind rostral series of 177 patients that followed.

Cerebral haemorrhage was the most frequent surgical or neurological complication.

Of the 220 patients who were alive more than 18 months after surgery, 7% were observed to have had seizures in the postoperative period. Incontinence was reported to have recurred in 10% of leucotomees.

Two further complications that might be included under personality, behavioural or social deficits were "hypomania" and "disinhibition." Hypomania, a less intense form of mania, was observed in ten patients who had been operated on for "depressive illness"; most of these had been diagnosed as suffering from recurrent endogenous depression. This hypomanic condition is apparently similar to "disinhibition" observed in other patients by Pippard (1955a). In his more extensive investigation of "personality changes after rostral leucotomy," Pippard (1955b) noted a reduction in "drive" in one third of the patients and that half suffered detectable affective deficits.

Memory difficulties were, however, more common among the 120 patients investigated more fully by Pippard. Altogether 16 patients experienced "patchy" or "Lacunar" memory, in which whole sequences of past experience were vague or missing. A further 36 leucotomees had difficulties with retention and recall. Many complained of being more absent minded.

With regard to cognitive or abstract impairment, Pippard (1955b) reported disturbances of conceptual thinking in 26 of 120 patients. Several distinct disturbances were identified; these included loss of ability to plan work or deal with more than one thing at a time, comprehension and calculating difficulties as well as an inability to do crossword puzzles. Altogether Pippard (1955b) reported that "half the patients had some intellectual impairment, but rarely of more than academic interest" (p. 787).

Knight's stereotaxic tractotomy, "which is probably most accurately designated a sub-caudate tractotomy" (Bridges *et al.*, 1973, p. 663), has been described by Bridges (1972) as "an effective treatment associated with side effects which are usually absent or only slight" (p. 1105). A cursory glance at Tables 5.2 and 5.4 does, indeed, reveal only minimal untoward sequelae associated with this form of operation. Only one patient has been described as worse following the operation. Furthermore, only one death attributable to operation (associated with a major seed displacement) was reported in the series of 750 cases reviewed by Ström-Olsen and Carlisle (1971), and this was blamed on an assistant's error (Knight, 1973). Surgical or neurological complications do not appear to be common (Ström-Olsen and Carlisle, 1972), and the incidence of patients developing seizures appears to be low (Göktepe *et al.*, 1975; Ström-Olsen and Carlisle, 1971).

Lasting urinary incontinence has been reported as absent following tractotomy (Knight, 1972; Ström-Olsen and Carlisle, 1971, 1972), although weight gains have been noted (Ström-Olsen and Carlisle, 1971).

Untoward personality, social or behavioural changes appear to be decidely less frequent with stereotactic tractotomy than with the older operations (Ström-Olsen and Carlisle, 1972). Knight (1972) reported "the total absence of the so-called 'leucotomy syndromes' " (p. 273). Nevertheless, less marked changes were noted. Those that occurred in the 150 more fully investigated patients have been listed by Ström-Olsen and Carlisle (1971) and have included "tiredness and lethargy," "irritability," "outspokenness" and "volubility," with both "excessive sexual demands" and "frigidity since tractotomy" also being noted (cf. descriptions by Bridges, 1972; Bridges *et al.*, 1973; Göktepe *et al.*, 1975). A further complication, especially in the elderly, was the presence of temporary confusion in the immediate postoperative period (Bridges, 1972; Knight, 1965).

Finally, there has been little systematic exploration of changes in intellectual functioning following tractotomy. Only two complaints of cognitive deterioration were recorded by Ström-Olsen and Carlisle (1971); "difficulty in remembering" in one case and "difficulty in concentrating" and "could not find the right words" (p. 149) in another.

As can be seen from Table 5.1, very few studies have reported patients deteriorating as a result of cingulectomy. However, with many accounts it is impossible to make a determination here. Of the four papers that admitted to patients having deteriorated, only one indicated more than one operatee affected. In this paper, Meyer *et al.* (1973) revealed that the four "therapeutic failures" were all diagnosed as alcoholics; two died of self-inflicted gunshot wounds, one of a self-administered barbiturate overdose and the fourth "died under mysterious circumstances" (p. 48). The deterioration observed in one patient in Richardson's (1972) series was the result of "destruction of more medial frontal lobe than necessary" (p. 122); severe "frontal lobe syndrome" occurred.

The highest incidence of operative mortality (Table 5.2) was reported by Gaches *et al.* (1972), although they did note that two of the three deaths were an indirect result of the operation. Bailey *et al.* (1977) reported on operative death that occurred as a result of cerebral haemorrhage and oedema. The two patients who died in Le Beau's (1954b) series were both children exhibiting "extreme mental retardation with uncontrollable agitation"; the main difficulty disclosed here was the need for "prolonged general anaesthesia" (pp. 269–270). Two further patients suffered transient hemiparesis, and in another intense anaemia developed. Laitinen and Vilkki (1972) reported vomiting in the early postoperative period: "Sickness, vomiting and headaches sometimes hid the immediate (anxiolitic) effect" (p. 246) (cf. Whitty *et al.*, 1952).

As revealed by Table 5.4 the incidence of postoperative seizures for cingulectomy is relatively low. Investigations of postoperative EEG changes with regard to seizures revealed that any abnormalities usually disappeared within three months and "in a few cases after a year" (Gaches *et al.*, 1972, p. 238), and that in the main, postoperative records were more characteristic of the normal EEG (cf. Laitinen and Vílkki, 1972).

Incontinence does not appear to be a serious complication of cingulectomy, although it appears to be quite common in the early postoperative period and may be linked to a generally poor immediate postoperative state, including "mental apathy" (Richardson, 1972) or postoperative confusion (Brown and Lighthill, 1968). Finally, temporary incontinence of both urine and faeces has also been recorded (Whitty *et al.*, 1952; Tow and Armstrong, 1954).

Weight gains following cingulectomy have received little comment, although Whitty *et al.* (1952) formally recorded that they were less marked than after prefrontal leucotomy. Other somatic changes (e.g. in pulse rate and blood pressure) were also noted by Whitty *et al.* (1952).

One of the major advantages claimed for cingulectomy over the older forms of operation is the lowered incidence of severe adverse personality, social or behavioural changes (e.g. Balasubramaniam *et al.*, 1973; Whitty *et al.*, 1952). However, some impairment especially in the early postoperative period, has been recorded and has included "a state of anergia and lack of drive," initially followed by "some increased irritability and verbal aggressiveness" (see reports by Bailey *et al.*, 1973; Gaches *et al.*, 1972; Richardson, 1972). Le Beau (1954b), however, denied any adverse changes. Laitinen and Vilkki (1972) reported that one of their operatees was arrested for theft. Changes in sexual behaviour after cingulectomy have been reported as variable (Bailey *et al.*, 1973; Richardson, 1972; Tow and Armstrong, 1954).

Impairment of memory after cingulectomy has not been extensively investigated, although some reports attest that it is not significant (Ballantine *et al.*, 1977; Laitinen and Vilkki, 1972). However, Paillas *et al.* (1971) noted memory deficits linked to postoperative confusion, including "the full-blown Korsakoff syndrome" (p. 946). Whitty *et al.* (1952) also listed confusion among the postoperative effects of cingulectomy (cf. reports of Brown and Lighthill, 1968, and Mingrino and Schergna, 1972).

Of the studies that have reported using formal psychometric tests, no significant impairment of intellectual functioning has been evidenced (Le Beau, 1954a; Brown and Lighthill, 1968; Paillas *et al.*, 1971; Bailey *et al.*, 1973). Indeed, Ballantine *et al.* (1977) claimed that some patients demonstrated performance improvements, while Meyer *et al.* (1973) argued that even for patients who showed a decline, there was no "evidence that the decline in IQ score was attributable to the surgery" (p. 56). Teuber *et al.* (1977) suggested that such data reflected a complex interaction of subtests, age of operatees, number of ECTs prior to surgery and time of testing after operation.

As can be seen from Table 5.3 no patient is reported to have deteriorated as a result of thalamotomy, and only one death was recorded. However, other less traumatic complications have been noted and have included impairments of upward movements of the eyes (Spiegel *et al.*, 1953) and some unilateral weakness in the face and limbs.

Epilepsy has not been reported as a frequent effect of thalamotomy. Spiegel *et al.* (1965) claimed only "one instance in which only a single convulsion occurred" (p. 389). The EEG of operatees failed to show any increase in convulsive reactivity.

Transient urinary incontinence was observed in 15 out of 41 operatees described by Spiegel and Wycis (1949). However, a definite increase in appetite and weight was observed in only three patients. Other side effects included transitory change in glucose tolerance curves and decline in blood pressure.

Personality, social or behavioural deficits after thalamotomy have been reported as less marked than after prefrontal leucotomy. However, while Spiegel *et al.* (1953) noted only some diminution of initiative in four cases, Nádvornik *et al.* (1973) claimed that these adverse sequelae of thalamotomy were such as to force them to abandon this form of operation.

Although Wycis (1972) claimed that there were not "amnestic reactions" and no "evidence of confusion" (p. 115) after thalamotomy, this is in contrast to his earlier reports of memory deficits and his own previous observation of postoperative confusion (Spiegel and Wycis, 1949; Spiegel *et al.*, 1953). The earlier reports also described disturbances such as somnolence, disorientation (particularly for a time), memory defects, inertia, apathy and psychomotor retardation as similar to those observed after prefrontal leucotomy. Memory impairment, in some cases severe, has also been reported by Andy (1975) as well as by Hassler and Dieckmann (1973). Impairment of intellectual functioning, sometimes long lasting, has also been recorded (Spiegel and Wycis, 1949; Spiegel *et al.*, 1953), although they suggested in their later report that such deficit might "at least be due partly to the underlying psychosis" (p. 389).

Hypothalamotomy is currently a more popular procedure than thalamotomy. It is particularly preferred by some psychosurgeons for the treatment of "sexual disorders" and occasionally applied for control of "behaviour disorders."

In only three studies summarized in Table 5.3 were patients reported to have been worse off after operation. In one of these the postoperative course of an operatee was marked by severe adverse sequelae. A death occurred in each of the other two reports.

Many studies have, however, reported surgical and neurological complications, which in some cases were severe. One of the cases reported by Nádvornik *et al.* (1977) developed bronchopneumonia, and another suffered haemorrhage after the removal of the electrode from the site of coagulation (Nádvornik *et al.*, 1973). Vomiting of blood (haematemesis) was an unusual complication described by Balasubramaniam *et al.* (1973). Further, distonic movements in upper limbs as well as akinetic mutism have also been reported (Arjona, 1974; Rubio *et al.*, 1977). Oculomotor disturbances were noted by Obrador *et al.* (1967) and hyperthemia by several surgeons (Arjona, 1974; Rubio *et al.*, 1977; Schvarcz, 1977).

No data regarding the incidence of seizures after hypothalamotomy have been reported, although Rubio *et al.* claimed that for those patients with epilepsy prior to surgery the rate of seizures declined postoperatively. Sano *et al.* (1972) similarly announced decrease in postoperative epileptic attacks and only temporary slowing of EEG activity. Obrador *et al.* (1967) also recorded EEG activity and described postoperative changes, which included large bilateral delta waves on the sixth day after operation.

Urinary incontinence, but in only one case (lasting four days), was observed by Schvarcz (1977), and Balasubramaniam *et al.* (1971) noted temporary increase in urinary output in two cases. Weight changes have been a far more commonly reported side effect of hypothalamotomy. Increase in appetite, often accompanied by gain in weight, has been recorded in several reports (Sano *et al.*, 1972; Balasubramaniam *et al.*, 1971; Dieckmann and Hassler, 1975; Nádvornik *et al.*, 1977). Sano *et al.* (1972), however, reported that such changes were within normal limits. Further, Roeder *et al.* (1972) and Black *et al.* (1975) claimed to have observed no gains in weight or appetite.

Other somatic changes have also been recorded. Tachycardia, with normal blood pressure, has been noted (Schvarcz, 1977; Schvarcz *et al.*, 1972). Glycaemia rising from 30 to 60 mg% (p. 447) was observed by Nádvornik *et al.* (1977). Transient diabetes insipidis occurred in two patients (Balasubramaniam *et al.*, 1973), although Dieckmann and Hassler (1975) reported that this was not a complication in their series.

A number of surgeons have claimed that no significant adverse personality, social or behavioural changes have taken place after hypothalamotomy (Roeder *et al.*, 1972; Nádvornik *et al.*, 1973; Black *et al.*, 1975). However, lethargy and hypersomnia after operation, especially in the immediate postoperative period, were observed by Schvarcz (1977) and Schvarcz *et al.* (1972). Some mild euphoria (Quaade *et al.*, 1974; Schneider, 1977; Nádvornik *et al.*, 1977) and disinhibition (Schneider, 1977) have also been described.

Since hypothalamotomy is addressed to very specific forms of sexual "deviance," the presence of fairly general changes in sexual behaviour should be monitored. Clearly, gross alterations must be regarded as adverse indications, since specific adjustments are intended. Roeder *et al.* (1972) have, in fact, reported a general decline in sexual behaviour after both unilateral and bilateral hypothalamotomy. Reduction in sexual drive was also recorded by Dieckmann and Hassler (1975) and in one case "an increasing loss of sexual drive to the point of his asserted impotence after 2.5 years" (p. 184). Hormonal changes were noted not to have occurred. Similar reductions in sexual behaviour have also been reported by other authorities (Müller *et al.*, 1973; Dieckmann and Hassler, 1977; Schneider, 1977).

Significant disturbances in memory have not been reported after hypothalamotomy. Obrador *et al.* (1967) described a postoperative confusional state which included "complete disorientation, amnesia, confusion and fabulation" (p. 286). This state, they noted, was similar to that of the Korsakoff syndrome (p. 279).

A number of authorities have claimed that significant impairment of cognitive or abstract functioning does not occur after hypothalamotomy (Sano *et al.*, 1972; Schvarcz, 1977; Schvarcz *et al.*, 1972; Black *et al.*, 1975). More subtle changes included disturbances of "visual organization" and "structure of thought," as well as "increased tendency to stereotypy" and a "diminution of thought content" (p. 466).

While Nádvornik *et al.* (1973) detailed their generally negative experiences with amygdalectomy, the experience of other surgeons would appear to have been more fortuitous, as revealed by the number of operatees designated "worse" in Table 5.3. The study of Balasubramaniam *et al.* (1970), however, constitutes an exception, since nine operatees are included in the "worse" category. All of these patients died after surgery, although it is not clear from the report whether this was invariably as a direct result of surgery. This doubt is signalled by a query in the "dead" column of the table. In a later report, Balasubramaniam *et al.* (1972) revealed that "one case had a fatal hematemesis after bilateral amygdalectomy" (p. 159).

A commonly reported complication is the complete or partial loss or weakening of the nervous function of some part of the body (Hitchcock *et al.*, 1972; Kiloh *et al.*, 1974; Sawa *et al.*, 1954; Williams and Freeman, 1951). Schaltenbrand, in a discussion of Vaernet's (1972) report, addressed the following question to Vaernet:

> We had one curious side effect and I want to know whether you have seen it too. For some weeks after operation, particularly when you coagulate Turk's bundle, there may be temporarily a certain tonic weakness of one side of the body. (p. 181)

The incidence of postoperative seizures occurring after amygdalectomy has not received extensive investigation. Kiloh *et al.* (1974) noted that four of their 13 non-epileptic patients suffered seizures after surgery. Transient incontinence was recorded by both Sawa *et al.* (1954) and by Balasubramaniam *et al.* (1973).

In Chapter 1, the five major behavioural changes that comprise the "Klüver–Bucy syndrome" were listed. It would appear that some of the side effects of amygdalectomy ("misrecognition of persons and objects," "phagomania" and "heterophagia," "hyperkinesis," "changefulness of mood" and "excessive friendliness" and finally "acceleration of sexual impulse") noted by Sawa *et al.* (1954) correspond to elements of the syndrome. Further, Narabayashi and Uno (1966) recorded the following case in their series:

> This case showed the partial Klüver–Bucy syndrome one week after bilateral amygdalotomy, consisting of unsteadiness, oral tendency, hyper-sexual behavior and relative hypermetamorphosis; it lasted for about two months and could finally be controlled by high doses of chlorpromazine. (p. 170)

However, the behaviour characteristic of amygdalectomized laboratory animals are, it would seem, only rarely observed in human operatees. Some of the possible reasons for this are discussed in Chapter 8.

Although various reports of amygdalectomy confirm that some standard psychometric tests reveal no significant impairment of memory or intellectual functioning (Narabayashi *et al.*, 1963; Balasubramaniam *et al.*, 1970; Vaernet, 1972; Hitchcock *et al.*, 1972, 1973; Kiloh *et al.*, 1974), more specific deficits, such as failure to recognize faces or objects, have been reported (Sawa *et al.*, 1954; Hitchcock and Cairns, 1973; Hitchcock *et al.*, 1973). The misrecognition of objects has been more systematically examined and confirmed by Andersen (1972), employing various psychometric tests. Mark *et al.* (1972) noted that one patient indulged in over-eating ("hyperphagia," pp. 148–149) for about 3½ months after bilateral amygdalectomy and gained 35 pounds in weight during this time. "Phagomania" (p. 312) and sometimes "heterophagia" (p. 312) were reported in all five operatees by Sawa *et al.* (1954). Mempel (1971), on the other hand, recorded that half of 16 patients suffered some transient loss of appetite after amygdalectomy. Hitchcock *et al.* (1972) noted that two patients showed signs of hormone imbalance postoperatively (p. 170), and Kiloh *et al.* (1974) recorded variable changes in autonomic nervous system activity. No other evidence of "strong oral changes" or "hypermetamorphosis" have been noted.

With regard to personality, social and behavioural impairment after surgery, Vaernet (1972) noted that following surgery, amygdalectomy patients were "less tense with a dampening of their emotions" (p. 179). Andersen (1972), in a discussion of behavioural changes apparent during learning tasks following amygdalectomy, indicated the appearance of inertia and emotional blunting; disinhibition has also been recorded (Andersen, 1972; Sawa *et al.*, 1954). Siegfried and Ben-Shmuel (1973) noted that "in two cases, aggravation of the aggressivity was observed in the first post-operative weeks" (p. 215) (cf. Narabayashi and Uno, 1966). Mempel (1971) reported that two out of 16 patients suffered slight depression for up to four days, and in one operatee, euphoria and moria (folly) lasting for four weeks occurred. Phrases such as "infantization of emotion and action," "poly-phrasia," "hyperkiresia," "increase of friendliness," and "acceleration of sexual impulse" were applied to most of the patients in the series of Sawa *et al.* (1954). Balasubramaniam *et al.* (1970) and Hitchcock and Cairns (1973) noted no adverse changes in sexual behaviour after amygdalectomy, while Mark *et al.* (1972) reported a case of impotence lasting two years after surgery.

Apart from the casual revelation that one patient deteriorated as a result of surgery (Cox and Brown, 1977, p. 477), descriptions of postoperative complications of multitarget limbic leucotomy in the United States have been limited to the following very uninformative submission:

> No mortality was experienced. There have been no problems with post-operative epilepsy and no wound infections using the plaster helmet for security. (p. 191)

In the preliminary account of 40 patients in Britain, Kelly *et al.* (1973c) reported that no patients deteriorated postoperatively (6 weeks). However, when 34 of these operatees were evaluated at 17 months (on average), three patients attracted the label "worse" (Kelly and Mitchell-Heggs, 1973). The rate for the first 66 consecutive patients was one deterioration at 6 weeks and seven at 16 month follow-up (Mitchell-Heggs *et al.*, 1976, 1977).

Headache has been reported as a common consequence of limbic leucotomy, and "the patient is retained in bed for 47 hours" (Kelly *et al.*, 1973a p. 138). Postoperative epilepsy, however, was not encouraged, although anticonvulsant medication had been administered (Kelly and Mitchell-Heggs, 1973). Transient incontinence and weight gain appear to be a fairly frequent consequence of surgery (Kelly and Mitchell-Heggs, 1973).

With regard to behavioural side effects, only transient inertia and mild depression (Kelly, 1973) and transient changes in sexual behaviour have been recorded (Kelly and Mitchell-Heggs, 1973).

Only occasional memory impairment was noted at 16 month follow-up by Mitchell-Heggs *et al.* (1977), although the majority of patients did suffer some degrees of confusion and disorientation in the immediate postoperative period (Kelly *et al.*, 1973c). However, marked and sustained intellectual deterioration has not been noted after limbic leucotomy (Mitchell-Heggs *et al.*, 1977).

With regard to adverse sequelae, capsulotomy could be considered as a safer operation than many of the older psychosurgical procedures (Table 5.4); no patients are reported to have died as a direct result of surgery. However, Herner (1961), in his extensive evaluation, indicated that some 15 patients out of 116 (13%) deteriorated following capsulotomy. Nevertheless, with respect to specifically surgical complications, Herner (1961) reported that "there were hardly any postoperative complications" (p. 38). Although transient hemiparesis was observed in two cases by Bingley *et al.* (1973), it was not considered to be a particular feature in a subsequent report (Bingley *et al.*, 1977).

Postoperative convulsive seizures were not reported to be a frequent consequence of capsulotomy in Herner's (1961) series and, apart from the one patient in the series of Bingley *et al.* (1973), postoperative epilepsy was not associated with more recent capsulotomies. In addition, postoperative

EEG recordings did not reveal any epileptogenic activity (Bingley *et al.*, 1977).

Both urinary and faecal incontinence were observed in Herner's (1961) more extensive examination of 44 cases out of the original 116 capsulotomees. Sixteen cases of urinary incontinence (p. 100) and five of faecal incontinence (p. 101) were recorded, which they related to mental confusion. The incidence of incontinence in the later series was not reported.

Some patients have gained considerable weight after capsulotomy, according to Bingley *et al.* (1977). Lopez-Ibor Aliño and Burzaco (1972) recorded dramatic changes in appetite behaviour. Finally, one female patient in Herner's (1961) series developed peptic ulcers after capsulotomy.

Untoward changes in personality and social behaviour were observed by Herner (1961) in about half of the 44 patients subjected to more extensive examination and have included fatigue (23 cases), emotional blunting (15 cases), emotional incontinence (five cases), volitional torpor (14 cases), impaired sense of judgement (five cases), disinhibition (five cases). Herner, reviewing the total complement of 116 operatees, described six instances of grossly pathological behaviour following capsulotomy:

> Of the above six cases, then, four showed *sexual asocialism;* five *addiction to alcohol*; and four signs of *criminality*. In one of these cases, the abnormal behaviour (addiction to alcohol) was temporary, but in the others it was apparently more or less permanent. (p. 51, italics in original).

Other researchers have noted some loss of initiative, diminution of inhibition and elevation of mood (Bingley *et al.*, 1973; Kullberg, 1977; Lopez Ibor and Lopez-Ibor Aliño, 1977).

Bingley *et al.* (1973) recorded some immediate postoperative confusion and memory deficits. Herner (1961) similarly reported some subjective and objective impairment of recent memory of his 44 cases. However, tests of longer-term memory revealed no noteworthy postoperative deficits for 22 of these patients. Performances on tests of attention and concentration, in contrast, declined significantly following capsulotomy. Tests of general intelligence were also administered in the assessment and some impairment recorded for the early postoperative period. While the other researchers have claimed no significant decline in general intelligence functioning after capsulotomy, their claim has been cased on less detailed and systematic observation than that carried out by Herner.

Anterior mesoloviotomy is an even less frequently performed operation than anterior capsulotomy. However, Laitinen and Vílkki have presented a number of reports on this procedure. Although no patients were reported by Laitinen and Vílkki (1973a) to have deteriorated after mesoloviotomy, in a later account, Vílkki (1977) described two patients as "worse" (p. 258). No operative deaths have been recorded and only one surgical complication (haemorrhage) noted (Laitinen and Vílkki, 1973a).

Laitinen and Vílkki (1972) claimed that in the first mesoloviotomy series there were "no signs of emotional blunting, disorientation or euphoria" (p. 473). No other information regarding the presence or absence of behavioural side effects has been presented – clearly an unsatisfactory state of affairs.

It is apparent from our fairly extensive account of adverse operative sequelae that the different psychosurgical procedures have been subject to widely varying investigation, both in terms of the quantity and quality of study. While some procedures have been examined fairly thoroughly for possible untoward side effects, others have attracted only the most meagre and perfunctory scrutiny. Clearly, this makes comparison between procedures extremely difficult, and in particular the comparison of older and newer procedures. While the latter are commonly considered to occasion a lower incidence of adverse sequelae and non-specific effects, this may simply reflect less exhaustive investigation. In addition, contemporary surgical candidates are generally less disturbed preoperatively than their earlier counterparts; less in the way of apparent side effects may reflect, in part, the better overall prognosis of contemporary patients. Furthermore, rarely have the newer operations been subjected to protracted follow-up investigations; it is possible that in some cases, adverse sequelae might only become apparent with longer follow-up (see Chapter 7).

However, what can be concluded from our present survey is that where sensitive and comprehensive examination has been undertaken, whether of older or newer procedures, a wide range of postoperative deficits and non-specific effects have been revealed. The range of side effects revealed seems mainly to reflect the comprehensiveness of the scrutiny, and to a lesser extent the size and location of the lesion and the technical sophistication of the operation – the focus of the next chapter.

6

Accuracy of operative techniques

It is undoubtedly the case that the success or failure of any surgical operation (i.e. the presence or absence of either good results or adverse side effects) will be markedly influenced by the successful achievement of the specified surgical objectives. The aim of any psychosurgical procedure would appear to be to lesion a specified amount of tissue in a specified location. Any deviation in accuracy might be expected to detract from the success of the operation. Traditional wisdom had it that too extensive a lesion would produce side effects likely to outweigh any benefits gained from the operation. If surgery were too cautious, the operation, while avoiding the more severe side effects, would not occasion sufficient improvement.

There are, however, a number of factors that can prevent the surgical objectives of psychosurgery from being adequately realized. Apart from the skill of the surgeon, the most important of these would seem to be technical limitations on the ability of the surgeon to correctly place a lesion and excise the desired mass of tissue. Further, however accurate the lesion and however exact the tissue destruction, there still remains the possibility that the lesion might have inadvertent effects on the surrounding areas of the brain. Finally, even if acceptable accuracy is achieved without the unintentional disruption of neighbouring tissue, errors can arise in regard to the exact brain site chosen for surgery. The validity of the choice of location for psychosurgery necessarily impinges on the business of surgical accuracy. However, this issue will receive only cursory consideration in the present chapter. A fuller discussion will be presented later.

Since the early days of psychosurgery, concern has been voiced about the inaccuracy of psychosurgical procedures. The older forms of operation are regarded by most commentators as imprecise and inaccurate. Aside from inaccuracy, the psychosurgical operations of the "first wave" have been criticized for excising too much tissue. It has been argued that postoperative improvement was consequently marred by adverse side effects accruing from the massive disruption of the frontal lobes. In contrast, the newer psychosurgical procedures are usually presented as more restrained and accurate affairs. Indeed, the history of psychosurgery can be characterized as a development towards the more precise placement of increasingly circumscribed lesions. The trend towards more selective operations and especially towards target sites lying more deeply within the brain has been associated with the appearance of more sophisticated methods of inspecting the extent and nature of the lesion.

The "precision" technique of leucotomy, described by Freeman and Watts (1950), represented an attempt to produce a selective operation. The particular procedure used (whether "standard," "minimal" or "radical") was selected on the basis of the patient's apparent condition. The criterion was straightforward: the more disturbed the individual, the more extensive the lesion. Radically disturbed behaviour, it was argued, demanded radical surgery. The risk of adverse sequelae was thought to be easily compensated by the substantial scope for improvement with extensively disturbed patients. With less disturbed individuals, a more restricted operation was preferred, since the scope for improvement was less and the potential for debility correspondingly greater (Freeman, 1949).

However, the "precision" technique of leucotomy which Freeman and Watts described was still noticeably imprecise. It was performed "blind," and the only control over the extent of the lesion was derived from calculations of how far the calibrated leucotomes penetrated the skull.

Transorbital leucotomy was developed as an "easy-to-perform" replacement. However, this form of operation can hardly boast greater precision. It was often carried out in the psychiatrist's office, where the only control over the accuracy of the incision was a visual or photographic inspection of the leucotome in position. Understandably, this style of surgery was viewed with alarm. Mention has already been made of Watts' general disquiet regarding transorbital leucotomy.

The subsequent "open" forms of operation were seen as an improvement. Here the surgeon could gain a better idea of the extent of a lesion, although, as McKissock (1943) observed, this benefit had to be weighed against the dangers that could result from making too large a hole in the skull. Similarly, Kalinowsky and Hoch (1952) argued that the "open" method of psychosurgery could lead to a higher incidence of postoperative seizures due to the wider area of the operation.

Apart from the "open" method of surgery or the use of bony landmarks as reference points, the most common method of inspecting the area of operation was by means of X-ray photography. In the older forms of operation this was generally carried out after the lesion had been effected. In order to identify lesioned areas in an X-ray photograph, it is necessary to introduce some foreign substance as a contrast medium. In the series of operations using the Moniz technique of excising cores of white matter, Freeman and Watts (1937) reported the introduction of a method to reveal the location of the cores. This involved the injection of a contrast medium (thorium dioxide) through a brain cannula along the needle tract of the leucotome. Alternative methods have included placing silver clips around the site of lesion. However, as Le Beau (1954b) pointed out, clips cannot be easily positioned with deep-sited lesions. Thin strips of tantalum wire have also been used but were soon abandoned in favour of other techniques. Tantalum power shows up fairly clearly on X-ray photographs and has been favoured by many psychosurgeons. Mention has already been made in Chapter 2 of the use of Lipiodol (poppy-seed oil containing iodine) as a contrast medium. However again, as Le Beau (1954b) noted, this substance can diffuse too easily into the ventricles causing side effects. As an improvement, he and Pecker (1950) introduced a new technique involving the use of gelatine infused with Lipiodol. This more viscous substance was less likely to diffuse into the ventricles and had the added advantage of being absorbed in a matter of weeks or months. Complications caused by having reserves of such foreign matter in the brain were thus considerably lessened. Recently, Hypaque and Pantopaque have been used as contrast media.

At present, however, X-ray visualization is frequently carried out before lesioning takes place. As early as 1918, Dandy devised a method of introducing air into the lateral ventricles of the brain through burr holes in the skull. Ventriculography, as this procedure is called, permits visualization of the ventricles. These can be then used as reference points for the correct placement of lesions. Encephalography or pneumoencephalography was a further procedure. This technique involved introducing air such that it travelled along the spinal canal towards the brain. Subarachnoid spaces as well as ventricles could then be visualized.

The preference for X-ray photography before lesioning takes place stemmed primarily from the dissatisfaction of some surgeons with the use of exterior bony landmarks. Broager (1947), for example, explained why he and his colleagues favoured X-ray techniques:

> As the human skull shows very great variation in shape and size, we ... abandoned this schematic, exterior method of measurement. Nowadays we preferably operate only patients who have been encephalographed, and we place the burr holes so that the frontal incision in the white matter runs just in front of the anterior horns. (p. 346)

Here the operation under consideration was the bilateral frontal leucotomy of Freeman and Watts, although similar X-ray procedures and reference points have been used in more selective operations. As Spiegel *et al.* (1952) pointed out, the use of such techniques is even more important when the structures to be lesioned lie deep within the brain:

> If one plans operations on subcortical structures of the human brain by means of mechanically guided electrodes or needles (stereoencephalotomy) it does not suffice to determine the coordinates of the areas in question in relation to parts of the skull. The great variability in the shape and the dimensions of the human skull precludes such a simple method as used by Horsley and Clarke in their stereotaxic method in animals such as cats and monkeys. In the human it is necessary to use intracerebral reference points that serve as centres of the coordinate system. (p. 121)

The use of air has since been superseded by other media, since it does not provide a particularly clear picture of all the ventricles and is frequently associated with side effects such as nausea and severe headaches. Pantopaque has been employed instead. However, Kandel and Chebotaryova (1972) have claimed that it, too, has unpleasant side effects, and it is not a very good contrast medium when used in "positive ventriculography". They have, instead, preferred to use Conray. Conray is a "60% aqueous solution of Meglumine Jothalamate and contains 28% iodine" (p. 35), and it has a lower toxicity than the alternatives. Nevertheless, headaches and nausea still appear as occasional side effects. The primary advantage of Conray seems to be that it permits a considerably clearer inspection of reference points than traditional pneumoencephalography.

Alongside the use of X-ray photography, the improved accuracy evident in contemporary psychosurgery owes much to the development of sophisticated stereotactic procedures. However, a number of commentators have observed that inaccuracies can still occur. Schaltenbrand *et al.* (1974) noted discrepancies between their results and those of other researchers with regard to thalamic stimulation. They commented that great care must be taken when stereotactic atlases are used for such stimulation studies.

Nevertheless, the use of stereotactic procedures allied with X-ray photography can greatly benefit the standardization and general accuracy of psychosurgical procedures. Unfortunately, however, such standardization can overlook important individual differences in brain anatomy and consequently jeopardize precise lesion placement. The importance of individual differences has been stressed by various researchers. Despite this, a review of the literature reveals that, in many cases, such differences appear to have been ignored.

By extensively investigating the brains of deceased leucotomized patients, Beck, McLardy and Meyer have shed light upon issues of anatomical precision in psychosurgery. Most of their work has been concerned with the older forms of operation. In one of their accounts (Beck *et al.*, 1950), they commented on the problems associated with using X-ray photography in leucotomy, noting that "post-operation contrast radiograph still gives information on the position of the cuts in relation to skull bearings" (p. 158). Because of individual anatomical differences, such a procedure could in certain cases lead to inaccuracies in lesion placement:

> In a case ... an X-ray photograph was taken after a metal clip had been left in each cut. It showed the marker to be in front of the coronal suture. Dissection of the brain five months later showed that they were still situated in the leucotomy scars, but that these involved structures as far back as the putamen, one marker clip actually lying within putamen, internal capsule and caudate nucleus. This is an example of the variability of the position of the coronal suture in relation to the underlying brain. (p. 158)

As Newcombe (1973) observed, stereotactic surgery has still not resolved this problem adequately. Bartlett and Bridges (1977) illustrate:

> The method of determining the target site depends on measurements taken from bony landmarks and the ventricular outline. The anatomical variation from one brain to another implies that the precise location of the lesion in relation to the nuclear masses and grey matter of the cortex is likely to vary, albeit to a small degree. (p. 388)

Three techniques have been employed to overcome the problems of imprecision due to anatomical variation. All three were described recently by Haaijman *et al.* (1977). First of all, the use of a large number of intracerebral depth electrodes increases the probability of hitting the target.

Serial coagulations constitute the second technique (devised by Crow and associates and described more fully in Chapter 2) used to reduce the consequences of an imprecisely placed electrode. Here, if an initial lesion is judged unsuccessful, a further coagulation can then be performed. These two techniques might be described as the "blunderbuss" approach to the problem of ensuring ablation of the specified site. They both appear to work on the premise that through trial and error the correct site and amount of tissue will eventually be lesioned.

The third technique described by Haaijman and his associates to offset difficulties in precisely hitting surgical targets was also based upon the work of Crow and colleagues. Crow and Cooper (1972) noted two major impediments to producing satisfactory circumscribed lesions in target sites deep within the brain:

> There are two fundamental difficulties in this quest for improved techniques. The first is individual variation in the anatomy of the brain. The second is the serious lack of knowledge concerning the anatomical

and physiological basis of mental events and psychiatric syndromes. (p. 93)

The uncertainty of surgical outcome, it was argued, could be attenuated by prior electrical stimulation of the proposed site. Such stimulation would produce a temporary disruption of the behavioural functions linked with the site.

However, a number of investigators have criticized this practice. The results of several experiments cast doubt upon the use of electrical stimulation in the prediction of permanent lesion effects. For example, Stevens *et al.* (1969) observed the results of depth stimulation in man and noted variability in the behaviour elicited on different occasions.

The general problems associated with data derived from electrical stimulation of the brain will be discussed further in Chapter 8. However, a brief summary here should help underline the difficulties involved in using electrical stimulation to locate target sites for subsequent surgery. First of all, electrodes cannot be located with perfect accuracy because of individual anatomical differences. Second, it is highly likely that the same complex behavioural function is organized differently in different individuals. Third, there is a great deal of experimental evidence (cf. Valenstein, 1973a, b) to suggest that stimulation rarely produces specific goal-directed behaviour. Rather, it evokes a more general motivational state to which individuals respond depending on their own particular propensities. Finally, it is clear that both time and situation influence the nature of stimulation effects.

Thus, it would appear that even in modern stereotactic operations, accuracy of surgical intervention cannot always be guaranteed. Indeed, although it is impossible to derive an *inaccuracy quotient*, there is evidence that in both the older and newer varieties of operation, lesions have been incorrectly placed and an inappropriate amount of tissue excised. While there are few directly pertinent investigations available, such studies as there are indicate that serious inaccuracies have taken place and, in all possibility, still do.

Autopsy reports provide the most searching test of whether the anatomical objectives of surgery have been achieved. Meyer and Beck (1954) investigated the brains of 102 patients who had undergone psychosurgery and had subsequently died. All operations had been addressed at the frontal lobes, and most had been of the "standard" type. Meyer and Beck noted considerable variation in both size and location of the lesions.

Commenting on these indications of inaccuracy in early psychosurgical procedures, Beck *et al.* (1950) wrote:

> It is the *blindness* of the usual operation that must be held responsible for the unintentional variability in the surgical cuts so consistently demonstrated in our large number of brains derived from leucotomised patients. (p. 157, italics in original)

They argued that the high proportion of surgical inaccuracies could not be exclusively accounted for by more obvious factors, such as different techniques of operation, different neurosurgeons or "deliberate intention". They reported on 21 cases operated by the same surgeons, "whose technique is highly standardized and whose skill is beyond question" (p. 158). In ten cases the cuts were too posterior, while in a further two they were placed in a more anterior location than they should have been. They noted that in some of these cases the inaccuracies were serious and potentially dangerous.

As indicated previously, the inaccuracy of lesions has been cited as a major cause of poor clinical results. While it seems reasonable to presume that surgical imprecision is, in fact, implicated in adverse postoperative effects, it does not necessarily follow that results deemed satisfactory reflect the accurate achievement of surgical objectives, i.e. reflect the precise ablation of a specified anatomical target. As Sykes and Tredgold (1964) concluded, following their assessment of a series of patients who had undergone restricted orbital undercutting:

> ... even if it be concluded that these results are clinically satisfactory, it does not, of course, inevitably follow that they were due to the direct cutting of certain fibres. (p. 636)

Analogously, Meyer and Beck (1954) noted of one of their recovered leucotomized patients, "In one of the four recovered cases the lesion was surprisingly incomplete and circumscribed" (p. 441).

Eie's (1954) remarks, based on a careful examination of the brains of 29 patients who had undergone frontal leucotomy, provide a suitable conclusion to the preceding discussion:

> The results of these investigations corroborate the conception already prevalent, that the original and still employed leucotomy procedure is no ideal surgical method for the treatment of mental cases, besides it so frequently produces different anatomical, and consequently different functional results, from those intended by the surgeon. (p. 39)

While Eie was specifically addressing the "first wave" of psychosurgical operations, similar criticisms might be levelled at modern stereotactic procedures. For example, Meyer *et al.* (1973) reported the incorrect placement of a cingulum lesion despite sophisticated stereotactic technology and the use of stimulation of the target site prior to lesioning. Similarly, Corsellis and Jack (1973) noted the variability in lesions produced in stereotactic tractotomy. In addition, Newcombe (1975) observed "slight deviations in the final position of the yttrium implants" (p. 488). Indeed, Göktepe *et al.* (1975) reported one death due to a major seed displacement.

The major displacement of radioactive seeds marks one of the more disastrous mishaps in psychosurgery. A slight deviation in the final position of seeds represents a less dramatic but still serious hazard. Any deviation can, in fact, affect tissue not intended as the focus for destruction.

With any lesioning technique it is always difficult to control with precision the amount of tissue destroyed. Even with precision, some undesired changes must be expected in tissue surrounding the target of operation. This is an inevitable outcome of interrupting histologically normal tissue. Usually such changes are not regarded as significant, but they may have undesirable consequences.

The particular technique used to produce a lesion can substantially influence the extent of peripheral tissue disturbance. Walder and Jaspar (1970) investigated the effects of different methods of producing lesions on the tissue surrounding the area destroyed. Although they were specifically interested in the treatment of Parkinsonism by thalamotomy, their findings can be generalized to psychosurgery. They listed "a few criteria which these lesions should meet in order to achieve their purpose":

1. It should be possible to make the lesion without inflicting undue damage to adjacent structures.
2. The lesions should have a predictable shape.
3. Their extent should be predictable within a certain margin of error.
4. Complication factors (haemorrhages, oedema) should be minimised.
5. If possible, the effect should be tested first by causing a reversible change in the cerebral tissue. (p. 353)

Walder and Jaspar's investigations clearly revealed that most of the techniques for producing lesions do not fulfil these criteria adequately. With the development of more sophisticated instruments for producing lesions, the extent of peripheral tissue complications and destruction decreased.

Walder and Jaspar (1970) indicated that of all the methods for producing lesions, electrocoagulation and freezing appeared to fulfil their criteria most adequately. They did, however, note that even these were not without risks.

The tissue most closely adjacent to the site of operation is undoubtedly most at risk; a "Lückenzone" or "margin zone" of adversely affected brain tissue can result. Here, adverse accumulation of fluid in tissue spaces (oedemas) occurs and makes the estimation of the true extent of the lesion difficult. There are now methods available for detecting such problems. In a study of the long-term effects of stereotactic anterior capsulotomy, Bingley *et al.* (1977) observed:

> Lately, with the availability of an EMI scanner, it has been possible in some cases to verify the lesions with computer-assisted tomography. ... These investigations were performed about 1 week after the operation. The area of decreased attenuation seen bilaterally close to the frontal horns reveals that there was still a considerable oedema surrounding the lesions, the true size of which, therefore, was difficult to estimate. (p. 288)

In summary, the effects of psychosurgery are not merely limited to the area of excision but involve the surrounding brain mass as well. In addition to the complications already mentioned, extensive atrophy of surrounding tissue may occur. This cerebral atrophy can take the form of cysts, as Stjernberg (1947) and Robin and MacDonald (1975) observed. More common seems to be the degeneration of nerve-fibre tracts. The uncertainties arising from secondary lesions may be considerably aggravated by inaccuracies in the operation. Robin and MacDonald (1975) indicated that such complication can arise even in stereotactic operations:

> In an apparent paradox, small lesions in some sites are followed by extensive secondary degeneration. Because the target areas for stereotaxic surgery tend to be in the deeper parts of the brain where many different tracts, connections and nuclei are in close proximity and from which fibre radiations emerge, despite improved overall accuracy in placing lesions, a small variation in either the location or size of a primary lesion may produce correspondingly large variations in the extent and pattern of the secondary lesion. (p. 44)

An early description of secondary lesions was provided by Freeman and Watts (1947a). They described four cases in which retrograde degeneration of the thalamus had taken place following frontal leucotomy. One of these four cases had been classified as a successful outcome. Degeneration of other pathways and areas of the brain following psychosurgery has been the subject of several investigations (cf. Robin and MacDonald, 1975).

Clearly, a number of factors continue to conspire against surgical precision; individual anatomical variation, surgical complications and secondary degeneration are among the most intractable problems. While many impressive technological advances have been made over the years, exactitude remains an unrealized goal.

Further, the finding that cases of cerebral atrophy after psychosurgery are not necessarily associated with poor clinical results is of some consequence. This, together with the observation that clinical outcomes regarded as successful can occur despite inaccuracy of operation, inevitably generates scepticism about the basis of psychosurgery. The lack of consensus among psychosurgeons regarding the importance of site choice reinforces concern. On the one hand, Kalinowsky (1973) favoured the thesis that different psychiatric conditions can be specifically localized within the brain. Obrador (1972) would appear to support this view and even included a diagram to show "preferential" areas of excision. Scoville (1972), on the other hand, argued that different locations of lesions were not necessary. As has already been noted, Pool (1949, 1951) believed that site or location of lesion was of less importance than amount of tissue excised.

Such disagreement suggests that psychosurgery lacks a concerted and consistent theoretical rationale. Where to place lesions and how much brain tissue should be excised frequently appear to be very much a matter of the subjective judgement of each surgeon. Given such conceptual uncertainties, the issue of surgical accuracy would seem to recede into insignificance.

7

Design and assessment of psychosurgical studies

The following amusing episode from the early days of American medica practice was recently related by Lee Birk (1973):

> On a panoramic hilltop one rainy afternoon in colonial America, about 200 years ago, perhaps during one of the dread yellow fever epidemics, Benjamin Rush, signer of the Declaration of Independence, framer of the Constitution and "Father of American Psychiatry", is said to have emerged inexplicably from his horse-drawn carriage, suddenly overcome with a sense of his healing mission and his therapeutic method; in this mood with a burst of zealotry, he is said to have shaken his cane at the city below while uttering the words: "Bleed and purge all the city!" This done, he got back in the carriage and drove on to see his next case.

While purging and bleeding have long since passed from the medical scene, there is a lesson of continuing significance to be gleaned from this anecdote. As Birk indicated

> It can be all too easy to become fervently fascinated with a treatment method, caught up in a kind of *furor therapeuticus* the practice and technology of which leaves little time and energy either for careful empirical evaluation of therapeutic efficacy, or for the analysis of underlying psychopathology. (p.l, italics in original)

Certainly, psychosurgeons have been major offenders in this regard. Rarely have reports of psychosurgical treatment conformed to even the most modest criteria necessary for a proper clinical analysis of efficacy. Further, Birk's *"Furor therapeuticus"* was not just confined to the early halcyon days of psychosurgery; it persists obstinately as a feature of modern practice. Throughout, untempered enthusiasm and unwavering conviction have generally substituted for careful evaluation; they are clearly, however, poor substitutes.

It should be conceded, nevertheless, that much of the opposition to psychosurgery embodies similar characteristics. Here again we frequently witness substantial departures from objectivity. However, the onus of proof, we insist, invariably lies with the innovators of a new therapy. It is they who must muster unequivocal and unambiguous evidence of validity and efficacy. Earnest testimonials, even from men of the highest integrity and intent, that reflect essentially subjective intuitions will continue to prove insufficient surety. Recognition of therapeutic efficacy can come only from evidence that satisfies the most rigorous conditions of scientific method, where the power of experimental design and control and the objectivity and thoroughness of the assessment procedures leave no room for doubt.

In the present chapter, then, we shall look closely at the experimental design and assessment procedures used in psychosurgical studies. The pervading issue is whether the methodology is sufficiently rigorous to permit clear and confident determination of efficacy. Our analysis of psychosurgical data in Chapter 3 largely ignored methodological considerations; data were presented and described with little reference to their scientific status. In the present chapter, we shall closely examine their scientific credentials. In Chapter 4 we did review the so-called "controlled" studies in a more critical fashion, pointing out some of the methodological inadequacies. At the end of the present chapter, we shall briefly return to these studies. The bulk of this chapter, then, will be taken up with a detailed comparison of the methodological characteristics and shortcomings of the studies sampled in Chapter 3. As in previous chapters, the relevant information for consideration will be displayed in tabular form.

The present analysis can be conveniently divided into three sections, the first concerned with experimental design, the second with matters of clinical and behavioural assessment and the third with the scientific value and status of different types of study. The first section, that of design, can be further subdivided into two aspects. Two sets of tables (three tables per set, one for each "period" or "wave" or psychosurgery) deal with the first of these aspects: the patient populations subjected to psychosurgery (Tables 7.1–7.6). Three tables (7.7, 7.8 and 7.9) are devoted to the second aspect of the design, i.e. the operations themselves. The second section focuses on assessment. This section contains tables that deal with the various assessment procedures used in psychosurgical studies (Tables 7.10–7.18) and also examines the treatment of psychosurgical data (Tables 7.23–7.25). The final section (Tables 7.26–7.30) considers the general nature of both controlled and uncontrolled psychosurgical studies as well as their status in the psychosurgery debate.

The first set of tables (7.1–7.6) allows the reader to assess the extent to which reports include (√), omit (–), or give inadequate information (?) on significant details about patient samples. Such details are frequently important in predicting the patient's likely prognosis in the absence of surgical intervention, as well as comprising essential information for comparison between studies (see Chapter 4). Inspection of these tables reveals that many psychosurgical studies are pitifully short of important information; the large number of dashes in the tables is staggering. Nor can comfort be drawn from modern psychosurgical reports, for in many cases (as can be seen from the tables), omissions and shortcomings are, if anything, more frequent than in first wave procedures.

As can be seen from Tables 7.1–7.3, even such basic "physical" details as the patient's age and sex have in many cases been omitted. Often, especially in contemporary reports, such details that are given are extremely sketchy and consist merely of a brief statement about the average age of the patient sample (at operation, although this is often not stated and must be presumed), sometimes, but not always, embellished with the range of ages present. Clearly, this sort of information affords only limited experimental replication. Further, average age data do not allow the reader to assess whether and how age interacts with success or failure for a particular operation, as well as permitting an estimate of how patients might have fared without surgery. Although many of the studies listed in the table as providing full details of this variable intimate that age does not appear a good indicator of outcome, some of the earlier studies implied age effects (cf. Chapter 4).

It must be noted, however, that such variables as age and sex may not be important in themselves but may exert an effect only insofar as they reflect the operation of other, fairly pervasive social factors. A good illustration of this point comes from two early psychosurgical studies. The Board of Control (1947), commenting on their findings of higher discharge rates for males, asked:

> ... was it perhaps easier to place men out in employment than it was to place women at a time when the records were compiled, so that proportionately more men than women were classed as recovered? (p. 12)

Freeman and Watts (1950) attributed their contrasting better discharge rates for females similarly to social circumstances, citing the greater protection afforded women in the home.

In some cases, age and sex effects may interact with diagnosis, i.e. the influence of age and sex on outcome may depend on the particular psychiatric

Table 7.1 Background data on patient populations used in "first-wave" studies

Study	*Age*	*Sex*	*Race*	*Family background*	*S.E.S.*	*Civil status*	*Occupation*	*Education*	*Premorbid personality*	*Morbid Personality*	*Type*	*Sub-type*	*Duration*	*Age of onset*	*Frequency*	*Average duration*	*Precipitating factors*	*Details*	*Confounding diagnoses*	*Mixed diagnoses*	*No. of diagnosticians*	*Status*	*Country*	*Period*	*System*	*Criteria*	*Symptoms*	*Inventory*	*Name*	*Data*
Rao and Govindaswamy (1944)	√	√	–	–	–	–	√	–	–	√[1]	√	√[2]	√[2]	–	–	–	–	–	?[3]	–	–	–	–	–	–	–	–	–	–	–
Board of Control (1947)	√[4]	√	–	–	–	–	–	–	–	–	√	–	?[5]	–	–	–	–	–	?[6]	–	–	–	–	–	–	?[6]	?[7]	–	–	–
Freeman and Watts (1950)	–	–	–	–	–	–	–	–	–	–	√	–	–	–	–	–	–	–	–	–	–	–	–	–	–	–	–	–	–	–
Hohman *et al.* (1951)	–	–	–	–	–	–	–	–	–	–	√	√	?[5]	–	–	–	–	–	–	–	–	–	–	–	–	–	–	–	–	–
Moore (1952)	√[8]	√[9]	–	–	–	√	–	–	–	–	√	–	?[10]	–	–	–	–	–	–	–	–	–	–	–	–	–	–	–	–	–
Tooth and Newton (1961)	√	√	–	–	–	√	–	–	–	–	√	–	√	–	–	–	–	–	–	√[6]	–	–	–	–	–	?[6]	–	–	–	–
Jones and Shanklin (1950)	√	√	–	–	–	–	–	–	–	–	√	√	√	–	–	–	–	–	–	–	–	–	–	–	–	–	–	–	–	–
Freeman and Watts (1950)	–	–	–	–	–	–	–	–	–	–	√	–	–	–	–	–	–	–	–	–	–	–	–	–	–	–	–	–	–	–
Wilson *et al.* (1953)	√[11]	√	?[12]	–	–	–	–	–	–	–	√	√	–	–	–	–	–	–	–	–	–	–	–	–	–	–	–	–	–	–
Fleming and Baker (1972)	√	√	–	–	–	–	–	–	–	–	√	√	–	–	–	–	–	–	–	–	–	–	–	–	–	–	–	–	–	–
Bernstein *et al.* (1975)	√	√	–	√	–	–	?[13]	–	–	–	√	√	√	–	–	–	–	–	–	√[14]	–	–	–	–	–	–	–	–	–	–
Tow and Lewin (1953)	?[15]	?[16]	–	–	–	–	–	–	–	–	√	√	√	–	–	–	–	–	–	–	–	–	–	–	–	–	–	–	–	–

Ström-Olsen and Northfield (1955)	?[17]	?[16]	–	–	–	–	–	–	–	–	√	√	√	–	–	–	–	–	–	√	–	–	–	–	–	–	–	–	–	–
Knight and Tredgold (1955)	√	–	?[18]	–	–	–	–	–	–	–	√	√	√	–	–	–	–	–	–	–	–	–	–	?[19]	–	√	–	–	–	–
Sykes and Tredgold (1964)	?[20]	?[16]	–	–	–	?[21]	–	–	–	–	√	√	?	–	√[22]	√[22]	–	–	–	–	–	–	–	–	–	√	–	–	–	–
McKissock (1951)	–	–	–	–	–	–	–	–	–	–	√	√	–	–	–	–	–	–	–	–	–	–	–	–	–	–	–	–	–	–
Pippard (1955a)	–	–	–	–	–	–	–	–	–	–	√	√	–	–	–	–	–	–	–	–	–	–	–	–	–	–	–	–	–	–

[1] Described as "Mental state before leucotomy" (p. 216)
[2] Details given for most of the leucotomees
[3] In one case a diagnosis was not given and a query (?) inserted in the table
[4] 6 age bands given
[5] Only numbers of cases in each duration band given
[6] See text
[7] Effect of leucotomy on particular symptoms given
[8] Average ages given
[9] Only sex ratio for schizophrenics given
[10] Only average duration of illness given
[11] Only average ages of diagnostic groups given
[12] Only race ratio (white/black) given
[13] Occupation at time of testing (postleucotomy) or death given
[14] Mixed diagnoses with psychotic patients given
[15] Numbers in age bands given
[16] Only sex ratio given
[17] Numbers in age bands given
[18] Only race ratios (British/Polish) given
[19] Diagnoses had "been labelled under the existing nomenclature" (p. 984)
[20] Age bands given for only some diagnostic categories
[21] Only rough proportions of married to unmarried given
[22] Only periods given for recurrent depression

Table 7.2 Background data on patient populations used in "mid-period" studies

Study	*Age*	*Sex*	*Race*	*Family background*	*S.E.S.*	*Civil status*	*Occupation*	*Education*	*Premorbid personality*	*Morbid personality*	*Type*	*Sub-type*	*Duration*	*Age of onset*	*Frequency*	*Average duration*	*Precipitating factors*	*Details*	*Confounding diagnoses*	*Mixed diagnoses*	*No. of diagnosticians*	*Status*	*Country*	*Period*	*System*	*Criteria*	*Symptoms*	*Inventory*	*Name*	*Data*
Ström-Olsen and Carlisle (1971)	?[1]	?[2]	–	–	?[3]	–	–	–	–	–	√	√	√	–	√[4]	√[4]	–	–	–	–	–	–	–	–	–	√	–	–	–	–
Göktepe *et al.* (1975)	?[5]	?[2]	–	?[6]	–	√	–	–	–	–	√	–	√	–	–	–	?[7]	?[7]	–	–	–	–	–	–	–	–	√	√	√	√
Whitty *et al.* (1952)	√	√	–	–	–	–	–	–	–	–	√	√	√	–	–	–	–	–	–	√	–	–	–	–	–	–	–	–	–	–
Le Beau (1954b)	–	–	–	–	–	–	–	–	–	–	√	–	–	–	–	–	–	–	–	√	–	–	–	–	–	–	–	–	–	–
Tow and Armstrong (1954)	√[7]	√	–	√	–	√	√	√	√	√	√	√	–	?[8]	–	–	–	–	–	–	–	–	–	–	–	–	√	–	–	–
Sano (1962)	√	√	–	–	–	–	–	–	–	–	√	–	–	–	–	–	–	–	–	–	–	–	–	–	–	–	–	–	–	–
Brown and Lighthill (1968)	?[9]	?[2]	–	–	–	–	–	–	–	–	?[10]	–	–	–	–	–	–	–	–	–	–	–	–	–	–	–	–	–	–	–
Paillas *et al.* (1971)	?[9]	?[2]	–	–	–	–	–	–	–	–	√[11]	–	–	–	–	–	–	–	–	–	–	–	–	–	–	–	–	–	–	–
Gaches *et al.* (1972)	?[9]	?[2]	–	–	–	–	–	–	–	–	√[12]	–	?[13]	–	–	–	–	–	–	–	–	–	–	–	–	–	–	–	–	–
Laitinen and Vilkki (1972)	?[14]	?[2]	–	–	–	–	–	–	–	–	√	–	–	–	–	–	–	–	–	√	–	–	–	–	–	–	–	–	–	–
Mingrino and Schergna (1972)	?[1]	?[2]	–	–	–	–	–	–	–	–	√[15]	–	–	–	–	–	–	–	–	–	–	–	–	–	–	–	–	–	–	–
Richardson (1972)	–	–	–	–	–	–	–	–	–	–	–	–	–	–	–	–	–	–	–	–	–	–	–	–	–	–	–	–	–	–

Balasubramaniam *et al.* (1973a)	?[5]	–	–	–	–	–	–	–	–	–	√	√	?[16]	–	–	–	–	–	–	–	–	–	–	–	–	–	–	–	–	–
Meyer *et al.* (1973)	?[17]	√	?[18]	–	–	–	–	?[19]	–	–	√	–	–	–	–	–	–	–	–	–	–	–	–	–	–	√	–	–	–	–
Ballantine *et al.* (1977)	–	–	–	–	–	–	–	–	–	–	√[20]	–	–	–	–	–	–	–	–	–	√	–	–	–	–	√	–	–	–	–
Martin *et al.* (1977)	–	–	–	–	–	–	–	–	–	–	√	–	–	–	–	–	–	–	–	–	–	–	–	–	–	–	–	–	–	–
Bailey *et al.* (1977)	√	√	–	–	–	–	–	–	–	–	√	–	–	–	–	–	–	–	–	√	–	–	–	–	–	–	–	–	–	–

[1] Only numbers and % in age bands given
[2] Only sex ratio given
[3] Only number for social class given
[4] For recurrent depression
[5] Only number in age bands given
[6] Only relationship with parents and family psychiatric history
[7] All details given in individual case histories
[8] Details given in only some case histories
[9] Only average age and age range given
[10] Only numbers and percentage in each diagnostic category given
[11] All were diagnosed as obsessional neuroses
[12] All were diagnosed as having severe obsessive syndromes
[13] Only average duration given
[14] Only age range given
[15] All patients described as aggressive
[16] Only numbers for each period of addiction given
[17] Only numbers in decades of life given
[18] Only race ratio given
[19] Only mean education level given
[20] Different groups were used

Table 7.3 Background data on patient population used in "second-wave" studies

Study	*Age*	*Sex*	*Race*	*Family background*	*S.E.S.*	*Civil status*	*Occupation*	*Education*	*Premorbid personality*	*Morbid personality*	*Type*	*Sub-type*	*Duration*	*Age of onset*	*Frequency*	*Average duration*	*Precipitating factors*	*Details*	*Confounding diagnoses*	*Mixed diagnoses*	*No. of diagnosticians*	*Status*	*Country*	*Period*	*System*	*Criteria*	*Symptoms*	*Inventory*	*Name*	*Data*
Spiegel *et al.* (1953)	–	–	–	–	–	–	–	–	–	–	√	–	–	–	–	–	–	–	–	–	–	–	–	–	–	–	–	√	√	√
Andy and Jurko (1972)	?[1]	–	–	–	–	–	–	–	–	–	?[2]	–	–	–	–	–	–	–	–	–	–	–	–	–	–	–	–	–	–	–
Schvarcz *et al.* (1972)	–	–	–	–	–	–	–	–	–	–	?[3]	–	–	–	–	–	–	–	–	√	–	–	–	–	–	–	–	–	–	–
Sano *et al.* (1972)	?[4]	?[5]	–	–	–	–	–	–	–	–	–	–	–	–	–	–	–	–	–	–	–	–	–	–	–	–	–	–	–	–
Müller *et al.* (1973)	–	–	–	–	–	–	–	–	–	–	√	√	√	–	–	–	–	–	–	–	–	–	–	–	–	–	–	–	–	–
Balasubramaniam *et al.* (1971)	–	–	–	–	–	–	–	–	–	–	–	–	–	–	–	–	–	–	–	–	–	–	–	–	–	–	√	–	–	–
Balasubramaniam *et al.* (1973b)	?[6]	–	–	–	–	–	–	–	–	–	√[7]	–	–	–	–	–	–	–	–	–	–	–	–	–	–	–	–	–	–	–
Dieckmann and Hassler (1975)	√[8]	√[9]	–	–	–	–	–	–	–	–	√[10]	–	√	–	–	–	–	–	–	–	–	–	–	–	–	–	–	–	–	–
Dieckmann and Hassler (1977)	√[9]	√[9]	–	–	–	–	–	–	–	–	√[11]	–	–	√	–	–	–	–	–	–	–	–	–	–	–	–	–	–	–	–
Schvarcz (1977)	–	–	–	–	–	–	–	–	–	–	–	–	–	–	–	–	–	–	–	–	?[12]	–	–	–	–	–	–	–	–	–
Nádvornik *et al.* (1977)	√	√	–	–	–	–	–	–	–	–	√[11]	–	–	–	–	–	–	–	–	–	–	–	–	–	–	–	–	–	–	–
Rubio *et al.* (1977)	?[13]	?[5]	–	–	–	–	–	–	–	–	–	–	–	–	–	–	–	–	–	–	–	–	–	–	–	–	–	–	–	–
Narabayashi and Uno (1966)	?[13]	–	–	–	–	–	–	–	–	–	√[11]	–	–	–	–	–	–	–	–	–	–	–	–	–	–	–	–	–	–	–
Balasubramaniam *et al.* (1970)	?[14]	?[5]	–	–	–	–	–	–	–	–	√[11]	–	–	–	–	–	–	–	–	–	–	–	–	–	–	–	–	–	–	–
Vaernet and Madsen (1970)	√[15]	√[16]	–	√[16]	√[16]	√[16]	√[16]	√[16]	√[16]	√[16]	√[16]	√[16]	–	–	–	–	–	–	–	√	–	–	–	–	–	–	–	–	–	–

Kiloh *et al.* (1974)	√	√	–	–	–	–	–	–	–	√	√	–	–	–	–	–	–	–	–	–	–	–	–	–	–	–	–	–	–	–
Mitchell-Heggs *et al.* (1977)	?[13]	?[5]	–	–	–	–	–	–	–	–	√	–	?[17]	–	–	–	–	–	–	–	–	–	–	–	–	–	√	–	–	–
López Ibor and López-Ibor Aliño (1977)	√	–	–	–	–	–	–	–	–	–	–	–	√	√	–	–	–	–	–	–	–	–	–	–	–	–	–	–	–	–
Bingley *et al.* (1977)	?[13]	?[5]	–	–	–	–	–	–	–	–	√[18]	–	–	–	–	–	–	–	–	–	–	–	–	–	–	–	–	–	–	–
Laitinen and Vilkki (1973a)	?[13]	?[5]	–	–	–	–	–	–	–	–	√	–	√[19]	–	–	–	–	–	–	–	–	–	–	–	–	–	√	–	–	–

[1] Only age range given
[2] All diagnosed as having "hyperresponsive syndrome"
[3] All diagnosed as having "behaviour disorders"
[4] Only number of children under 15 yrs. given
[5] Only sex ratio given
[6] Only numbers in age band given
[7] All diagnosed as having "behaviour disorders"
[8] All operatees were male
[9] Details in case histories
[10] All diagnosed as sexual delinquents
[11] All diagnosed as having "aggressive behavior" or behaviour "disorders"
[12] At least 2 psychiatrists
[13] Only mean age and/or age range
[14] Only nos. in age bands
[15] All women
[16] For only 6/12 full details given
[17] Only average duration and illness range given
[18] All "obsessive compulsive"
[19] Only nos. for each duration of illness

disorder (cf. Board of Control, 1947; Freeman and Watts, 1950; Tooth and Newton, 1961).

A further complication is that the same variables can have different effects upon different outcome measures. Thus, for example, while increased age might be associated with good outcomes on one measure, it might not on another. Tooth and Newton's (1961) results indicated this sort of interaction between age effects and outcome measure. While they observed little overall association between age *per se* and outcome (although their data do intimate a marginally worse prognosis for older patients), there was a much higher risk of relapse with younger patients and a much greater likelihood of adverse sequelae appearing with older patients (cf. Partridge, 1950).

The operation of extraneous factors might also underlie the association between outcome and race postulated in early accounts (Freeman and Watts, 1950; Jackson and Jaco, 1954). However, few subsequent studies give details of patients' racial origins (Tables 7.1–7.3) and no study affords direct correlation between race and outcome. Only anecdotal information based upon casual observation and few patients is available (cf. Chapter 4).

The family background of psychosurgical candidates has been largely ignored in reports; few provide even minimal details, despite Greenblatt *et al.* (1950) and Freeman and Watts' (1950) suggestions that a good family background was likely to yield a more favourable result. In the absence of reliable and detailed information, these contentions must remain unsubstantiated.

The socio-economic status (S.E.S.) of patients has not been described save in one study, although even here only the number in each class is given. This particular omission is surprising, since S.E.S. has been thought to be of importance in prognosis generally. Individuals from the higher socio-economic levels are more likely to attend private hospitals (especially in the United States). Private institutions are usually considered to be linked with better outcomes than their public counterparts. Bernstein *et al.* (1975), in their report of lobotomy in private practice, noted, "There is a general agreement that high social class is a favourable prognostic feature" (p. 1042).

As shown by Tables 7.1–7.3, a few reports give details of civil status. However, either numbers are too small or not enough information is provided to enable any useful conclusion to be drawn on the possible association between civil status and outcome. Nevertheless, Greenblatt *et al.* (1950) and Jackson and Jaco (1954) have suggested that married individuals fared better in psychosurgery. Sykes and Tredgold (1964) have indicated a confounding factor here, namely that any marital status effect may simply have reflected better outcomes for women *per se*, since housewives predominated in married samples of operatees.

In many cases, operatees do not have a recognized occupation in the period immediately before surgery; they are registered simply as hospital inpatients. Freeman and Watts (1950) represented these patients as "failures in occupational adjustment" (p. 208) and recorded that the proportion of them commencing useful active work postoperatively would seem to be negligible.

In contrast, Freeman and Watts (1950) reported that there were some notable successes among professional individuals; however, those whose personality had deteriorated were not considered as good candidates for psychosurgery. This reveals again the interaction of general prognostic indicators in psychosurgery and again commends that studies include wide-ranging background information on surgical candidates. While Freeman and Watts (1950) stressed the positive advantages of professional status, they indicated at the same time that the prospects for returning to preoperative working capacity were exceedingly bleak for some professional occupations (physicians, dentists, artists, musicians and writers are specifically mentioned). In general, they observed that "the simpler occupations witness a greater resumption of useful activity" (p. 269). Jackson and Jaco (1954) largely echoed this view. In some cases, though, whether or not a patient has regained his or her *previous* occupational status is not considered in assessing general postoperative adjustment and operative success. Rao and Govindaswamy's (1944) study provide us with an example. One of their cases is introduced as a 25-year-old female agriculturist. Following surgery she was described as:

> Quiet and co-operative. Reported to be attending to her household tasks without difficulty. Recovered. (p. 217)

In the same series a farmer was described postoperatively as:

> Friendly and co-operative. Works hard in the hospital kitchen. (p. 217)

No indication is given in either case whether there was a return to previous employment. For any proper evaluation of outcome, such details are essential. Further, if we assume in such cases that the omission of specific postoperative occupational information conceals a failure to regain previous employment status, then inferences such as "recovered" are wholly unjustified. The capacity of a professional agriculturist to perform household tasks is a naive and insufficient index of her occupational rehabilitation.

While only a fraction of psychosurgical reports present information about the preoperative educational status of surgical candidates, there is reason to suspect from those reports that have considered this factor that it is not inconsequential to outcome. Several authorities attest that those patients with higher educational attainment have a better chance of a recovery (Bailey *et al.*, 1977; Freeman and Watts, 1950; Greenblatt *et al.*, 1950; Jackson and Jaco, 1954; Meyer *et al.*, 1973). Greenblatt *et al.* (1950) have suggested that this advantage for the highly educated reflected their greater "measure of maturity before illness".

Developing such lines of argument, it is possible to subsume many of the prognostic indicators discussed above under the general rubric of preoperative personality. It is widely assumed that a stable preoperative personality signifies a successful postoperative outcome and vice versa. For example, Greenblatt *et al.* (1950) confidently announced that:

> ... the individual who is most likely to fail with lobotomy indicates a lesser level of personality development preoperatively. (p. 294)

Despite the general presumption of importance, it has, as Tables 7.1–7.3 clearly reveal, received little attention in practice. Few studies have bothered with even the most subjective and casual personality assessments; fewer still have attempted more rigorous and objective testing.

It is obvious that premorbid personality as an index or predictor of outcome following psychosurgery will be affected by the nature of the psychiatric "disorder" exhibited. Stated simply, a stable or good premorbid personality will undergo more severe disruption during a major psychotic breakdown than during a minor neurotic episode. Thus the utility of this index is limited within specific diagnostic categories. It will be substantially confounded if applied across categories.

The general importance of the type of psychiatric "disorder" for psychosurgical outcome has already been discussed in Chapters 3 and 4, as has the interaction between the nature of the "disorder" and the type of operative procedure. Fortunately, in most studies, sufficient details of diagnosis are provided to permit estimations of comparative "improvement rates" for each diagnostic category (see Tables 7.1–7.3; also cf. Tables 3.1–3.13). Even here, however, there are substantial omissions of potentially important detail.

Generally, studies have included patients described as suffering from a variety of specified conditions, although a number of endeavours have confined themselves to more particular "abnormalities" such as schizophrenia, behavioural disorders and, more rarely, obsessional neuroses. Thus, while general diagnostic categories are presented, few reports go on to specify the subtypes of such gross diagnostic categories. Tables 7.1–7.3 indicate that it is generally only studies from the "first wave" of psychosurgery that offer such detail. Here the subtype of schizophrenia (whether "paranoid," "simple," "hebephrenic," etc.) or of depression (whether "recurrent," "reactive," "endogenous," etc.) is specified.

The subtypes of disorder may in some cases be almost as important a signal of prognosis, with or without psychosurgery, as the major diagnostic category itself. Detailed examination of Tables 3.1–3.13 also confirms the fact of different outcomes associated with different subdiagnoses. Hohman *et al.* (1951), however, expressed some scepticism about the reliability of their own results for different subcategories of schizophrenia. They indicated some confounding factors in the diagnosis of schizophrenic subtypes, noting that the choice of diagnosis "is often determined by when in the course of the illness the diagnosis is made, or by whether the observer is struck more by one than another feature of the case" (pp. 531–532).

Duration of disorder has been generally regarded as interacting with outcome of psychosurgery. It has been commonly asserted that patients with shorter illness duration will fare better than those who have been disabled for more protracted periods (Board of Control, 1947; Greenblatt *et al.*, 1950; Jackson and Jaco, 1954; Rao and Govindaswamy, 1944; Ström-Olsen and Northfield, 1955; Tooth and Newton, 1961) although some evidence no relationship at all (Bernstein *et al.*, 1975; Jones and Shanklin, 1950; López Ibor and López-Ibor Aliño, 1977; Tow and Lewin, 1953; Whitty *et al.*, 1952). While the balance of the data available would seem to indicate a modest relationship between surgical outcome and illness duration, it should be stressed that the relationship could well be artificial. Rees (1978) has indicated that duration of illness is a predictor of general prognosis, and thus psychosurgery patients of short illness duration may fare better simply because they would have had a better chance of improvement anyway.

Rees (1978) also suggested that age of onset of illness was associated with general prognosis, with early onset attracting the more unfavourable prognosis. Only the study by López Ibor and López-Ibor Aliño (1977) provided a specific test of this thesis, and their results indicate that the younger the age of onset of illness, the better the prognosis following surgery. However, it is possible that the operatees in this study, since they were fairly advanced in years when their illness started, were already characterized by poorer premorbid personalities.

For recurrent illness, such as certain depressive states, the frequency at which the attacks or episodes occur and their average duration could be pertinent to prognosis. Rees (1978) suggested that "a history of previous attacks from which the patient has made a complete recovery" (p. 179) was an indicator of good general prognosis. Sykes and Tredgold (1964), as well as Ström-Olsen and Carlisle (1971), presented details of the patterning of recurrent depressive episodes in diagrammatic form. From both sets of diagrams it is apparent that surgery was performed when attacks were at their most frequent. In both reports, recurrent depression was regarded as commanding a particularly good prognosis with surgery. However, Robin and Macdonald (1975) offered the following analysis of the Sykes and Tredgold data:

> As by definition the cases are recurrent ... it can be assumed that a bad patch could be followed by improvement. To compare the patient's condition at the time of operation with the period immediately following it, as the authors have done, is then illogical. If a comparison is made between the patients in the second year after operation and 5 to 3 years before operation, using the Wilcoxon Matched Pairs Sign Ranks Test ... their conditions are shown to be comparable. (p. 16)

Finally, the presence of clear precipitating factors for the illness has been seen as a good indicator for psychosurgery (Greenblatt *et al.*, 1950) as well as for general prognosis (Rees, 1978), although due to the absence of specific data, no definite analysis is possible.

Details of the diagnostic practices encountered in psychosurgical studies are depicted in Tables 7.1–7.3, general inspection of which reveals a lamentable sparsity of essential information. Two columns of the main body of the table, i.e. "Confounding Diagnoses" and "Mixed Diagnoses," recount two specific problems in diagnostic categorization that serve to compromise efforts to relate diagnosis to outcome.

Fortunately, most studies seem to avoid "Confounding Diagnoses". The study by Rao and Govindaswamy (1944), however, includes one patient (among a group of schizophrenics) for whom no diagnosis was presented. This is signified by a query (?) in the table. More serious difficulties arise in the Board of Control (1947) study. Inherent in the survey method used here is the problem of having to accommodate a wide variety of diagnostic labels and idiosyncracies. The Board of Control received nearly 60 different labels and attempted to fit them into broad groups. In their second largest group, for example, a variety of diagnostic descriptions was accommodated under the rubric of manic-depressive anxiety. It is more than possible that this aggregate, far from defining a uniform disability, embraced a wide range of disorders, many of which may well have had substantially different general prognostic characteristics.

Tooth and Newton's (1961) survey illustrates the more frequently encountered problem of "Mixed Diagnoses," where a patient has been assigned more than one diagnostic label. While this practice may well comply with the principles of *ICD-9* (World Health Organization, 1977), it does render interpretation of treatment data difficult. In some instances only a few patients may be involved (Ström-Olsen and Northfield, 1955; Whitty *et al.*, 1952). However, in other cases, "Mixed Diagnoses" are a general feature of the study (cf. Le Beau, 1954b; Bernstein *et al.*, 1975).

Finally, there are several reports in which a highly specific behavioural symptom has been declared as the primary target for surgery. Vaernet and Madsen (1970) and Schvarcz *et al.* (1972) have both addressed surgery at aggressive or violent behaviour. For Laitinen and Vílkki (1972), anxious behaviour constituted the major focus; surgery was aimed at producing an anxiolytic effect. Any conventional diagnostic label is clearly a secondary embellishment in such enterprises.

Reliability constitutes a major problem in diagnosis (cf. Chapter 4). To what extent is a patient population assigned a particular diagnosis in one report equivalent, with respect to disorder, to a population similarly defined in another report? It was noted in Chapter 4 that diagnostic criteria had varied over time, had varied with geography and could vary among psychiatrists working in the same institution at the same time. Some of the dubiety that understandably ensues from such considerations could be moderated in psychosurgical endeavours were details forthcoming on the origins of diagnostic pronouncements. However, as can be seen from Tables 7.1–7.3, details of this kind are almost invariably omitted from psychosurgery reports.

There is a similar paucity of information on the status of the diagnostician in psychosurgery reports. Rarely can one unequivocally determine whether diagnosis was made by the psychosurgeons, as one suspects in some cases, or, if made by a referring psychiatrist whether he was of junior or senior status; such factors are likely to colour the reliability of diagnosis.

While it is possible to reliably infer the geographical origins of diagnoses in psychosurgery reports, locating the approximate time period of diagnoses can be fraught with difficulties. For example, the diagnoses attached to a particular group of psychosurgery candidates may have been assigned some years ago by the original referring agency. Even more problematically, the group may comprise patients whose diagnostic descriptions were allocated at very different periods; e.g. the study of Bernstein *et al.* (1975), which was a follow-up "of 43 psychiatric patients referred for open bimedial prefrontal lobotomies between 1948 and 1970" (p. 1041).

This highlights a major problem with almost all psychosurgery studies: the failure to specify the diagnostic classification system used. Only the reports of Laitinen and Vilkki (1973a) and Mitchell-Heggs *et al.* (1977) specifically list the *ICD-8* codes. Knight and Tredgold (1955) rather vaguely referred to the "existing nomenclature," although they did discuss the difficulties associated with psychiatric diagnosis. Göktepe *et al.* (1975) also rehearsed some of these problems and opted for deciding diagnosis on the basis of the presenting symptoms. The outcome data of Göktepe *et al.* were listed for the various presenting disorders (see Table 3.6). In addition, they employed two standard questionnaires to provide a more objective measure of symptom severity after operation.

The inclusion of such standard inventories clearly marks an attempt at a more objective and quantifiable evaluation of the severity of any presenting problem(s) before and after operation. Typically, their use involves scoring a number of items presumed either to exclude or to indicate a particular problem; the total score is computed to provide an overall grade of problem severity. This can be seen from Tables 7.1–7.3, however, very few studies appear to have methodically applied instruments of this sort.

It should be noted that most of the studies that have investigated the effects of psychosurgery on specific symptoms or particular presenting problem(s), rather than on gross diagnostic categories, have proclaimed that "anxiety" and "depression" are the symptoms most favourably influenced by surgery (cf. Board of Control, 1947; Knight and Tredgold, 1955; Ström-Olsen and Northfield, 1955; Sykes and Tredgold, 1964). Hallucinations, on the other hand, have been reported as a singularly intractable symptom and usually resistant to surgery (cf. Board of Control, 1947; Sykes and Tredgold, 1964), although some success with amygdalectomy has been claimed (Freeman and Williams, 1952).

As was noted in Chapter 4, length of hospitalization has generally been considered to be inversely related to postoperative improvement rates. Unfortunately, however, few details of hospitalization(s) have been offered in most reports (Tables 7.4–7.6). Only a handful of studies even bother to

Table 7.4 Details of previous psychiatric hospitalization(s) and treatment(s) of patient populations in "first-wave" studies

Study	*Referral status*	*Duration of present hospitalization*	*Age at first hospitalization*	*Frequency of hospitalization*	*Average duration*	*Type of treatment*	*Frequency*	*Dosage*	*Duration*	*Reaction to*	*Complications with*	*Time elapsed since*
Rao and Govindaswamy (1944)	–	–	–	–	–	√	–	–	?[1]	√	–	–
Board of Control (1947)	–	–	–	–	–	–	–	–	–	–	–	–
Freeman and Watts (1950)	–	–	–	–	–	–	–	–	–	–	–	–
Hohman *et al.* (1951)	?[2]	–	–	–	–	–	–	–	–	–	–	–
Moore (1952)	–	–	–	–	–	–	–	–	–	–	–	–
Tooth and Newton (1961)	–	–	–	–	–	–	–	–	–	–	–	–
Jones and Shanklin (1950)	√	√	–	–	–	–	–	–	–	–	–	–
Freeman and Watts (1950)	–	–	–	–	–	–	–	–	–	–	–	–
Wilson *et al.* (1953)	–	–	–	–	–	–	–	–	–	–	–	–
Fleming and Baker (1972)	–	–	–	–	–	√[3]	–	–	?[4]	√[5]	–	–
Bernstein *et al.* (1975)	?[6]	–	–	–	–	–	–	–	–	–	–	–
Tow and Lewin (1953)	√	–	–	–	–	–	–	–	–	–	–	–
Ström-Olsen and Northfield (1955)	–	–	–	–	–	–	–	–	–	–	–	–
Knight and Tredgold (1955)	–	–	–	–	–	√	–	–	√	–	–	–
Sykes and Tredgold (1964)	?[7]	?[8]	–	–	–	–	–	–	–	–	–	–
McKissock (1951)	–	–	–	–	–	–	–	–	–	–	–	–
Pippard (1955a)	–	–	–	–	–	–	–	–	–	–	–	–

[1] In some cases year of administration given
[2] Most of patients were inmates of two hospitals
[3] Only general description for group given
[4] Only average duration and range given
[5] Described as "without benefit" (p. 325)
[6] Described as "private patients" (p. 1041)
[7] Only numbers of hospitalized, "under close medical supervision at home" and "unsupervised" given
[8] Only number for different periods of hospitalization given

give the referral status of patients, i.e. whether outpatient or inpatient, although most probably assume inpatient status. Duration of present hospitalization has been similarly ignored. Not one study details the circumstances of the patient's first hospitalization.

An individual admitted a large number of times prior to operation may be in hospital only for extremely short periods of time. It is difficult to match

Table 7.5 Details of previous hospitalization(s) and treatment(s) of patient populations used in "mid-period" studies

Study	*Referral status*	*Duration of present hospitalization*	*Age at first hospitalization*	*Frequency of hospitalization*	*Average duration*	*Type of treatment*	*Frequency*	*Dosage*	*Duration*	*Reaction to*	*Complications with*	*Time elapsed since*
Ström-Olsen and Carlisle (1971)	–	–	–	–	–	?[1]	?[1]	–	–	–	–	–
Göktepe *et al.* (1975)	–	√	–	√	√	√	√	–	–	√	–	–
Whitty *et al.* (1952)	√	√[2]	–	–	√[2]	?[3]	–	–	–	–	–	–
Le Beau (1954b)	–	–	–	–	–	–	–	–	–	–	–	–
Tow and Armstrong (1954)	–	–	–	–	–	√[4]	√[4]	√[4]	–	–	–	–
Sano (1962)	–	–	–	–	–	–	–	–	–	–	–	–
Brown and Lighthill (1968)	–	–	–	–	–	–	–	–	–	–	–	–
Paillas *et al.* (1971)	–	–	–	–	–	–	–	–	–	–	–	–
Gaches *et al.* (1972)	–	–	–	–	–	–	–	–	–	–	–	–
Laitinen and Vilkki (1972)	–	–	–	–	–	?[3]	–	–	–	–	–	–
Mingrino and Schergna (1972)	–	–	–	–	–	–	–	–	–	–	–	–
Richardson (1972)	–	–	–	–	–	?[5]	?[5]	–	–	–	–	–
Balasubramaniam *et al.* (1973a)	–	–	–	–	–	–	–	–	–	–	–	–
Meyer *et al.* (1973)	–	–	–	–	–	–	–	–	–	–	–	–
Ballantine *et al.* (1977)	–	–	–	–	–	?[3]	–	–	–	–	–	–
Martin *et al.* (1977)	–	–	–	–	–	?[3]	–	–	–	–	–	–
Bailey *et al.* (1977)	–	–	–	–	–	–	–	–	–	–	–	–

[1] Only number given
[2] Impossible to say which referred to in report
[3] Only vague description for whole group given
[4] Details given in only some case histories
[5] Details given in only some of the case histories of 12 patients

Table 7.6 Details of previous hospitalization(s) and treatment(s) of patient populations used in "second-wave" studies

Study	*Referral status*	*Duration of present hospitalization*	*Age at first hospitalization*	*Frequency of hospitalization*	*Average duration of hospitalization*	*Type of treatment*	*Frequency*	*Dosage*	*Duration*	*Reaction to*	*Complications with*	*Time elapsed since*
Spiegel *et al.* (1954)	–	–	–	–	–	?[1]	–	–	–	–	–	–
Andy and Jurko (1972)	–	–	–	–	–	–	–	–	–	–	–	–
Schvarcz *et al.* (1972)	–	–	–	–	–	–	–	–	–	–	–	–
Sano *et al.* (1972)	–	–	–	–	–	–	–	–	–	–	–	–
Müller *et al.* (1973)	–	–	–	–	–	–	–	–	–	–	–	–
Balasubramaniam *et al.* (1971)	–	–	–	–	–	–	–	–	–	–	–	–
Balasubramaniam *et al.* (1973b)	–	–	–	–	–	–	–	–	–	–	–	–
Dieckmann and Hassler (1975)	–	√[2]	–	–	–	–	–	–	–	–	–	–
Dieckmann and Hassler (1977)	–	√[2]	–	–	–	–	–	–	–	–	–	–
Schvarcz (1977)	–	–	–	–	–	–	–	–	–	–	–	–
Nádvornik *et al.* (1977)	–	–	–	–	–	–	–	–	–	–	–	–
Rubio *et al.* (1977)	–	–	–	–	–	–	–	–	–	–	–	–
Narabayashi and Uno (1966)	–	–	–	–	–	–	–	–	–	–	–	–
Balasubramaniam *et al.* (1970)	–	–	–	–	–	–	–	–	–	–	–	–
Vaernet and Madsen (1970)	–	√[2]	–	–	–	–	–	–	–	–	–	–
Kiloh *et al.* (1974)	–	–	–	–	?[3]	–	–	–	–	–	–	–
Mitchell-Heggs *et al.* (1977)	–	–	–	–	–	–	?[4]	?[4]	–	–	–	–
López Ibor and López-Ibor Aliño (1977)	–	–	–	–	–	–	?[4]	–	–	–	–	–
Bingley *et al.* (1977)	–	–	–	–	–	–	?[4]	–	–	–	–	–
Laitinen and Vílkki (1973a)	–	–	–	–	–	–	–	–	–	–	–	–

[1] Only vague details of the group were given
[2] All imprisoned
[3] Mean number of hospitalizations given
[4] Only general details about previous treatment for the group given

or compare this sort of record with a contemporary admission who remained in hospital from initial entry to the time of operation. Both variables are investigated by Göktepe *et al.*, who noted that while the number of admissions prior to operation was not associated with improvement, the mean duration of preoperative admissions did appear to be marginally related to outcome: the longer the periods, the poorer the outcome.

Even in the very few studies that provide an account of the therapeutic interventions prior to surgery, the extent of the information leaves much to be desired (Tables 7.4–7.6). The studies of Rao and Govindaswamy (1944), Knight and Tredgold (1955) and Göktepe *et al.* (1975) are unusual in that they provide details of what previous treatments were administered and the effect they had.

Some of the early rationales prescribed for many of the operations seem to imply that the administration of ECT should mimic some of the effects of later surgery. Freeman's advocacy of ECT administration immediately prior to transorbital leucotomy was essentially governed by this sort of notion (cf. Freeman and Watts, 1950). However, the results of Knight and Tredgold (1955) indicated that response to ECT did not predict the outcome of subsequent psychosurgery.

Göktepe *et al.* also contest a relationship between improvement following ECT and progress after surgery. However, they unfortunately omitted important details, such as the frequency of ECT administration, dosage, duration, subsequent complications and time since administration. These may all have complex interactional effects. For example, although temporary improvement following a limited number of ECT administrations might conceivably influence progress favourably, with an extensive series of ECTs the opposite might hold, since temporary improvement in the latter case could imply that any improvement following surgery would also be temporary. Jackson and Jaco (1954), in fact, contended that operatees who had received less than ten ESTs (electroshock therapy) were more likely to improve after transorbital leucotomy. A further complicating factor here is that the previous administration of treatment may well influence the results of surgery directly. A person suffering severe complications following, say, an extended bout of ECTs might well constitute a far from ideal candidate for psychosurgery. As will be seen later, the administration of certain drugs before operation may predispose the operatees to epileptic seizures after psychosurgery, either indirectly, by affecting general prognosis without operation, or directly, by altering the operatee's response (whether psychological or physical or both) to the operation.

As with ECT, temporary improvement following an earlier psychosurgical operation might be considered a favourable prognostic indicator for subsequent surgery. However, frequent or extensive prior incisions, even where temporary benefit appears to follow, could have detrimental consequences; for instance, exposure to previous surgery could well have an important

Table 7.7 Details of previous, present and subsequent operations reported in "first-wave" studies

Study	*No. of previous*	*Type of previous*	*Length of time*	*No. of reoperations*	*Type*	*Duration*	*Neurosurgery*	*Confounding operations*	*Bilateral*	*1 Stage*	*2 Stage*	*Left or right side first*	*Unilateral*	*Left or right*	*Multi-serial*	*Duration*	*Description*	*Record*	*Complications*	*Stereo*	*Blind*	*Open*	*Accuracy prior*	*Accuracy during*	*Accuracy after*	*Stimulation*	*Amount*	*Postmortem*
Rao and Govindaswamy (1954)	?[1]								✓	✓							✓		✓		✓		✓	✓				
Board of Control (1947)									?[2]				?[2]				✓		?[3]		✓							
Freeman and Watts (1950)	?[4]	?[4]		?[4]	?[4]				✓								✓	?[4]			✓			✓	✓			
Hohman *et al.* (1951)									✓								?[4]					✓		✓				
Moore (1952)								✓	✓																			
Tooth and Newton (1961)	✓[1]							✓																				
Jones and Shanklin (1950)				✓	✓				✓	✓							✓		✓		✓							
Freeman and Watts (1950)	?[4]	?[4]		?[4]	?[4]				✓	✓							✓		✓		✓			✓	✓			
Wilson *et al.* (1953)	✓	✓		✓	✓				✓												✓							
Fleming and Baker (1972)				✓	✓				✓								?[4]				✓							

Bernstein *et al.* (1975)					√	√	√									
Tow and Lewin (1953)	√[1]	√				√	√	√		√		√	√		√	√
Ström-Olsen and Northfield (1955)			√	√		√	√	√	?[3]	√		√		√		√
Knight and Tredgold (1955)	√[1]					√	√	√				√				
Sykes and Tredgold (1964)	√	√				√	√									
McKissock (1951)						√	√	√		√	√	√		√		
Pippard (1955a)						√	√	√		√	√	√				

[1] Those having more than one operation were excluded from the study
[2] Some sparse details, but difficult to distinguish who had what
[3] For only some patients
[4] Insufficient details given

bearing on the nature and severity of adverse sequelae resulting from a subsequent ablation. In addition, at a psychological level, it is probable that the repeated application of such drastic procedures, without permanent benefit, leaves the patient, as well as his/her family or guardians, extremely distrustful and discouraged – attitudes likely to colour the effectiveness of any future intervention.

Unfortunately, as can be seen from Tables 7.7–7.9, very few reports indicate whether or not previous psychosurgery has been carried out on the patients comprising their samples. It is quite possible that omissions here signify no previous psychosurgery, since surgeons could hardly fail to notice and register signs of colleagues' earlier endeavours. However, their recognition of previous surgery may not always be formally recorded. Furthermore, when previous psychosurgical treatment has been encountered and recorded, it has often occasioned a patient's exclusion from the results reported for a subsequent operation, although not, it appears, from the operation itself (e.g. Tooth and Newton, 1961; Tow and Lewin, 1953). It is possible that the timing of the earlier operation constitutes a further complicating factor, although undoubtedly time will interact to some extent with the type of operation conducted. However, given the same previous procedure applied in two cases, differences in time could be important.

Sometimes subsequent surgery is not a new or different procedure but rather an extension of the earlier lesion. As has been discussed in the previous chapter, sometimes the target site will not have been accurately located in the first intervention or the amount of tissue excised will have been in error and a second operation will be conducted for correction. This immediately poses the question of whether patients undergoing subsequent corrective surgery can be directly compared to those satisfactorily lesioned the first time. One would suspect not. Further, subsequent extension lesions always increase the possibility of excising too much tissue. Bartlett and Bridges (1977), discussing extended subcaudate tractotomy lesions, commented:

> While long-term side effects have not been a significant problem, the transient disinhibition that followed the lesion enlargement in every case may be the clinical warning that, despite the benefits to these particular patients, the safe limits of lesion size has been reached. (p. 393)

Discussion so far is premised on the assumption that a standard lesion is generally appropriate. However, several authorities have stressed that lesion size and location should be tailored to a patient's particular condition (cf. Chapter 2). This necessarily complicates the issue even further.

Obviously interwoven with the problem of previous operations is the matter of surgery subsequent to the operation that forms the major focus of the report. Patients may well press for a further operation, especially if there has been at least some temporary improvement after the first (cf. Bartlett and Bridges, 1977). An important consideration here is whether the assess-

Table 7.8 Details of previous, present and subsequent operations reported in "mid-period" studies

	No. of previous	*Type of previous*	*Length of time*	*No. of reoperations*	*Type*	*Duration*	*Neurosurgery*	*Confounding operations*	*Bilateral*	*1 stage*	*2 stage*	*Left or right side first*	*Unilateral*	*Left or right*	*Multi-serial*	*Duration*	*Description*	*Record*	*Complications*	*Stereo*	*Blind*	*Open*	*Accuracy prior*	*Accuracy during*	*Accuracy after*	*Stimulation*	*Amount*	*Postmortem*
Ström-Olsen and Carlisle (1971)	?[1]	?[1]		√	√																							
Göktepe *et al.* (1975)																												
Whitty *et al.* (1952)	√	√		√	√	√			√	√							√					√		√			√	√
Le Beau (1954b)									√	√							√					√			√			
Tow and Armstrong (1954)	√	√	√	√	√	√																						
Sano (1962)									√	√																		
Brown and Lighthill (1968)				?[1]					√	√							√					√	√	√		√		
Paillas *et al.* (1971)																												
Gaches *et al.* (1972)				?[1]	?[1]	?[1]		√																				
Laitinen and Vilkki (1972)									√	√		√					√		√				√	√		√		
Mingrino and Schergna (1972)									?[2]	?[2]	?[2]		?[2]				√		√				√	√				
Richardson (1972)																			√									
Balasubramaniam *et al.* (1973a)																												
Meyer *et al.* (1973)				√	√	√			√	√									√				√	√		√		√
Ballantine *et al.* (1977)																												
Martin *et al.* (1977)																												
Bailey *et al.* (1977)				√	?[1]				√	√						√					√			√				

[1] Insufficient details given
[2] Only very scant details given

Table 7.9 Details of previous, present and subsequent operations reported in "second-wave" studies

Study	*No. of previous*	*Type of previous*	*Length of time*	*No. of reoperations*	*Type*	*Duration*	*Neurosurgery*	*Confounding operations*	*Bilateral*	*1 stage*	*2 stage*	*Left or right side first*	*Unilateral*	*Left or right*	*Multi-serial*	*Duration*	*Description*	*Record*	*Complications*	*Stereo*	*Blind*	*Open*	*Accuracy prior*	*Accuracy during*	*Accuracy after*	*Stimulation*	*Amount*	*Postmortem*
Spiegel *et al.* (1953)	–	–	–	?[1]	?[1]	–	–	?[1]	√	?[1]	?[1]	–	–	–	–	–	?[1]	–	–	√		–	√	–	√	–		√
Andy and Jurko (1972)	–	–	–	–	–	–	–	?[1]	√	√	√	–	√	√	–	√	?[1]			√	–		√	–	–	–		
Schvarcz *et al.* (1972)	–	–	–	–	–	–	–	–	√	?[2]	?[2]	–	?[3]	?[3]		?[4]				√			√			√		
Sano *et al* (1972)	–	–	–	–	–	–	–	–	?[5]		–	–	?[5]	–	–	√[6]	?[1]	–		√	–		–			√	–	–
Müller *et al.* (1973)	–	–	–	–	–	–	–		√	–	–	–	√	√	–		√	–		√			–					√
Balasubramaniam *et al.* (1971)	√	√		–	–	–			?[2]		√	?[2]	?[2]			√	√			√	–		√	√		√		
Balasubramaniam *et al.* (1973b)	–	–	–	–	–	–	–	?[1]	?[1]	–	√	?[1]	?[1]	–	–	√	√			√	–					√		
Dieckmann and Hassler (1975)	–	–	–	–	–	–	–	–	–	–	–	–	√	√	–	–				√	–		√			√	–	
Dieckmann and Hassler (1977)	–	–	–	–	–	–		√					√	√			√	√	√	√			√	√		√		
Schvarcz (1977)	?[1]	?[1]		?[1]	?[1]				?[1]		√	–	?[1]			√	√			√			√	√		√		
Nádvornik *et al.* (1977)	–	–	–	–	–	–		–	√	√	–	√	–		–		√			√			√	√		√		
Rubio *et al.* (1977)	√	√	–	–	–	–	–	–	√	–	√	–	?[1]	–	–	√	–	–	–	√	–	–	–	–	–	–	–	

Narabayashi and Uno (1966)								?[1]											√							
Balasubramaniam *et al.* (1970)			?[1]	?[1]			?[1]	√	√							√			√			√				
Vaernet and Madsen (1970)	√	√	√	√	√			√	√	√	√				√	√		√	√			√	?[7]			
Kiloh *et al.* (1974)	√	√						√		√	√	√	√		√	√			√			√	√			
Mitchell-Heggs *et al.* (1977)	?[1]	?[1]												√					√			√				
López Ibor and López-Ibor Aliño (1977)																			√							√
Bingley *et al.* (1977)	?[1]	?[1]						√								√			√			√	?[7]	√	?[8]	
Laitinen and Vilkki (1973a)							?[1]	√								√			√			√			√	√

[1] Insufficient details given
[2] Impossible to tell how many were bilateral
[3] 1 patient received a right hypothalamotomy
[4] "With an average interval of 10 days" (p. 357)
[5] "Usually bilaterally' (p. 59)
[6] "An interval of 7 10 days" (p. 59)
[7] Depth electrode recordings made in some operatees
[8] In some cases

ment presented in the report was carried out before or after reoperation. Unfortunately, in many cases it is difficult to tell (Tables 7.7–7.9). Once again, data on the comparative effects of subsequent relative to initial operation are insufficient for a proper assessment; either the numbers of patients are insufficient or the details provided are inadequate, or different combinations of operative procedures are involved. Considerations rehearsed before, such as length of time between serial operations, discussed previously in relation to the interaction between previous and present surgery, clearly bear on the present matter.

A related factor that seems to have been completely ignored in reports is the patient's previous "non-psychosurgical" operative history, particularly his/her neurosurgical history. The anatomical focus of neurosurgery implies that its potential interactive influence (whether carried out prior to or subsequent to psychosurgery) could, in some respects, be similar to psychosurgery.

Finally, it must be conceded that it is difficult even to discern the incidence of patients receiving more than one operation, let alone specify the biological and psychological significance of the practice. From Tooth and Newton's (1961) survey it would appear that just over 4% of the total sample had experienced subsequent operation(s). Subsequent changes in the character of psychosurgery and its candidates may well have profoundly affected the incidence of reoperation (cf. Vaernet and Madsen, 1970); for some psychosurgeons a hierarchy of operations almost constitutes standard practice (Balasubramaniam *et al.*, 1971; Balasubramaniam and Kanaka, 1975).

The problems encountered in attempting to decipher the effects of a particular operation given the confounds of previous or subsequent psychosurgical treatment are similar in some respects to difficulties that attend evaluation of a group of patients that have not been uniformly treated. Fortunately, the applications of different operations within the one study has not been too typical a practice (Tables 7.7–7.9). Nevertheless, it should be appreciated that each study listed in the tables has been allocated to a particular category of operative procedure, and in some cases, allocation merely selects the *majority* operation performed.

The case of prefrontal leucotomy is especially complicated, as sometimes the term is used to indicate the "standard" operation and at other times it encompasses such variations as topectomy and bimedial leucotomy as well as "standard," "minimal" and "radical" leucotomy. The term has also been applied to describe operations that necessarily appear as separate categories in the present tables.

In general, few reports give sufficient details to afford a comparison between different procedures within the same study. The present tables reveal only three comparison studies: Laitinen and Vilkki (1972), who compared anterior cingulectomy with mesoloviotomy; Sano (1962), in which comparison can be made between cingulectomy, thalamotomy, fornicotomy, upper mesencephalic reticulotomy and posteromedial hypothalamotomy; Freeman and Watts (1950), in which the results of transorbital leucotomy and the "standard" operation are presented separately. In effect, these studies provide a more legitimate basis for assessing the relative efficacy of different operative procedures than that derived from comparing different studies. The manifold sources of experimental error and bias that variously effect psychosurgical studies presumably exert a more constant influence within the same study, i.e. while error and bias will vary between studies, it should be relatively constant between conditions within the same study. It is, of course, still possible that procedural shortcomings are sufficiently fundamental to undermine comparison even within one study.

Comparable difficulties attend the question of whether an operation is bilateral or unilateral. Several researchers have suggested that in certain cases a unilateral procedure could be clinically effective (Greenblatt and Solomon, 1953; Lyerly, 1939; Ody, 1938; Scarff, 1950; Smolik, 1950).

Despite its importance, some reports actually fail to record whether an operation was carried out bilaterally or unilaterally (Tables 7.7–7.9). Table 7.7 reveals that reports from the first wave usually did include information of this sort. Bilateral procedures seem to have been preferred.

As to the preferred hemisphere of ablation in unilateral procedures, Greenblatt and Solomon (1953) indicated that they opted for the right hemisphere. Dieckmann and Hassler (1975) likewise reported that all their operations were directed at the right hemisphere. In some studies, however, a unilateral operation was not originally intended, and therefore the side receiving ablation would appear to be a random matter (e.g. Kiloh *et al.*, 1974).

To some extent the issues surrounding whether an operation is carried out in one or two stages have already been discussed under the rubric of successive operations or reoperation. Many of the reports summarized in Tables 7.7–7.9 do in fact specify whether surgery was completed in one or two sessions, although many neglect to mention which hemisphere was lesioned first.

Procedures that involve serial coagulations may confound two important areas of difficulty discussed earlier. First, because this form of operation involves the successive ablation of brain material, it may give rise to some of the problems that attend both reoperation and two-stage procedures discussed earlier. Second, because the lesion sites may be somewhat scattered, the problems that stem from the confounding of different operations could arise here. This complication also occurs with the multitarget procedures, especially when these involve the lesioning of diverse brain structures at a single session. Fortunately, reports of the results of serial coagulations and multitarget operations do explicitly state the nature of the procedure (Table 7.9).

Finally, an issue worthy of mention in relation to both two-stage procedures and serial coagulations is the interval between ablations. With brief intervals, a two-stage procedure can be considered more akin to a one-stage operation, whereas with longer intervals the second stage can be seen as more analogous to a reoperation or an extension of the first operation. Consequently, the outcome of the two-stage operation may be differentially affected with short and long interoperation intervals.

Many of the above criticisms can be subsumed under the general rubric of "failure to provide adequate details of the operative procedure". Although many reports do indeed provide some sort of general description of how the surgery was performed (Tables 7.7–7.9), in a substantial number of cases it would seem far too sketchy for the practical purpose of replication. Often procedures are merely listed on the presumption that all are familiar with the intricacies. In other instances, reference is made to an earlier account in which the method of surgery is fully described. While this style of reporting may prevent redundancy, it can be exceedingly frustrating for the reviewer and, more importantly, may conceal technical modifications. Only occasionally are adequate descriptions easily accessible (cf. Freeman and Watts, 1950). Further, very few reports present a record of individual operations. Such information could be important, particularly when an individual intervention deviates in some way from usual practice. Of those that provide individual protocols, some merely offer a selection as sample case histories (Ström-Olsen and Northfield, 1955; Tow and Lewin, 1953) and accordingly provide little concerted information, while others present only the most meagre details in tabular form (Balasubramaniam *et al.*, 1973a; Dieckmann and Hassler, 1975; Spiegel *et al.*, 1953). Similarly, any complications arising during surgery should be formally recorded. Whenever no complications are apparent, a simple explicit statement of "no complications" would certainly decrease ambiguity at the cost of little additional journal space.

An account of surgery should also specify the methods used to ensure accuracy of incision. The method of lesioning (stereotactic, blind or open) should be indicated. Here, most reports are commendably explicit. In Chapter 6 we described a number of methods for assessing the accuracy of psychosurgical incisions. However, few reports indicate their application.

Only one report in the series presented in the tables has produced postmortem data to indicate whether or not the desired location and amount of tissue had been lesioned (Spiegel *et al.*, 1953). Indeed, very few studies do actually reveal the amount of tissue lesioned (Tables 7.7–7.9). Our previous discussions (cf. Chapters 2, 5 and 6) intimate the possible importance of determining exactly the size of a lesion as well as its location. Consequently, it is unfortunate that rarely are details presented of how much brain matter was lesioned, either in terms of area or weight.

The second section of the present chapter deals with matters surrounding assessment. As Tables 7.10–7.12 intimate, a wide variety of factors need to be considered here. Undeniably the most crucial of these is the nature of the measure(s) used to evaluate the outcome of a psychosurgical procedure. While the results of the studies listed in the present tables were summarily classified in Chapter 3 according to a single classification scheme (i.e. improvement categories I, II, III, and IV), the original reports were characterized by a range of different outcome measures. Comparison among studies and psychosurgical procedures is obviously made easier if common outcome measures have been used. It might be countered that there is likely to be a high correlation between different outcome measures. However, this is not necessarily the case, since factors other than postoperative clinical conditions influence the different outcome measures, and such extraneous effects may be far from uniform across measures.

Table 7.10 Type of outcome measures and method of data collection used in "first-wave" studies

Study	*Gainful employment*	*Work adjustment*	*Discharge*	*Psychiatric ratings*	*Other measures*	*Relapse*	*Time*	*Psychiatric interview*	*Visit*	*Phone call*	*Letter/card*	*Questionnaire*	*Hospital record*
Rao and Govindaswamy (1944)	?[1]	–	?[1]	√	?[1]	–	–	–	–	–	–	–	–
Board of Control (1947)	?[2]	–	√	√	√	–	–	–	–	–	–	√	√
Freeman and Watts (1950)	√	–	√	√	√	–	–	√	–	–	–	–	–
Hohman *et al.* (1951)	?[1]	–	√	–	–	–	–	–	–	–	√	–	–
Moore (1952)	√	–	√	√	–	√	–	?[1]	–	–	?[1]	–	–
Tooth and Newton (1961)	?[3]	–	√	√	–	√	–	–	–	–	–	√	√
Jones and Shanklin (1950)	√	–	√	√	–	–	–	√	–	–	–	–	–
Freeman and Watts (1950)	√	–	√	√	–	–	–	√	–	–	–	–	–
Wilson *et al.* (1953)	–	–	√	√	–	√	–	√	–	–	–	–	–
Fleming and Baker (1972)	√	–	–	√	√	√	–	√	–	–	–	–	–
Bernstein *et al.* (1975)	√	–	√	√	√	√	–	√	–	–	–	√	√
Tow and Lewin (1953)	–	–	√	√	√	√	–	–	–	–	–	–	–
Ström-Olsen and Northfield (1955)	–	–	√	√	–	–	–	√	√	–	–	–	–
Knight and Tredgold (1955)	–	–	√	√	–	–	–	√	–	–	–	–	√
Sykes and Tredgold (1964)	–	√	√	√	–	√	–	?[1]	–	–	–	–	–
McKissock (1951)	–	–	–	–	–	–	–	–	–	–	–	–	–
Pippard (1955a)	–	?[4]	–	√	–	–	–	√	–	–	–	–	√

[1] Details given for only some patients
[2] "Habit of work" (p. 16)
[3] Difficult to extract from general psychiatric ratings
[4] Insufficient details given

F*

Table 7.11 Type of outcome measures used in "mid-period" studies

Study	*Gainful employment*	*Work adjustment*	*Discharge*	*Psychiatric ratings*	*Other measures*	*Relapse*	*Time*	*Psychiatric interview*	*Visit*	*Phone call*	*Letter/card*	*Questionnaire*	*Hospital record*
Ström-Olsen and Carlisle (1971)	√	√	–	√	√	√	–	√[1]	√[1]	–	–	–	√[1]
Göktepe *et al.* (1975)	–	√	–	√	√	√	–	√[1]	√[1]	–	–	–	–
Whitty *et al.* (1952)	–	–	–	√[2]	–	√	–	–	–	–	–	–	–
Le Beau (1954b)	–	–	–	√[3]	√	–	√	–	–	–	–	–	–
Tow and Armstrong (1954)	√[4]	√[4]	√[4]	–	√[4]	√[4]	√[4]	–	–	–	–	–	–
Sano (1962)	–	–	–	√[5]	–	–	–	–	–	–	–	–	–
Brown and Lighthill (1968)	–	–	–	√[3]	–	–	–	√	–	–	–	–	–
Paillas *et al.* (1971)	–	–	–	√	–	√	–	–	–	–	–	–	√
Gaches *et al.* (1972)	–	–	–	√	–	–	–	–	–	–	–	–	–
Laitinen and Vilkki (1972)	–	–	–	√[3]	–	–	–	–	–	–	–	–	–
Mingrino and Schergna (1972)	–	–	–	√[3]	–	–	–	–	–	–	–	–	–
Richardson (1972)	–	–	–	√[6]	–	–	–	√	–	–	–	–	–
Balasubramaniam *et al.* (1973a)	–	–	–	√[7]	√	–	–	–	–	–	–	–	–
Meyer *et al.* (1973)	–	–	–	√	√	–	–	√	–	–	√	–	–
Ballantine *et al.* (1977)	–	–	–	√	√	–	–	√	–	√	–	√	√
Martin *et al.* (1977)	–	–	–	√	√	–	–	√	√	–	–	–	–
Bailey *et al.* (1977)	–	–	–	√	√	–	–	–	–	–	–	–	–

[1] Depending on the group
[2] "Improvement," etc.
[3] "Good" results, etc.
[4] In case reports
[5] "Effective," etc.
[6] "Excellent," "good", etc.
[7] "Successes," etc.

Whether a person had resumed gainful employment would, on face value at least, appear to be a satisfactory index of success. It implies that the operatee has recovered sufficiently to both find and keep a job; we would expect him/her to have a high psychiatric improvement rating. There are, however, indications that gainful employment as a measure may in practice be somewhat independent of estimated postoperative psychiatric status. First of all, the term "gainful employment" is itself ambiguous, as a variety of occupational experiences have been subsumed under this heading, ranging

Table 7.12 Type of outcome measures used in "second-wave" studies

Study	*Gainful employment*	*Work adjustment*	*Discharge*	*Psychiatric ratings*	*Other measures*	*Relapse*	*Time*	*Psychiatric interview*	*Visit*	*Phone call*	*Letter/card*	*Questionnaire*	*Hospital record*
Spiegel *et al.* (1953)	–	–	–	√	√	–	–	–	–	–	–	–	–
Andy and Jurko (1972)	–	–	–	√	√	–	–	–	–	–	–	–	–
Schvarcz *et al.* (1972)	–	–	–	–	–	–	–	–	–	–	–	–	–
Sano *et al.* (1972)	–	–	–	–	√[1]	–	–	–	–	–	–	–	–
Müller *et al.* (1973)	–	–	–	–	√[1]	–	–	–	–	–	–	–	–
Balasubramaniam *et al.* (1971)	–	–	–	√	–	–	–	–	–	–	–	–	–
Balasubramaniam *et al.* (1973b)	–	–	–	–	–	–	–	–	–	–	–	–	–
Dieckmann and Hassler (1975)	–	–	–	–	√[2]	–	–	–	–	–	–	–	–
Dieckmann and Hassler (1977)	–	–	√[3]	–	√[4]	√[5]	–	–	–	–	–	–	–
Schvarcz (1977)	–	–	–	√	–	–	–	–	–	–	–	–	–
Nádvornik *et al.* (1977)	–	–	–	–	√[6]	–	–	–	–	–	–	–	–
Rubio *et al.* (1977)	–	–	–	–	√[1]	–	–	–	–	–	–	–	–
Narabayashi and Uno (1966)	–	–	–	√	–	–	–	√	–	–	√	–	–
Balasubramaniam *et al.* (1970)	–	–	–	√	–	–	–	√	–	–	–	–	–
Vaernet and Madsen (1970)	–	–	–	–	√[7]	–	–	–	–	–	–	–	–
Kiloh *et al.* (1974)	–	–	–	√	–	–	–	√	–	–	–	√	√
Mitchell-Heggs *et al.* (1977)	–	–	–	√	√	–	–	√	–	–	–	√	–
López Ibor and López-Ibor Aliño (1977)	–	–	–	√	√	–	–	√	–	–	–	–	–
Bingley *et al.* (1977)	√	√	–	√	–	–	–	√	√	–	–	–	–
Laitinen and Vilkki (1973a)	–	–	–	√	√	–	–	–	–	–	–	–	–

[1] Excellent, etc.
[2] Good, etc.
[3] Released from jail, etc.
[4] In case reports
[5] No instances of relapse reported
[6] Normal life, etc.
[7] Marked improvements   no aggression

from attendance at Occupational Therapy to the return to a full-time professional career.

A simple count of return to qualified employment is clearly an insufficient index here. Further, can a patient previously engaged in a professional occupation be regarded as fully gainfully employed if he/she has returned to a decidedly more routine job (the earlier discussion concerning the female agriculturist is certainly of relevance here)? A further difficulty arises in the case of female operatees (who, as will be recalled, constitute about two thirds of all psychosurgery candidates). Many of them will formerly not have had occupations (in the sense of formally paid work). Again, is it satisfactory to compare these operatees with other female patients who previously held occupations but were unable to return to them postoperatively? Is successful rehabilitation as a "housewife" an appropriate measure of vocational re-adjustment for women who had been actively pursuing a career prior to surgery?

Ström-Olsen and Carlisle (1971) indicated certain specific extraneous factors that could influence operatees' ability to return to and hold down a job postoperatively. The capacity to continue working through their illness seemed to be especially important (Ström-Olsen and Carlisle, 1971; Sykes and Tredgold, 1964). Further, ex-psychiatric patients are undoubtedly more likely to obtain work in a prosperous area during a boom than in poor regions in times of recession. Thus, a simple-minded comparison of postoperative employment rates reported in studies from different regions, countries and periods, could prove a far from legitimate index of comparative operative success. An allied issue relates to how much the hospital encourages and trains leucotomees for employment. Those institutions or agencies that operate more training and rehabilitation programmes are more likely to produce higher ex-patient workrates than those that do not (cf. Miller, 1948).

To offset some of the difficulties of this general form of assessment, Ström-Olsen and Carlisle (1971) developed a "working capacity" rating scale. Further, they excluded from such ratings patients aged 70 or over, the physically infirm and those for whom there was a complete lack of information. While a scale of this sort may appear to be a considerable advance in that it overcomes some of the difficulties associated with the use of a simple "gainful employment index", it suffers from all the problems that generally surround rating scales. These will be discussed below.

Rate of discharge has been a more common measure of outcome than employment, especially during the first wave of psychosurgery. Once again it would appear, at face value, to constitute a reasonable measure of therapeutic success. Again, one might assume that operatees discharged from hospital would be those with the highest psychiatric rating. However, as with "gainful employment," there are reasons for challenging this assumption.

First of all, we can detect systematic biases in the manner in which discharge criteria have been applied in some studies (see discussion of the West Virginia Lobotomy Project in Chapter 4). Further, close inspection of discharge practices alerts us to a range of additional extraneous influences. First, in some instances patients have either been retained in hospital in spite of a recommendation for discharge (Landis *et al.*, 1950) or have been discharged against advice (Ström-Olsen and Northfield, 1955). Second, the role of the family as a variable affecting both discharge and relapse rate has already received some attention (Brown *et al.*, 1962; Copas *et al.*, 1974). Factors other than family circumstances also can affect the possibility of discharge. The attitudes of the general community and the after-care provisions that such attitudes have inspired (e.g. the availability of group homes) may also play an important role.

Another aspect of the importance of family and particularly community attitudes is apparent. This concerns the difficulties of comparing rates of discharge between reports. If the chances of leaving hospital depend partially on the attitudes of family and community, the attitudinal variation across families, communities and countries makes if difficult to directly compare discharge rates (cf. Lewis, 1967; Robin and MacDonald, 1975). Shifts in attitudes over time add to the problem (cf. Scheff, 1966).

However, the major stumbling block to comparing rates of discharge between studies arises from indications that different hospitals have different discharge machinery and criteria. (Here it must be mentioned that some operatees had never been in hospital, a factor that complicates matters further – cf. Hohman *et al.*, 1951, p. 531.) Enormous discrepancies exist between different institutions; in addition, discharge policy varies markedly with locale and time.

In summary, discharge rate, as a dependent measure in psychosurgery studies, is not without problems. It is subject to bias and to geographic and temporal variability, and it has, in general, been applied insensitively with little regard for the conceptual complexities involved.

The most common outcome measure following psychosurgery has been some form of psychiatric rating. The popularity of the rating approach can be attributed to its two apparent advantages over other styles of evaluation. First of all, it permits relatively easy compilation of results. At its simplest, a rating scale of psychiatric improvement consists of four categories, ranging from category 1 (recovered or markedly improved) down to category 4 (worse). The rater assigns each operatee to one of these. The total number of patients in the first two categories combined is taken as an indication of the success of surgery. The second advantage of psychiatric ratings is that they seem to offer an easy means of comparing results from different studies.

In Chapter 3, we dubbed this method of evaluating therapeutic success the "head-counting approach". Apart from being an extremely uncritical means of assessing outcome, there are certain particular problems associated with the use of psychiatric rating scales.

First of all, different versions of rating scales have been employed. These encompass a wide range, beginning with the simple variety, where the patient is rated after psychosurgery on a scale of one through four – category 1 for "recovered," category 4 for worse or "deteriorated." Here, no formal criteria for group allocation are given (cf. Rao and Govindaswamy, 1944). At its most complex, the scale encompasses a series of subscales of particular variables. Separate ratings are first made on the subscales and then an overall grade is obtained by compiling the subscale scores (e.g. Pippard, 1955a).

Clearly, different problems are associated with different sorts of rating scales. However, a major weakness with all types of scales is the substantial subjectivity involved in the assignation of a patient to a particular category; the simpler type of rating scale may be more liable in this respect. What is rated as marked improvement by one assessor on his/her own scale may not necessarily bear a great deal of relation to the patient's status as revealed by other methods of evaluation.

However, even the complicated device used by Pippard (1955a), mentioned above cannot be exempt from the problem of subjectivity. More importantly perhaps, Pippard's scheme assumes that subscale scores can be simply combined to provide the overall rating. However, the variables underlying the scales may be far from equally predictive, i.e. some form of differential weighting of subscale scores may be necessary. Pokorny and Faibish (1968) proposed instead the application of multivariate analysis to identify the most salient variables and the relationships between them. While this approach certainly constitutes an advance in terms of sophistication and objectivity, it, too, has its limitations. It should be emphasized that for each region, time and even diagnostic category, different outcome variables may assume different relative weightings with regard to therapeutic success.

These considerations direct us to another problem complicating the use of rating scales: the degree of variability in their use. Clearly, the more liable the scale to subjective bias, the lower will be the reliability both within and between studies (the discussion of reliability of psychiatric diagnosis in Chapter 4 is of relevance here). This difficulty is compounded where different rating scales are employed between studies. (In Tables 3.1–3.13 we indicated just how we had accommodated the original categories into our own rating scale.)

Clinical rating scales have also been used (e.g. Sands and Malamud, 1949), although infrequently. They pose their own particular problems. In addition to sharing some of the general difficulties associated with global psychiatric rating scales, clinical rating scales are liable to most of the pitfalls and dangers that attend the rating and assessment of individual clinical symptoms (cf. Chapter 4). Further, clinical rating scales have attracted the criticism that by concentrating exclusively on symptom relief, they may ignore other significant variables such as social functioning (cf. Pokorny and Faibish, 1968). The "continuing need for medication" item used in some clinical rating scales has been specifically criticized in this respect. Bridges (1973) announced a modification to his own method of assessment "to emphasize social functioning rather than continuing need for treatment as medication sometimes continues to be taken without clear justification" (p. 342).

For those operations aimed at specific psychiatric or behavioural "disorders," specially-tailored outcome measures or rating scales have been applied especially for depression, anxiety and obsessionality. There are, however, few scales available for rating outcome after surgery for "aggressive" behaviour. Further, those scales and tests developed for this purpose are often based upon a "personality type" perspective and fail to acknowledge the manifest situational specificity of what is deemed "aggressive behaviour". Hitchcock *et al.*'s (1973) efforts indicate the "state of play" in this area of assessment. They presented details of three specific tasks: mirror image drawing, pursuit rotor tracking and a modification of the Gibson spiral maze (Gibson, 1965). They observed of these tasks:

> The aim of these three techniques is to put the patient in mildly frustrating or stressful situations. It was not considered desirable to create situations of a severely stressful nature as it was felt that this would have immediate repercussions in terms of patient management, and would also be likely to preclude any further co-operation in future testing. (p. 151)

Hitchcock *et al.* clearly presume that if the operatee's "abnormal" responses (or pattern of responses) on these tasks are controlled by surgery, then "naturally" occurring "aggressive" behaviour (i.e. outside the experimental situation) should also be curbed. Clearly, this may not be so. For any individual, the occurrence of "aggressive" behaviour may well be specific to certain particular environmental circumstances. These may be far removed from the artificial situations engineered by Hitchcock *et al.* An additional difficulty with this sort of assessment is that it may fail to distinguish between specific effects (aggression) and general effects (sedation). What is recorded in these tasks as a diminution in aggression may, in fact, be nothing short of a general disability in responsiveness, i.e. psychosurgery may have effected sedation rather than caused any specific decline in aggression. The present style of assessment lacks the sensitivity necessary for differentiation here. (The general issue of the specificity of psychosurgical effects is treated in subsequent chapters.)

Other methods of evaluation have included the comparison of photographs taken before and after surgery (Freeman and Watts, 1950), the ease with which the patient could be managed in the hospital (Hohman *et al.*, 1951), the patient's capacity for pleasure (Ström-Olsen and Carlisle, 1971) and the use, or rather "abuse," of "one tablet or one injection in the post-operative period" (Balasubramaniam *et al.*, 1973a p. 64).

Finally, two other associated outcome measures are worth mentioning: rate of relapse and time of relapse after surgery. As Tables 7.10–7.12 show, very few studies appear to have used these. Of those that have, readmission rate to psychiatric hospital as an index of the rate of relapse is the most common measure. This lack of information is clearly a matter of significance; permanent rehabilitation is obviously better than a brief and unsuccessful return to the community. Consequently, it is unfortunate that comparison between reports here is vitiated by the lack of appropriate follow-up data.

While the absence of data here may reflect a negligible incidence of readmission, this may not necessarily be the case. It is possible that the information was not available, was not made available or was passed on too late for inclusion in the report. Further, the operatee may have been admitted to another hospital (cf. Board of Control, 1947; Moore, 1952; Wilson *et al.*, 1953), a fact that may never have reached the authors of the original report. Once again it should be noted that rate of readmission is unlikely to be a simple index of general psychiatric condition. Rather, it will reflect the same matrix of influences that affects discharge rate. Heath *et al.* (1949), for example, reported that one patient "remained institutionalized for sociological reasons" (p. 417). She had been discharged, but –

> One day following release she was returned by a drunken husband who found her too much trouble – an impediment to his new and freer life. (p. 417)

Occasionally, residents are "paroled" after surgery, rather than fully discharged. Jones and Shanklin (1950) listed the date of "parole" followed by the dates of any subsequent readmissions. The time between release and relapse is, however, rarely furnished (Tables 7.10–7.12).

In summary, therefore, outcome measures have on the whole been somewhat crude and fraught with difficulties. Many of them have been highly subjective or at least susceptible to factors other than improvement after surgery. Social, temporal and cultural effects render the comparison of even the same outcome measures from different reports difficult. Clearly, more objective, comprehensive and realistic measures are needed.

Tables 7.10–7.12 also list the means by which information was accessed. As can be seen from these tables, the most common method of access was the interview. This would appear to be the most sensitive and practical form of gaining information; the results revealed by postsurgery psychiatric interview can be readily compared to those recorded before surgery during a similar encounter. A number of points should, however, be made. First of all, interviews are necessarily highly subjective affairs. Much of the discussion in Chapter 4 concerning the issues surrounding psychiatric diagnosis is of relevance here. The style and direction of the interview and hence the nature of the information disclosed is likely to depend very much on the interviewer. Inter-interviewer reliability is rarely satisfactory. In addition, the interviewer will almost certainly harbour particular expectancies derived from the knowledge that the patient has undergone psychosurgery. These expectancies may interfere with the conduct of the interview and colour the results derived from it in subtle and covert ways. Inconsistency between pre- and posttreatment interviews is another problem. This is especially likely where the two sessions are conducted by different interviewers. All in all, an interview panel (cross disciplinary) would seem an appropriate solution. It would circumvent many of the difficulties mentioned.

The second approach is less satisfactory than the psychiatric interview: this is what can only be described as the "brief visit." Here, the ex-patient and the data collector meet only briefly; sparse data are gathered in an invariably unsystematic fashion. Either the operatee merely "pops in" to see the assessor or a brief "home visit" is made. This approach has little to commend it; it lacks the potential sensitivity of the protracted interview but still suffers from all the problems of subjectivity.

Even further along a decreasing scale of patient–assessor contact are the telephone call and the solicited (or even unsolicited) letter or postcard – even Christmas cards have been included as sources of information! (e.g. Freeman and Watts, 1950). The nature of such contact will ensure only scanty, selective and ambiguous data.

Questionnaires certainly constitute a more structured method of information gathering. Two sorts of questionnaire approach have been in evidence in psychosurgery. The first consists of a series of questions posed directly to the operatee by the assessor in a letter. Unfortunately the rate of return can be low (less than half in the Ballantine *et al.*, 1977, study). A further difficulty is that of comparing results derived from questionnaires that may be different in both form and content. In the second approach, questionnaires are distributed by the assessor to various agencies requesting details about the patients with whom they have had some contact (e.g. Board of Control, 1947; Tooth and Newton, 1961). While a higher return rate is likely, problems of subjectivity and between-study comparability remain.

Hospital records provide another source of information. Usually, comparison is made of the operatees' "notes" before and after surgery. Once again this is often a very unsatisfactory means of gathering data. In the first place, the assessor may select only certain items of information from the records or interpret the patient's notes in a highly idiosyncratic fashion. There is the further difficulty that the reports themselves are likely to be an aggregate of highly subjective judgements, whether from nurses, medical officers, psychologists or other agencies. The validity of each contributory judgement will vary markedly, and the reliability between them may be extremely low.

Finally, it must be noted in passing that the various difficulties attending different approaches to evaluation are compounded in some studies by the use of different means of assessment with different patients. Bernstein *et al.* (1975) provide an example of this:

> Thirty-five patients were followed up to 1972: 29 with personal interviews, four with telephone interviews, and two with letter questionnaires. (p. 1042)

A structured interview of all operatees and significant others carried out by a multidisciplinary team, together with an assessment of functioning outside the hospital and the use of objective tests, would appear the most valid and reliable means of obtaining data.

Allied to the difficulties over the outcome measures used in psychosurgery and over the means of evaluation are issues concerning the assessor. Tables 7.13–7.15 display a variety of different agencies from which information about therapeutic outcome has been obtained. Obviously, it would be hoped that the data offered by the various sources listed would be compatible. Unfortunately, few studies have attempted precise comparison. While the data presented by Ballantine *et al.* (1977) do suggest some general agreement

Table 7.13 Agencies from whom outcome data was derived in "first-wave" studies

Study	*Psychosurgeon*	*Psychiatrist*	*Family doctor*	*Nurse*	*Psychologist*	*Social worker*	*Operatee*	*Relative*	*Friend*	*Other*	*Treatment assessor*	*Referral assessor*	*Hospital agency*	*Other*
Rao and Govindaswamy (1944)	?[1]	?[1]	–	–	–	–	–	–	–	–	?[2]	?[2]	?[2]	–
Board of Control (1947)	–	?[3]	–	–	–	–	–	–	–	–	–	–	–	–
Freeman and Watts (1950)	√	√	–	–	√	–	–	–	–	–	√	√	√	–
Hohman *et al.* (1951)	?[1]	?[1]	–	√[4]	–	–	–	√	–	–	?[2]	?[2]	√	–
Moore (1952)	–	√	–	–	–	–	–	?[5]	–	–	–	√	–	–
Tooth and Newton (1961)	–	?[3]	–	–	–	–	–	–	–	–	–	–	√	–
Jones and Shanklin (1950)	?	√[3]	√	–	–	–	–	–	–	–	?[2]	√	–	–
Freeman and Watts (1950)	√	–	–	–	√	–	–	–	–	–	√	–	–	–
Wilson *et al.* (1953)	?[1]	√	–	√	–	–	–	–	–	–	?[2]	√	√	–
Fleming and Baker (1977)	√	√	–	–	–	–	–	–	–	–	√	√	–	–
Bernstein *et al.* (1975)	?[1]	√	–	–	–	–	–	–	–	–	?[2]	√	–	–
Tow and Lewin (1973)	√	?	–	–	–	–	–	–	–	–	√	?[2]	–	–
Ström-Olsen and Northfield (1955)	√	√	–	–	√	√	√	√	–	–	√	√	–	–
Knight and Tredgold (1955)	√	√	–	–	–	–	√	–	–	–	√	√	–	–
Sykes and Tredgold (1964)	√	√	–	–	√	√	√	√	–	–	√	√	–	–
McKissock (1951)	√	–	–	–	–	–	–	–	–	–	√	–	–	–
Pippard (1955a)	–	√	–	–	–	–	√	√	–	–	–	–	√	–

[1] Difficult to tell from whom the data were derived
[2] Difficult to tell relationship of assessor to treatment process
[3] Hospital agencies (superintendent)
[4] Described as "attendant"
[5] Data probably not taken from every operatee's relative(s)

Table 7.14 Agencies from whom outcome data was derived in "mid-period" studies

Study	*Psychosurgeon*	*Psychiatrist*	*Family doctor*	*Nurse*	*Psychologist*	*Social worker*	*Operatee*	*Relative*	*Friend*	*Other*	*Treatment assessor*	*Referral assessor*	*Hospital agency*	*Other*
Ström-Olsen and Carlisle (1971)	–	✓	✓	✓	–	✓	✓	✓	✓	–	–	–	–	✓
Göktepe *et al.* (1975)	–	✓	✓	–	✓	✓	✓	✓	–	✓	–	–	–	✓
Whitty *et al.* (1952)	✓	✓	–	–	–	–	–	–	–	–	✓	?[1]	?[1]	–
Le Beau (1954b)	✓	–	–	–	–	–	–	–	–	–	✓	–	–	–
Tow and Armstrong (1954)	?[1]	–	–	–	–	–	–	–	–	–	?[1]	–	–	–
Sano (1962)	✓	–	–	–	–	–	–	–	–	–	✓	–	–	–
Brown and Lighthill (1968)	✓	✓	–	–	✓	–	–	–	–	–	✓	?[1]	?[1]	–
Paillas *et al.* (1971)	–	✓	–	–	–	–	–	–	–	–	–	–	–	✓
Gaches *et al.* (1972)	✓	–	–	–	–	–	✓	–	–	✓	–	–	–	?[1]
Laitinen and Vilkki (1972)	✓	–	–	–	–	–	–	–	–	–	✓	–	–	–
Mingrino and Schergna (1972)	✓	–	–	–	–	–	–	–	–	–	✓	–	–	–
Richardson (1972)	✓	–	–	–	–	–	–	–	–	–	✓	–	–	–
Balasubramaniam *et al.* (1973a)	✓	–	–	–	✓	–	–	–	–	–	✓	–	–	–
Meyer *et al.* (1973)	✓	✓	–	–	–	–	–	–	–	–	✓	–	✓	✓
Ballantine *et al.* (1977)	✓	✓	✓[2]	–	–	✓[2]	✓[2]	–	–	–	✓	–	–	✓
Martin *et al.* (1977)	✓	✓	–	–	✓	–	–	–	–	–	✓	–	–	✓
Bailey *et al.* (1977)	✓	✓	–	–	✓	–	–	–	–	–	✓	–	–	✓

[1] Insufficient details given
[2] Depending on group

between different evaluators, any conclusions must be tempered by the exceptionally poor rate of questionnaire return.

Thus, until more complete data are available, the suspicion that different evaluating agencies will arrive at different assessments must remain. There are reasonable *a priori* grounds for harbouring such a suspicion. The particular agencies (relatives, surgeon, psychiatrists, psychologists, etc.) are characterized by different sorts of training (or lack of it), criteria of success, expectancies for relief via psychosurgery and by different amounts and styles of contact with the patient.

In the usual format, the psychosurgeon operates, the psychiatrist evaluates and they jointly report the outcome (cf. Valenstein, 1977). Exceptions exist, however; there have been cases in which psychiatrists themselves have carried

Table 7.15 Agencies from whom outcome data was derived in "second-wave" studies

Study	*Psychosurgeon*	*Psychiatrist*	*Family doctor*	*Nurse*	*Psychologist*	*Social worker*	*Operatee*	*Relative*	*Friend*	*Other*	*Treatment assessor*	*Referral assessor*	*Hospital agency*	*Other*
Spiegel *et al.* (1954)	√[1]	–	–	–	–	–	–	–	–	–	√[1]	–	–	–
Andy and Jurko (1972)	√[1]	–	–	–	–	–	–	–	–	–	√[1]	–	–	–
Schvarcz *et al.* (1972)	√[1]	–	–	–	–	–	–	–	–	–	√[1]	–	–	–
Sano *et al.* (1972)	√[1]	–	–	–	–	–	–	–	–	–	√[1]	–	–	–
Müller *et al.* (1973)	√[1]	–	–	–	–	–	–	–	–	–	√[1]	–	–	–
Balasubramaniam *et al.* (1971)	√[1]	–	–	–	–	–	–	–	–	–	√[1]	–	–	–
Balasubramaniam *et al.* (1973b)	√	–	–	–	–	–	–	–	–	–	√[1]	–	–	–
Dieckmann and Hassler (1975)	√	–	–	–	–	–	–	–	–	–	√[1]	–	–	–
Dieckmann and Hassler (1977)	√	–	–	–	–	–	–	–	–	–	√[1]	–	–	–
Schvarcz (1977)	√	–	–	–	–	–	–	–	–	–	√		–	–
Nádvornik *et al.* (1977)	√	–	–	–	–	–	–	–	–	–	√[1]	–	√	–
Rubio *et al.* (1977)	√	–	–	–	√	–	–	–	–	–	√[1]	–	–	–
Narabayashi and Uno (1966)	√[1]	√	√	–	–	–	–	–	–	–	√[1]	–	–	–
Balasubramaniam *et al.* (1970)	√[1]	–	–	–	–	–	–	–	–	–	√[1]	–	–	–
Vaernet and Madsen (1970)	√[1]	–	–	–	–	–	–	–	–	–	√[1]	–	–	–
Kiloh *et al.* (1974)	–	√	–	–	√	√	√	–	–	–	–	–	–	–
Mitchell-Heggs *et al.* (1977)	√	√	√	√	√	–	√	√	–	√[2]	√	–	√[3]	–
López Ibor and López-Ibor Aliño (1977)	–	–	–	–	–	–	–	–	–	–	–	–	–	–
Bingley *et al.* (1977)	√[1]	√	–	–	–	–	–	–	–	–	√[1]	–	–	–
Laitinen and Vilkki (1973a)	√[1]	–	–	–	–	–	–	–	–	–	–	–	–	–

[1] Insufficient details as to status of other author(s)
[2] Psychologist
[3] Occupational therapist

out the surgery (cf. Spiegel *et al.*, 1953, p. 390). In other instances it is the surgeon who does the assessment (cf. McKissock, 1951; Richardson, 1972). Often it is difficult to determine who did what. Clearly, considerations of training, experience and opportunity commend assessments conducted by psychiatrists in the course of extensive interviews over cursory evaluations undertaken by specialist surgeons.

However, while psychiatrists are to be preferred to specialized surgeons in matters of psychological or behavioural evaluation, assessment by the psychiatrist is no automatic guarantee of comprehensiveness or accuracy. Much hinges on the nature of the psychiatrist's contact with the operatee. From our previous discussion, it is clear that the extent and circumstances of contact are often far from optimal.

Considerations of this sort suggest the involvement of diverse agencies (psychiatrists, psychologists, nurses, social workers, the operatee, relatives, friends, etc.) in assessment. Diversification would seem to offer several advantages. First of all, different styles of evaluation can be brought to bear, ranging from highly structured psychometric assessments to informal observations by relatives and the introspective judgements of the operatee him/herself. Second, the use of different agencies will ensure assessment in a wide variety of environmental contexts (not merely in the ward or in the psychiatrist's office). Third, such an approach would introduce into the evaluative process individuals (relatives, friends, etc.) who have had substantially more contact with the patient than the usual professional agencies. Fourth, diversification allows a wide range of perspectives to impinge on assessment. While these may give rise to differing judgements of outcome, a composite evaluation distilled from heterogeneous sources is likely to be considerably more accurate and realistic than one based on a single, particular perspective. Individual biases and expectancies should be counteracted and compensated where there is a wide range of input into the assessment process. Further, the strength of concurrence between diverse sources of judgement could not only be thoroughly examined if such an approach were adopted but could also be used as an index of the confidence that ought to be placed in any composite evaluation.

There is a final reason for advocating the multifarious approach to assessment: the matter of independence. It is generally conceded that it is good practice, particularly with unestablished or poorly established procedures, to have assessors that are independent from the treatment process. If the individual carrying out the assessment is also intimately involved in the treatment, it can be argued that objectivity may be compromised by vested interest. Valenstein (1977) indicated the consequences for psychosurgery's credibility of failing to incorporate independent assessment:

> Those opposed to psychosurgery are likely to discount these results entirely on the basis of the subjectivity of the ratings and the fact that the neurosurgeons and psychiatrists responsible for the patient's treatment have assigned the ratings in most cases. (p. 78)

Tables 7.13–7.15 indicate the assessor's involvement in the treatment process. It is clearly common in psychosurgery for the assessor to be involved in treatment.

However, Valenstein has argued that, in practice, objectivity is rarely undermined in such circumstances:

> ... it is not likely that many neurosurgeons would rate their results as excellent simply on the basis of the elimination of troublesome behavior without considering other aspects of the patient's overall adjustment. It would take overt deceit, not self-deception, to assign a rating of excellent to a patient who spends the days passively and unresponsively at home even if no longer a burden to anyone. (p. 78)

Valenstein's interpretation should not escape comment; two points must be made. First of all, as far as can be determined from published reports, those assessing psychosurgical outcome have often failed to consider "other aspects of the patient's overall adjustment" and have indeed based their judgement simply on the basis of the elimination of target symptoms or behaviour. Second, while it would be mischievous to suggest that assessors with a vested interest in a particular therapy suspend judgement entirely, there are very good grounds for believing that less spectacular adjustments occur.

The work of Rosenthal (1966) clearly reveals the intrusive effects of experimenter's beliefs and expectancies. Rosenthal's studies do not lead us to suspect that "totally passive and unresponsive" operatees will be rated "excellent." They do, however, warn us that "no change" may be occasionally elevated to "slightly better" and that "slightly improved" may be viewed as "markedly improved". In summary, more credence should always be given to independent evaluation, and one of the virtues of involving diverse agencies in assessment is that it provides for just such independence. It would seem unfortunate that the multifarious or multidisciplinary approach has rarely been used.

While the occurrence of inflated judgements of success from subjective and poorly controlled assessment procedures may be bad for science, it is often "good for business". Scheflin and Opton (1978) provided an illustration of this in their discussion of the funding of the Boston Violence Project (cf. Mark and Ervin, 1970):

> Unfortunately, government funding agencies had no information about the psychosurgical achievements of the group except what the physicians themselves provided. Later investigations showed that the data provided had been seriously incomplete and, to put the matter most charitably, subject to radically different interpretations. (pp. 295–296)

The case of "Thomas R", which will be discussed later (see Chapter 11), illustrates Scheflin and Opton's contention.

The timing and duration of assessment also deserve our attention. As can be seen from Tables 7.16–7.18, the lag between operation and evaluation varies considerably among studies. May and Van Putten (1974) pinpointed a major consequence of differences in the timing of assessment.

> Apparent conflict between the findings of different studies is sometimes attributable to failure to distinguish between immediate and long-term

results. For example, a study that examines patients 5 years after treatment was terminated is addressing a different focus than one that examines patients at the time of discharge. (p. 269)

Clearly, temporal variations in assessment complicate the comparison of psychosurgical studies.

However, May and Van Putten argued that an overall inspection of the variously timed evaluations arising from different studies could yield useful information on the time course of treatment effects. To facilitate an exercise of this sort, they proposed classifying the timing of assessment as immediate (within the first six postoperative months), short-term (six months to a year), intermediate (two to four years) and long-term (five or more years). The

Table 7.16 Details of follow-up in "first-wave" studies

Study	*Possible to relate length of follow-up to improvement*	*Details of follow-up*
Rao and Govindaswamy (1944)	√	Up to 7 years
Board of Control (1947)	–	Impossible to estimate
Freeman and Watts (1950)	–	Up to about 13–14 years
Hohman *et al.* (1951)	–	4–48 months
Moore (1952)	–	Average 25 months
Tooth and Newton (1961)	–	Up to 13 years
Jones and Shanklin (1950)	√	1–2 years
Freeman and Watts (1950)	–	Up to about 3–4 years
Wilson *et al.* (1953)	–	1 and 2 years
Fleming and Baker (1972)	–	Average 7 years (most 3½ years)
Bernstein *et al.* (1975)	√	1–25 years (average 9.7 years)
Tow and Lewin (1953)	√	1½–3 years
Ström-Olsen and Northfield (1955)	√	5 months–3¾ years (average 2½ years)
Knight and Tredgold (1955)	–	Less than 5 years
Sykes and Tredgold (1964)	–	Up to 10 years
McKissock (1951)	–	Less than 4 years
Pippard (1955a)	–	1½–5 years

Table 7.17 Details of follow-up in "mid-period" studies

Study	*Possible to relate length of follow-up to improvement*	*Details of follow-up*
Ström-Olsen and Carlisle (1971)	–	16 months–8 years
Göktepe *et al.* (1975)	–	At least 2½ years follow-up
Whitty *et al.* (1952)	√	½–3 years
Le Beau (1954b)	–	½–5½ years
Tow and Armstrong (1954)	–	–
Sano (1962)	√	Minimum follow-up of 1 month for patients for whom results reported
Brown and Lighthill (1968)	–	1–17 years
Paillas *et al.* (1971)	–	3–16 years
Gaches *et al.* (1972)	–	At least 5 years
Laitinen and Vilkki (1972)	–	Less than 2 years
Mingrino and Schergna (1972)	–	15–32 months (av. 27 months)
Richardson (1972)	–	–
Balasubramaniam *et al.* (1973a)	–	Less than 2 years
Meyer *et al.* (1973)	–	5 months–4½ years
Ballantine *et al.* (1977)	–	8 months–13 years
Martin *et al.* (1977)	–	Minimum 4 years
Bailey *et al.* (1977)	–	Up to 13 years

Table 7.18 Details of follow-up in "second-wave" studies

Study	*Possible to relate length of follow-up to improvement*	*Details of follow-up*
Spiegel *et al.* (1953)	–	½–4½ years
Andy and Jurko (1972)	√	8 months–10 years
Schvarcz *et al.* (1972)	–	6–18 months
Sano *et al.* (1972)	–	2–8 years
Müller *et al.* (1973)	–	–
Balasubramaniam *et al.* (1971)	–	–
Balasubramaniam *et al.* (1973b)	–	–
Dieckmann and Hassler (1975)	–	7 months–4 years
Dieckmann and Hassler (1977)	–	7 months–3 years, 4 months
Schvarcz (1977)	–	1–8 years
Nádvornik *et al.* (1977)	–	Less than 1 year–5 years
Rubio *et al.* (1977)		8 months–5 years
Narabayashi and Uno (1966)	–	3–6½ years
Balasubramaniam *et al.* (1970)	–	–
Vaernet and Madsen (1970)	–	1 month–3 years
Kiloh *et al.* (1974)	√	27 months–nearly 6 years
Mitchell-Heggs *et al.* (1977)	–	mean of 16 months
López Ibor and López-Ibor Aliño (1977)	–	–
Bingley *et al.* (1977)	–	4–55 months (35 mean)
Laitinen and Vilkki (1973a)	–	1–12 months

Board of Control (1947) recommended a similar scheme. Unfortunately, the majority of studies listed in Tables 7.16–7.18 do not provide nearly enough detail to apply such a scheme. In most cases the timing of evaluation varies considerably *within* a study, and the results are summarized without regard to time, making it impossible to plot outcomes reliably at different assessment lags. For example, Ballantine *et al.* (1977) lump together postoperative follow-ups ranging in time from eight months to 13 years.

As with other parameters of outcome, the time course of psychosurgical effects requires careful and controlled investigation. However, many of the psychosurgeons and psychiatrists engaged in assessing outcome seem to proceed on the assumption that the timing and duration of assessment are fairly inconsequential; that once surgery has effected changes in behaviour, then these remain constant over time. While few clear data exist, the observations of Staudt and Zubin (1957) and Zubin (1958) (see Chapter 4) that operatees displayed more variable behavioural profiles than untreated controls over the course of a five-year follow-up strongly suggest that this could be an unwarranted assumption. The scattered comments of other researchers similarly imply that the timing and duration of postoperative evaluation are important considerations. Bridges and Bartlett (1973), for example, insisted that "a final and reliable assessment of the result cannot be made in under 2 years" (p. 858). In the same vein, Ström-Olsen and Northfield (1955) claimed that "Experience has shown that improvement in social adaptation may continue up to two years after discharge" (p. 987). For limbic leucotomy, Kelly (1973) reported that the "reduction of symptoms occurs gradually and full improvement is often not reached until 9 months to 1 year after the operation" (p. 361).

In conclusion, standard and protracted follow-up practices would seem essential. The Board of Control (1947) suggested assessment at six months, one year, two years and five years as suitably comprehensive. While follow-up at five years may seem excessively elaborate given the likely practical difficulties, the possibility of relapse, the vicissitudes of spontaneous remission and the character of non-specific treatment effects (see Chapter 4) make it necessary. Finally, it goes without saying that in any optimally controlled study of psychosurgery, no-treatment and placebo control patients would be subject to the same extensive assessment regime.

Laitinen and Vílkki's accounts of mesoloviotomy well illustrate the case for longer term follow-up. They also indicate the problems that confront any review of the time course of operative effects. A vast amount of careful scrutiny and deduction is required to untangle the precise nature of the outcomes and their permanence. It will be recalled that Laitinen and Vílkki's data for a total of 38 patients receiving mesoloviotomy were classified by us as 58% "much improved" (category I), 21% "improved" (category II) and 21% "no improvement" (category III) (see Table 3.13). In Table 3.17 we placed mesoloviotomy joint fourth in terms of the rank order of psychosurgical procedures with respect to apparent efficacy.

Our classification of outcomes and our subsequent ranking of mesoloviotomy were based on the results presented at the Third International Congress of Psychosurgery in 1972 and reported by Laitinen and Vílkki (1973a). Comparison with two other contemporary reports are of interest here. Laitinen (1972) provided provisional information on the first 12 patients, but no detailed data were given. Laitinen and Vílkki (1973b) offered details of the outcomes for 28 operatees. In a subsequent account (a paper delivered to the Fourth World Congress of Psychiatric Surgery in 1975), Vílkki (1977) presented results for 31 patients examined before and after mesoloviotomy between 1970 and 1973 (Table 7.19).

Table 7.19 Details of the mesoloviotomy studies

Study	*Total no. of operatees*	*Total no. of schizophrenia*	*Total no. of affective psychosis*	*Total no. of neurosis*	*Follow-up*
Laitinen and Vilkki (1973b)	28	18	5	7*	"Follow up months . . . 6–14" (p. 258)
Laitinen and Vilkki (1973a)	38	17	5	10	"The follow-up time ranges from 1–12 months" (p. 78)
Vilkki (1977)	31	20	4	7	"The follow up time ranged from 9 to 40 months after mesoloviotomy" (p. 254)

* Includes what were termed "anxiety neurosis" but not one "obsessive-compulsive neurosis"

While a superficial inspection of these various reports would appear to indicate completely independent samples of operatees and an impressively large overall total, closer examination strongly suggests that the various accounts actually deal with largely the same core sample of patients, selected and evaluated at different postoperative periods, i.e. the majority of the patients included in the most recent were also featured in the earlier analyses. As indicated, the results presented by Laitinen and Vílkki (1973a) revealed a highly efficacious treatment.

However, the subsequent data reported by Vílkki (1977) tell a markedly different story and suggest that the positive effects of mesoloviotomy are decidedly short-lived (Table 7.20). Using "marked improvement" as the measure of clinical success, efficacy drops spectacularly from 82% to 15% for schizophrenia patients and from 58% to 16% for the total patient group (Table 7.21). Eliminating some of the operatees from the earlier report so that the two sets of outcome data reflect the same diagnostic categories, the comparison of early to late analyses is one of 63–16% improvement. These latter data relegate the mesoloviotomy to the lowest ranking for efficacy and, excluding thalamotomy and rostral leucotomy, make it the least indicated for schizophrenia (cf. Tables 3.17 and 7.21). This drastic decline in efficacy, interpreted here as reflecting the fact that mesoloviotomy produces only the most transient and fleeting gains which completely disappear with lengthier follow-up, attracted no particular comment from Vílkki (1977) and occasioned no mention of the earlier data.

Table 7.20 Comparison of the results of the mesoloviotomy studies

	Schizophrenics			*Total*		
Study	*Good*	*Fair*	*Poor*	*Good*	*Fair*	*Poor*
Laitinen and Vílkki (1973b)	84	8	8	64	14	22
	I & II	III	IV V	I & II	III	IV V
Laitinen and Vílkki (1973a)	82	12	6 –	58	21	21 –
Vílkki (1977)	15	45	35 5	16	42	36 6

Table 7.21 Comparison of overall efficacy of mesoloviotomy studies

	Schizophrenia		*Total*	
Study	*Marked improvement I & II*	*Improvement I & II & III*	*Marked improvement I & II*	*Improvement I & II & III*
Laitinen and Vílkki (1973b)	84	92	64	78
Laitinen and Vílkki (1973a)	82	94	58	79
Vílkki (1977)	15	60	16	58

A similar drop in improvement rates at long-term follow-up can be seen with amygdalectomy (Table 7.22). While this decline in outcome could reflect the subsequent inclusion of patients with a generally poorer prognosis in the Heimburger *et al.* (1966, 1978) studies, this would seen unlikely. In any case, Narabayashi's (1979) data are not confounded in this manner and clearly depict a marked decrease in substantive postoperative improvement with time.

Protracted follow-ups are likely to be crucial not only for proper assess-

Table 7.22 Comparison of short- and long-term results of amygdalectomy Percentage of operatees in each improvement category

<table>
<tr><th>Study</th><th>No.</th><th>Worse
4</th><th>No. imp.
3</th><th>Some imp.
2</th><th>Marked imp.
1</th><th>Follow-up</th></tr>
<tr><td>Heimburger et al. (1966)</td><td>25</td><td colspan="2">8</td><td>28</td><td>64</td><td>1–3 yrs.</td></tr>
<tr><td>Heimburger et al. (1978)</td><td>58</td><td>7</td><td>48</td><td colspan="2">45</td><td>1–11 yrs.
(average 6 yrs.)</td></tr>
<tr><td>Narabayashi (1979)</td><td>18</td><td></td><td>22</td><td>17</td><td>61</td><td>"immediate"</td></tr>
<tr><td>Narabayashi (1979)</td><td>18</td><td></td><td>39</td><td>22</td><td>39</td><td>5–17 yrs.</td></tr>
</table>

ment of efficacy but also for adequate determination of adverse sequelae. As indicated in Chapter 5, there appears to be a number of fairly immediate postoperative side effects that are largely transient in nature. This suggests that very short-term follow-ups may give rise to an unjustly unfavourable picture of psychosurgery. However, the incidence of some of the more drastic side effects may, in some instances, increase rather than decrease with time. As might be suspected from our earlier discussion of the time course of psychosurgical effects, it is not easy to decipher the temporal characteristics of adverse sequelae.

With regard to mortality, for example, it is difficult to determine whether a postoperative death, especially one occurring some time after surgery, was actually a direct consequence of surgery. One approach to this problem has been to compare the overall mortality rate of operatees with that found in similar, but untreated, patients. Thus, Robin (1958a) reported that there were no differences in death rates between operatees and untreated control patients. On the other hand, Staudt and Zubin (1967), comparing various somatotherapies (including psychosurgery), noted that, while the various treatment groups were not significantly different from the untreated control group in terms of clinical improvement, in general treatment was associated with a lower overall death rate. However, no specific case was presented for psychosurgery in this regard.

If one of the aims of psychosurgery is to "normalize" its clientele, then operatee mortality should be checked against comparable (age, sex, social class, etc.) non-psychiatric populations. Many psychiatric conditions are associated with higher death rates than occur in the general community (cf. Tsuang and Woolson, 1978). Higher rates of suicide have been held to account for much of this difference (Achté, 1973; Pokorny, 1964; Sims, 1973). In fact, risk of suicide has been frequently cited to justify psychosurgical intervention. It is now clear, though, that higher suicide rates cannot account for all the additional mortality associated with psychiatric patients (Tsuang and Woolson, 1978).

Similar problems attend postoperative estimates of epileptic seizure rate. Our previous analysis (see Chapter 5) indicated a higher incidence of convulsive seizures immediately after surgery relative to that apparent at later follow-up. However, there is evidence that in some patients seizure onset lags surgery by a considerable period of time and therefore studies that follow up patients for only a couple of years or so run the risk of underestimating the incidence of convulsive seizures by as much as one half (Logothetis, 1976; Paul *et al.*, 1956). Longer follow-ups are again indicated. In addition, the problems of attributing causality, mentioned earlier, commend an assessment of postoperative seizures that contrasts the overall rates for operatees with the rates apparent in appropriate patients and non-patient control groups (and with the preoperative incidence). Similarly, Smith (1964), reporting on a sample of leucotomized patients, indicated that intellectual impairment became apparent only a decade or so after surgery. The true incidence of adverse sequelae may only be evident with an extended follow-up of many years duration and in comparison with appropriate control subjects.

The next set of tables (Tables 7.23–7.25) is concerned with data handling. With regard to the data treatment, very few studies have employed formal and systematic methods of analysis. Some rely solely on a very casual description of individual cases.

Moore's (1952) attitude would appear to be fairly widely shared:

> Statistics are notoriously dull and unreliable, and to try and enliven this communication, I propose to give a brief thumb-nail sketch of a few patients from each group, and give the replies to my follow-up letter. (p. 121)

Unfortunately, this approach does not permit an adequate comparison between studies or even among cases within the same report.

The most common method of data report is, in fact, the summary table (Tables 7.23–7.25). This is the format that we ourselves adopted in Chapter 3 (see Tables 3.1–3.13). Typically, such tables list the different categories of improvement horizontally, the different diagnostic divisions vertically and display patient numbers or percentages with regard to diagnosis and outcome. This method readily enables comparison of outcome for different diagnostic groups. Further, it allows for comparison to be made between studies. In some reports, however, only outcome totals are given and no evaluation with regard to diagnosis is possible. In some other instances, the data have not been displayed in tabular or summary form but sufficient detail is provided to enable determination of clinical efficacy either for the various psychiatric conditions or for the total group. Reports of this sort have been indicated by a query (?) in the appropriate columns ("Diagnosis" and "Group").

However, while tabular presentation of data may intimate clinical improvement and/or differences in efficacy between diagnostic groups, it does not by itself allow unequivocal pronouncements. The improvement rates observed and the differences recorded for different psychiatric conditions may simply reflect chance variation. To arbitrate between real and chance variations, appropriate statistical analyses have to be undertaken. Unfortunately, very

Table 7.23 Treatment of outcome data in "first-wave" studies

Study	*By case reports*	*By individual tables*	*By diagnosis*	*By group*	*Statistics used*	*Statistical significance*	*Clinical significance*	*"Drop-outs"*	*Reasons*	*Inconsistencies/errors*
Rao and Govindaswamy (1944)	?[1]	√	?[2]	?[2]	–	–	–	–	–	–
Board of Control (1947)	?[1]	–	√	√	–	–	–	√	√[3]	–
Freeman and Watts (1950)	?[1]	–	√	√	–	–	–	√	√[4]	–
Hohman *et al.* (1951)	?[1]	–	√	√	–	–	–	√	√[5]	–
Moore (1952)	–	–	–	–	–	–	–	√	√[6]	–
Tooth and Newton (1961)	–	–	?[2]	√	–	–	–	√	√[7]	–
Jones and Shanklin (1950)	–	√	?[2]	?[2]	–	–	–	√	√[8]	–
Freeman and Watts (1950)	?[1]	–	√	√	–	–	–	√	√[9]	–
Wilson *et al.* (1953)	?[10]	–	√	√	–	–	–	–	–	–
Fleming and Baker (1962)	–	–	?[2]	√	–	–	–	√	√[11]	–
Bernstein *et al.* (1975)	?[1]	√	√	√	–	–	–	–	–	–
Tow and Lewin (1953)	?[1]	√	?[2]	√	–	–	–	√	√[12]	–
Ström-Olsen and Northfield (1955)	?[1]	√	?[2]	?[2]	–	–	–	–	–	–
Knight and Tredgold (1955)	?[1]	–	√	√	–	–	–	√	√[13]	–
Sykes and Tredgold (1964)	–	–	√	√	–	–	–	√	√[14]	√
McKissock (1951)	–	–	–	√	–	–	–	–	–	–
Pippard (1955a)	?[1]	–	√	?[2]	–	–	–	√	√[15]	–

[1] Only some case reports given
[2] Not actually given but can be derived from the data supplied in another form
[3] 3 institutions sent returns in too late and 1 did not send in a return
[4] 623 → 569 (excludes pain patients and operative deaths)
[5] 367 → 254 (30 pain patients excluded)
[6] 71 → 70 (1 patient untraced)
[7] 11 127 → 10 365 (300 forms incomplete or inconsistent and 462 more than 1 operation)
[8] 74 → 52 (less than 1 year follow-up excluded)
[9] 400 → 262 (pain patients and operative deaths excluded)
[10] Only 1 case report given
[11] 70 → 42 (2 lost to follow-up and 28 it was too short)
[12] 21 → 20 (1 had previous leucotomy)
[13] 59 → 52 (4 did not reply, 3 previous operation)
[14] 350 → 207 (others not fully assessed)
[15] 240 → 223 (4 case notes destroyed and 13 died)

Table 7.24 Treatment of outcome data in "mid-period" studies

Study	*By case reports*	*By individual tables*	*By diagnosis*	*By group*	*Statistics used*	*Statistical significance*	*Clinical significance*	*"Drop-outs"*	*Reasons*	*Inconsistencies/errors*
Ström-Olsen and Carlisle (1971)	–	–	√	√	–	–	–	√	√[1]	–
Göktepe *et al.* (1975)	–	–	√	√	–	–	–	√	√[2]	–
Whitty *et al.* (1952)	?[3]	√	?	?	–	–	–	√	√[4]	–
Le Beau (1954b)	–	–	√	?[5]	–	–	–	√	√[6]	–
Tow and Armstrong (1954)	√	–	?[5]	?[5]	–	–	–	–	–	–
Sano (1962)	–	√	?[5]	?[5]	–	–	–	–	–	–
Brown and Lighthill (1968)	?[3]	–	–	√	–	–	–	–	–	–
Paillas *et al.* (1971)	?[3]	–	√[1]	√[1]	–	–	–	√	√[8]	–
Gaches *et al.* (1972)	–	–	√[8]	√[8]	–	–	–	√	√[9]	–
Laitinen and Vilkki (1972)	–	–	√	√	–	–	–	–	–	–
Mingrino and Schergna (1972)	–	–	√[10]	√[10]	–	–	–	–	–	–
Richardson (1972)	?[3]	–	–	√	–	–	–	–	–	–
Balasubramaniam *et al.* (1973a)	–	–	√	√	–	–	–	–	–	–
Meyer *et al.* (1973)	–	–	√	√	–	–	–	√	√[11]	–
Ballantine *et al.* (1977)	–	–	√	√	–	–	–	√	√[12]	–
Martin *et al.* (1977)	–	–	√	√	–	–	–	√	√[13]	–
Bailey *et al.* (1977)	–	√	√	√	–	–	–	–	–	–

[1] 210 → 150 (29 not contacted, 2 not traced, 29 died)
[2] 208 → 134 (next series to above; 25 died, 49 incompletely assessed or not interviewed)
[3] Only some case reports given
[4] 29 → 24 (others excluded due to follow-up of less than 1½ years)
[5] Not actually given but can be derived from the data supplied in another form
[6] 50 → 30 (14 epileptics and 2 children died, other 4 patients no clear reason given)
[7] (Selected according to diagnosis)
[8] All diagnosed as obsessional
[9] 351 → 20 (selected according to diagnosis)
[10] All diagnosed as aggressive
[11] 75 → 68 (7 had too short follow-up)
[12] 238 → 149 (34 pain patients and 15 deaths excluded, no reason given for other 40)
[13] 68 → 67 (1 pain patient excluded)

Table 7.25 Treatment of outcome data in "second-wave" studies

Study	*By case reports*	*By individual tables*	*By diagnosis*	*By group*	*Statistics used*	*Statistical significance*	*Clinical significance*	*"Drop-outs"*	*Reasons*	*Inconsistencies/errors*
Spiegel *et al.* (1953)	–	–	√	√	–	–	–	√	√[1]	–
Andy and Jurko (1972)	–	√	?[2]	?[2]	–	–	–	–	–	–
Schvarcz *et al.* (1972)	?[3]	–	√[4]	√[4]	–	–	–	–	–	–
Sano *et al.* (1972)	–	–	√[4]	√[4]	–	–	–	√	√[5]	–
Müller *et al.* (1973)	–	√	√[2]	√[2]	–	–	–	–	–	–
Balasubramaniam *et al.* (1971)	–	–	√[4]	√[4]	–	–	–	–	–	–
Balasubramaniam *et al.* (1973b)	–	–	√[4]	√[4]	–	–	–	–	–	–
Dieckmann and Hassler (1975)	–	√	√[4]	√[4]	–	–	–	–	–	–
Dieckmann and Hassler (1977)	√	√	√[4]	√[4]	–	–	–	–	–	–
Schvarcz (1977)	?[3]	–	√[4]	√[4]	–	–	–	–	–	–
Nádvornik *et al.* (1977)	–	√	√[4]	√[4]	–	–	–	–	–	–
Rubio *et al.* (1977)	–	–	√[4]	√[4]	–	–	–	√	√[6]	–
Narabayashi and Uno (1966)	–	–	√[4]	√[4]	–	–	–	√	√[7]	–
Balasubramaniam *et al.* (1970)	–	–	√[4]	√[4]	–	–	–	–	–	–
Vaernet and Madsen (1970)	–	√	√[4]	√[4]	–	–	–	–	–	–
Kiloh *et al.* (1974)	–	√	√[4]	√[4]	–	–	–	–	–	–
Mitchell-Heggs *et al.* (1977)	–	–	√	√	–	–	–	√	√[8]	–
López Ibor and López-Ibor Aliño (1977)	–	–	√[4]	√[4]	–	–	–	–	–	–
Bingley *et al.* (1977)	–	–	√[4]	√[4]	–	–	–	–	–	–
Laitinen and Vilkki (1973a)	–	–	√	√	–	–	–	–	–	–

[1] 65 → 51 (2 operative deaths excluded and first-time operatees due to too small a lesion)
[2] Not actually given but can be derived from the data supplied in another form
[3] Only some case reports given
[4] All receiving a similar diagnosis
[5] 53 → 43 (others excluded due to too short follow-up)
[6] 31 → 24 (others excluded due to too short follow-up)
[7] 98 → 40 (20 excluded due to returns considered unreliable; the 40 here were in the first in the series)
[8] 120 → 66 (first 66 patients)

few studies have bothered (Tables 7.23–7.25). Accounts of statistical significance may be "dull," but they are necessary and far from "unreliable" when they reflect the appropriate application of statistical tools.

In considering the matter of statistics, it is important to distinguish between statistical significance and clinical significance; the latter is not an inevitable consequence of the former. Thus, a study may demonstrate that a particular treatment has an apparent ameliorative effect on one group of patients but not on another. The application of statistics may confirm that the results obtained are not easily attributable to chance variation and that the differential effect of treatment is real; thus, the difference in efficacy is statistically significant. However, the effect may not be clinically significant, i.e. the effect, although statistically reliable, may be slight in absolute terms, a matter of one point or less on a 10-point rating of improvement. Clearly, clinical significance is a complex matter and must be demonstrated in addition to statistical significance before unqualified assurances of relative efficacy can be accepted.

Finally, in this context, it is worth mentioning that assertions of statistical improbability have been applied to the distribution of favourable and unfavourable published reports dealing with psychosurgery. Proponents of psychosurgery often point to the greater number of favourable reports (i.e. those claiming clinical improvement following surgery) as evidence of efficacy. However, an index of this sort embodies a range of assumptions, many of them unjustified. For example, it assumes that there are no systematic biases operating either in what is submitted or what is accepted for publication. Several authorities have argued otherwise (e.g. Bakan, 1969; Lykken, 1968).

Tables 7.23–7.25 list data anomalies. Some of these can be discerned from Tables 3.1–3.13. Occasionally, the total number of operatees exceeds the number subsequently evaluated and/or reported on. In the present tables, discrepancies of this sort are graced by the term "drop-outs". In some cases, reasons have been provided for the shortfall, in others this is not so. Either way, one is invited to assume that the results of truncated groups are representative of the total pool of operatees.

If the "drop-out" rate is low and there are no grounds for suspecting bias, then this would seem a reasonable assumption. However, in some instances, particularly where extended follow-ups have been attempted, the "drop-out" rate is noticeably high. As time elapses, many patients are simply not able to be easily contacted. It is frequently presumed that such unavailability intimates recovery, i.e. that these "lost" operatees are unavailable because they no longer require assistance (Tooth and Newton, 1961). Tow and Lewin, who managed at follow-up to locate only just over a third of a total of 4768 discharges, concluded:

> By using the gradings of this follow-up group as the basis for estimating the condition of all discharged patients, it is thus likely that the

> proportion of those in less favourable grades has been over-represented. (p. 121)

Gaches *et al.* (1972) presented some anecdotal support for the assumption that unavailable discharges have fared better than those available for assessment. They had lost contact with 31 patients but subsequently re-encountered three of them:

> One of them said, "For ten years I never had to see a doctor." Another said, "It was ungrateful of us, but I was alright and we did not wish to disturb you." The third one said, "We left to live in the country, I have a lot of work to do at home, so I could not undertake a journey to Paris." (pp. 236–237).

In contrast, according to Gaches *et al.*, bad news travelled more quickly:

> On the other hand, we usually heard about our unsuccessful results. When patients were re-admitted elsewhere we were generally notified of this by physicians, most of whom were opposed to our methods, who sought information concerning the patients' previous history. Our statistics are, therefore, pessimistic rather than optimistic. (p. 236)

However, the results of some psychosurgeons cast doubt on the presumption that unavailability always means success. Sykes and Tredgold (1964), for example, were able to evaluate fully only 177 (Group A) out of a series of 320 operatees (Series A):

> A study of all cases in Series A (320) suggested that the findings on Group A (177) had a slight halo effect, since some of the reasons which prevented patients coming for interview indicated less satisfactory progress. Among these were the deaths (which were attributed to the operation) of 5 patients (1.5 per cent); 3 others had later committed suicide. (p. 360)

Ström-Olsen and Carlisle's (1971) data also imply that the unavailable discharges fare worse than those present for assessment. In the main contactable group, 73 out of 150 (almost 50%) achieved the rating of I and II, compared with 10 out of 29 (only just over 33% for the "lost" operatees. Similarly, Göktepe *et al.* (1975) reported that of the 23 operatees who declined to co-operate in their study "there was evidence from their letters that 8 had shown improvement, and 8 were unchanged, while 7 did not mention their progress" (p. 271). For the 134 that did co-operate in the follow-up, Göktepe *et al.* reported that only 17% failed to show improvement.

The reasons given for failure to include assessments for all patients vary (cf. Tables 7.23–7.25) and in most cases help us a little in identifying the extent and direction of possible bias. Lacking the necessary information, we can but occasionally suspect the subtle intrusion of bias, as in the case of Narabayashi and Uno's (1966) meagre account of how 20 of their operatees were excluded on the basis of replies to an "inquiry card".

> The cases, the family of which sent no answer at all and the cases, answers about which by the family were considered rather unreliable, were excluded from the study; the total number of cases excluded were 20. (p. 168)

This study brings us to the next area of interest regarding data handling, i.e. appearance of unexplained inconsistencies in the data (Tables 7.23–7.25). Narabayashi and Uno, for example, indicated that the total number of amygdalotomized cases "is 98 as May 1, 1965" (p. 168). From this total, 20 operatees were excluded (see above). However, they then revealed that "this paper is based on the observations in 40 cases" (p. 168). No account is given of the apparently 38 residual patients, and no reasons are supplied for the numerical inconsistency. While Narabayashi and Uno seem prone to subtraction, Sykes and Tredgold (1964) have difficulty with addition. Their table of patients unaccountably includes six patients more (two under "Anxiety" and four under "Involutional depression") than their total number of operatees.

The last set of tables in this series (Tables 7.26–7.28) deals with experimental design. As can be seen from these tables, most of the studies listed are "prospective"; very few are "retrospective". Feinstein (1973), however, has argued that the labels "prospective" and "retrospective", as generally applied, confuse approaches to the "collection of data" with the "direction of populational pursuit". Accordingly, he has coined two new terms, "prolective" and "retrolective", to clarify matters. "Prolective" (formerly prospective) denotes, according to Feinstein, that method of data collection whereby:

> the investigator makes special plans before hand for the techniques with which each person is to be examined and the data collected. (p. 292)

"Retrolective" (retrospective), on the other hand, describes the approach whereby:

> the person under study was originally observed by people who were not performing a specific investigation, and who reported the observation in routine records. Afterwards, to get the research data, the investigator extracts the information available in these records. (p. 292)

As might be surmised, there are a number of obstacles to comparing data derived from these two sorts of study. Prolective studies are generally to be preferred. Here measures, preselected in terms of their likely relevance, can be taken both before and after treatment; adequate baselines can be recorded and systematic follow-up assessments structured. Retrolective studies are usually much more haphazard affairs. The absence of *a priori* knowledge almost always ensures this; gaps and shortcomings in the data are inevitably more likely.

While very few of the studies listed appear retrolective at first glance, closer

Table 7.26 Design features of "first-wave" studies

Study	*Prospective*	*Retrospective*	*Single blind*	*Double blind*	*No-treatment control*	*Placebo control*	*Other treatment control*	*Within-subject control*
Rao and Govindaswamy (1944)	√	–	–	–	–	–	–	–
Board of Control (1947)	–	√	–	–	–	–	–	–
Freeman and Watts (1950)	√	–	–	–	–	–	–	–
Hohman *et al.* (1951)	√	–	–	–	–	–	–	–
Moore (1952)	√	–	–	–	–	–	–	–
Tooth and Newton (1961)	–	√	–	–	–	–	–	–
Jones and Shanklin (1950)	√	–	–	–	–	–	–	–
Freeman and Watts (1950)	√	–	–	–	–	–	–	–
Wilson *et al.* (1953)	√	–	–	–	–	–	–	–
Fleming and Baker (1972)	?[1]	?[1]	–	–	–	–	–	–
Bernstein *et al.* (1975)	?[1]	?[1]	–	–	–	–	–	–
Tow and Lewin (1953)	√	–	–	–	–	–	–	–
Ström-Olsen and Northfield (1955)	√	–	–	–	–	–	–	–
Knight and Tredgold (1955)	√	–	–	–	–		–	–
Sykes and Tredgold (1964)	√	–	–	–	–		–	–
McKissock (1951)	√	–	–					
Pippard (1955a)	–	√	–		–			–

[1] To some extent both prospective and retrospective

Table 7.27 Design features of "mid-period" studies

Study	*Prospective*	*Retrospective*	*Single blind*	*Double blind*	*No-treatment control*	*Placebo control*	*Other treatment control*	*Within-subject control*
Ström-Olsen and Carlisle (1971)	√	–	–	–	–	–	–	–
Göktepe *et al.* (1975)	√	–	–	–	–	–	–	–
Whitty *et al.* (1952)	√	–	–	–	–	–	–	–
Le Beau (1954b)	√	–	–	–	–	–	–	–
Tow and Armstrong (1954)	√	–	–	–	–	–	–	–
Sano (1962)	√	–	–	–	–	–	–	–
Brown and Lighthill (1968)	√	–	–	–	–	–	–	–
Paillas *et al.* (1971)	√	–	–	–	–	–	–	–
Gaches *et al.* (1972)	√	–	–	–	–	–	–	–
Laitinen and Vilkki (1972)	√	–	–	–	–	–	–	–
Mingrino and Schergna (1972)	√	–	–	–	–	–	–	–
Richardson (1972)	√	–	–	–	–	–	–	–
Balasubramaniam *et al.* (1973a)	√	–	–	–	–	–	–	–
Meyer *et al.* (1973)	√	–	–	–	–	–	–	–
Ballantine *et al.* (1977)	√	–	–	–	–	–	–	–
Martin *et al.* (1977)	√	–	–	–	–	–	–	–
Bailey *et al.* (1977)	√	–	–	–	–	–	–	–

Table 7.28 Design features of "second-wave" studies

Study	*Prospective*	*Retrospective*	*Single blind*	*Double blind*	*No-treatment control*	*Placebo control*	*Other treatment control*	*Within-subject control*
Spiegel *et al.* (1953)	√	–	–	–	–	–	–	–
Andy and Jurko (1972)	√	–	–	–	–	–	–	–
Schvarcz *et al.* (1972)	√	–	–	–	–	–	–	–
Sano *et al.* (1972)	√	–	–	–	–	–	–	–
Müller *et al.* (1973)	√	–	–	–	–	–	–	–
Balasubramaniam *et al.* (1971)	√	–	–	–	–	–	–	–
Balasubramaniam *et al.* (1973b)	√	–	–	–	–	–	–	–
Dieckmann and Hassler (1975)	√	–	–	–	–	–	–	–
Dieckmann and Hassler (1977)	√	–	–	–	–	–	–	–
Schvarcz (1977)	√	–	–	–	–	–	–	–
Nádvornik *et al.* (1977)	√	–	–	–	–	–	–	–
Rubio *et al.* (1977)	√	–	–	–	–	–	–	–
Narabayashi and Uno (1966)	√	–	–	–	–	–	–	–
Balasubramaniam *et al.* (1970)	√	–	–	–	–	–	–	–
Vaernet and Madsen (1970)	√	–	–	–	–	–	–	–
Kiloh *et al.* (1974)	√	–	–	–	–	–	–	–
Mitchell-Heggs *et al.* (1977)	√	–	–	–	–	–	–	–
López Ibor and López-Ibor Aliño (1977)	√	–	–	–	–	–	–	–
Bingley *et al.* (1977)	√	–	–	–	–	–	–	–
Laitinen and Vilkki (1973a)	√	–	–	–	–	–	–	–

inspection indicates that a number of non-retrolective enterprises fall short of true prolective status. For example, planning at the pretreatment stage seems to have been fairly rudimentary in several studies and was clearly completed only after surgery had been carried out. In such circumstances, part of the subsequent analysis was prolective but part was necessarily retrolective. The study of Bernstein *et al.* (1975) provides an example of this sort of approach. It is fairly apparent that the character of this study was not fully forged until the start of follow-up assessments some time after 1970. Follow-up outcomes were retrolectively compared to earlier observations: in one case, the data had been collected some 25 years previously. Further, in some instances, no comparative information is presented regarding preoperative condition; the report merely lists operatees' presurgical diagnoses. Studies of this sort are clearly not optimally prolective.

As indicated, bias is always a potential intruder in treatment evaluation. Both prolective and retrolective research are susceptible. Although the data in retrolective studies may have been provided by persons wholly unconnected with the final study, the form of that data may require extensive subsequent sifting, interpreting and summarizing into the desired format for analysis and report. While bias is invariably more of a potential problem in uncontrolled case studies, the addition of a control group is by itself an insufficient provision in this context; blind evaluation is essential. In single blind arrangements the evaluator(s) should be unaware of the treatment contingencies, i.e. who has or has not received treatment. This reduces the risk of bias; it does not, however, totally eliminate the possibility. In retrolective studies, for example, certain details in a patient's notes may hint at treatment status. Complete innocence may not always be realizable in practice. In prolective studies it is even more difficult to sustain experimenter ignorance when surgery is the treatment involved, and an unwitting "spotting" of operated subjects may occur.

Even if experimenter innocence is presumed here, unconscious contamination of results can still occur by awarding fairly invariant ratings across subjects. Thus a researcher sympathetic to psychosurgery may unwittingly "level" adverse sequelae ratings, while an unsympathetic experimenter might operate this "levelling" for ratings of clinical improvement. The ideal control for bias is generally considered to be the double-blind procedure. Here, both patient and evaluator are kept ignorant (or even misled) about whether treatment has or has not been carried out. Aside from the necessary issues of morality involved in inflicting treatment on unsuspecting patients or in withholding treatment where it is expected, and the problems of "spotting" and "levelling" mentioned above, it is extremely doubtful whether in practice patients' naiveté in psychosurgical studies could be sustained. Even a superficial perusal indicates that many psychosurgical studies to date have not taken the elementary precaution of single-blind assessment; there are, as one would expect, no convincing double-blind control studies.

The next three columns in Tables 7.26–7.28 deal with the type of experimental control used in studies: "no-treatment control", a "placebo control" and "other treatment control". In practice, "no-treatment control" subsumes a number of different conditions. First of all, there is what may be termed "no-involvement control"; here, a number of patients are merely subjected to a single assessment and their results compared to the experimental or treatment group. There is also the "assessment control", in which patients are assessed and then reassessed some time later to check the variations arising from assessment.

Next comes the "rejection control", in which the subjects that comprise the control group have for some reason or other been considered unsuited for psychosurgical treatment. As has been discussed in Chapter 4, the results of control studies can be biased either for or against psychosurgery, depending on the criteria employed for allocating subjects to groups. In some cases, however, as has been previously noted, the patient (or his/her family acting as guardian) refuses to undergo surgery; this "refusal" group may sometimes comprise patients whose families are not supportive and as such intimates a poor prognosis; the converse may also be the case. "Waiting-list control" presumes to comprise subjects suitable for psychosurgery who would consent to treatment. The researcher simply informs some of the subjects that they are to be put on a waiting list with a view to later treatment. The subjects are reassessed at some later stage and the results of the two assessments compared to the pre- and postoperative data of the operatees. The effect of being put on a "waiting list" may bias the results in either direction with regard to psychosurgery. For some individuals their second assessment may be artificially depressed through disappointment at not receiving the recommended treatment. For others, the renewed hope of finally receiving treatment may elevate this second evaluation. It must be noted that all the above groups might be generally denoted as "routine-treatment control" groups, since they usually continue to attract whatever non-surgical treatments (psychotherapy, chemotherapy, ECT or combinations of these, etc.) have been prescribed.

The next column in Tables 7.26–7.28 deals with "placebo control", which presumes to control for all possible variables other than the designated therapeutic one, i.e. the surgical interruption or destruction of tissue in a given region of the brain. Critics of psychosurgery have contended that some of these extraneous variables, in particular the positive expectations of the operatee, may well account for much if not all of any therapeutic benefit derived from the psychosurgical treatment complex. However, Brown and Lighthill (1968) rejected such contentions, offering two pieces of evidence in support.

First of all, they indicated that in some circumstances, patients have "needed" a second operation. If psychosurgery was pure placebo, they argued, then subjects should invariably improve after the first operation and should not need a second. They claimed that it was "only" after reoperation in seven of their 110 cases that benefit was noted. However, the intricacies and vagaries of placebo effects are still ill-understood. Nevertheless, it is clear that not everyone is equally susceptible to suggestion; some may require the additional persuasion of a second procedure (see Bartlett and Bridges, 1977, comments cited earlier).

Further, as indicated in the previous chapter when discussing postmortem data, recovery of improvement has been reported in some cases where post-mortem subsequently revealed an imperfect or erroneously sited lesion.

Brown and Lighthill offered a second and, in their opinion, a more telling piece of evidence: the research carried out by Livingston in 1953. Livingston's study has been widely cited as affording conclusive proof that psychosurgery has specific therapeutic effects and is not just an elaborate placebo.

> In 4 separate cases in this series we carried out a control procedure in which the skin incision is made and the bone button removed but no cerebral lesion produced. Each of these patients was included in a group of four operated on at one time, three of whom had a standard anterior cingulate isolation. The four patients were carried as a group through the entire post-operative routine without knowledge on the part of the patients or other hospital personnel that these control patients had not been subjected to the complete surgical procedure. None of these patients showed even slight improvement during their period of control study and all were subjected to cingulate isolation one to three months later. This group serves to some extent as a control for factors other than the surgical lesion itself. (p. 377)

However, several points need to be made. First, the number of placebo control subjects was exceedingly small; only four patients were exposed to the sham procedure. Second, we are provided with very little information on the preoperative status of these control patients. Both of these limitations conspire to mitigate direct and formal statistical comparison between the control and the experimental subjects. Without the confidence afforded by statistical confirmation of a difference, the suspicion of chance variation must remain. Third, we are offered little in the way of detail regarding criteria for group allocation. We need to be convinced that the control subjects did not differ in any substantial way from their experimental counterparts. Fourth, only three months had elapsed before these patients underwent a complete anterior cingulectomy. While we appreciate the ethical dilemma facing Livingston, many would argue that three months is an unsufficient period for proper evaluation (cf. earlier discussion). Finally, Livingston's role (either direct or indirect) in assessment has to be made explicit. While others may have been in the dark, Livingston would appear to have been clearly cognizant of the experimental contingencies and was presumably instrumental in the decision to reoperate.

More recently, Teuber *et al.* (1977) reported a placebo control subject, who received burr holes for a cingulectomy but no cingulectomy was performed. While this placebo patient was operated on for chronic pain, the reported finding of relief may have a general significance.

It should be conceded, however, that it is particularly difficult to determine whether or to what extent psychosurgical operations elicit a "placebo effect" in the absence of properly conducted controlled trials. There is certainly evidence of "placebo effects" in other forms of surgery. In the context of more general surgery, Rawlings (1972/1973) surveyed 235 women whose symptoms he considered primarily attributable to psychological factors. Altogether, some 453 operations had been performed on these women, and of those for whom operation notes were available, no disease could be demonstrated. Yet three-quarters of the patients considered their operations to have been a success. Beecher (1961, 1962) has also investigated the placebo effect in a variety of surgical procedures. His own studies as well as his review of those of others led him to identify factors other than the expectations of the patients as being important in the production of the placebo response. One important characteristic was the enthusiasm of the *surgeon* for the procedure. This is in line with the evidence from other forms of therapy addressed at psychiatric "disorders" (e.g. Shapiro, 1971; Tuma *et al.*, 1978). A whole host of non-specific factors have been identified to contribute to therapeutic improvement, either individually or in combination (Blanchard and Young, 1973; Davison and Neale, 1974; Frank, 1961; Shapiro, 1971).

One of these non-specific factors in psychosurgery may well be the actual opening of the skull itself. It should be recalled that trepanning has in the past been used as a treatment in its own right (see Chapter 1). Fielding (1978), advocating that trepanning should become freely available on demand from the British National Health Service, attributed its supposed beneficial effects to an increase in blood brain volume, by virtue of which "brain metabolism is restored to its youthful level" (p. 19).

At the psychological rather than the physiological level, it is possible that the increased attention accorded psychosurgery patients (especially those from more chronic wards) is responsible for some of the apparent improvement noted. It should be recounted that many psychosurgery programmes have specifically involved a long and intensive period of postoperative care, attention and rehabilitation as part of the overall therapeutic package.

Even at the height of the first wave of psychosurgery, many stressed the importance of rehabilitation programmes for positive results (cf. Burlingame, 1949; McKissock, 1951; Moore, 1952; Whitman, 1948). In some cases the operatees were transferred from the psychosurgical unit to the referring hospital for rehabilitation (cf. Bridges and Bartlett, 1973; Göktepe *et al.*, 1975; McKissock, 1951). Some have even urged that for maximal and sustained improvement the patient's relatives, friends and general environmental circumstances should be sensitized to the patient's rehabilitation needs (cf.

previous discussion concerning Tables 7.10–7.12, and also Laitinen and Vilkki, 1973a; Moore, 1952; Pippard, 1955a).

If, as has been suggested, environmental engineering is an important part of the psychosurgery treatment complex, possibly accounting for much of any sustained improvement, then it would seem reasonable to ask whether environmental manipulation by itself would be beneficial. Unfortunately, few studies have set out to compare directly psychosurgery with other, particularly environmentally based, methods of intervention (Tables 7.26–7.28). While it has often been claimed that all conventional treatments have been tried before a candidate was considered for surgery, the accuracy of such assertions has been challenged (cf. Valenstein, 1973a) and in any case, casual pronouncements about previous treatments do not afford a reasonable comparison between psychosurgery and alternative therapies. There are reasons for suspecting that a therapy carried out in the context of a formal study may be somewhat more effective than one administered routinely.

With regard to formal studies comparing psychosurgery with other therapies, Scherer and Trehub (1957), in a retrospective study, compared the efficacy of prefrontal leucotomy with other physical methods of treatment (insulin therapy, electroconvulsive therapy and chemotherapy) in the treatment of both acute and chronic schizophrenics. Psychosurgery did not appear to produce greater improvement than the other therapies for either acute or chronic cases (cf. Staudt and Zubin, 1957).

However, there are many other therapeutic alternatives to physical methods of treatment. Under the umbrella terms of "behaviour therapy" and "psychotherapy" exists a whole range of different procedures for a variety of disorders. Most, if not all, of the conditions that have attracted psychosurgery have been reported to have yielded successfully to these behavioural procedures. Thus, those "disorders" listed in Table 3.17 – sexual "deviation", obsessional neurosis, manic-depression, depression, anxiety/tension, aggression/hyperkinesis ("behaviour disorder") and schizophrenia – have all been subject to a variety of behaviour therapies, for example, with reported benefit (the references for behaviour therapy, and psychotherapy, are legion; the reader is therefore directed to journals such as *Behaviour Research and Therapy*, *Behavior Therapy*, *Journal of Applied Behavioral Analysis*, *Journal of Behavior Therapy and Experimental Psychiatry*, and *Journal of Consulting and Clinical Psychology*, as well as to reviews of the field as in Craighead *et al.*, 1976; Davison and Neale, 1974; Feldman and Broadhurst, 1978; Ullman and Krasner, 1975). Even some of the symptoms regarded as resistant to surgery have apparently been regarded as particularly intractable (it was the possibility of surgically excising hallucinations that prompted Burkhardt's unsuccessful initiative). However, recent evidence suggests that even hallucinations may respond to behavioural treatment (see Green *et al.*, 1979; Marzillier and Birchwood, 1980). It has, however, been claimed that in particularly difficult cases, psychosurgery in combination with such techniques can yield highly beneficial results. Haaijman *et al.* (1977) for example, combined serial coagulations with behaviour modification for five patients suffering from severe obsessive–compulsive neurosis. Surgery is undertaken to alleviate the patient's adverse emotional state, supposedly rendering him/her more amenable to further behavioural treatment (cf. Bridges and Bartlett, 1973; Laitinen and Vílkki, 1972; Mingrino and Schergna, 1972). Even in patients diagnosed as schizophrenic, Sykes and Tredgold (1964) suggested that surgically produced tension-reduction occasioned greater amenability to subsequent therapy with beneficial results.

At a more general level, a decrease in emotional tension has been frequently cited as the most visible benefit of psychosurgery (see Board of Control, 1947; Freeman and Watts, 1950). However, opponents of psychosurgery have interpreted this "beneficial" reduction in emotional tension somewhat differently, and indeed it is frequently a matter of value judgement whether a result is accorded the status of tension reduction or emotional blunting. With regard to the charge of emotional blunting, Sykes and Tredgold (1964) conceded:

> There is some blunting of emotional tone, and some reduction of standards, which is beneficial if they were previously abnormally high. (p. 639).

Later these authors elaborated:

> In this sense their "standards were reduced," but this was a return to normal from excessively scrupulous standards, not a lowering beneath that approved by society. (pp. 613–614)

With regard to this reduction in standards, and its evaluation as a positive characteristic, there seems to be a fair amount of consensus (Bailey *et al.*, 1977; Brown and Lighthill, 1968; Moore, 1952; Richardson, 1972). The cynic, however, can but harbour the suspicion that surgeons regard the social standards appropriate for patients as substantially different from those that pervade the social world of physicians and their ilk. The following admission by Balasubramaniam *et al.* (1971) illustrates the cynic's case:

> In assessing the usefulness of an operation like hypothalamotomy what should be taken into consideration is the manageability of the patient. Whereas previously the patient had to be tied to a post or kept in a cell, post operatively even a small relief is welcome. (p. 230)

Balasubramaniam and his associates are not alone in emphasizing manageability as a prime benefit of psychosurgery. It has been frequently delineated as a criterion for pronouncing success (cf. Board of Control, 1947; Hohman *et al.*, 1951; Moore, 1952).

The application of contentious social criteria of operative success, such as manageability, is exemplified by a case described by Freeman and Watts (1950). The patient was "a negress of gigantic proportions who, for years, was confined to a strong room at St. Elizabeth's Hospital" (p. 406). Freeman and Watts reported that "five attendants were required to restrain her while the nurse gave her the hypodermic" (p. 406), in order to prepare her for surgery. Following the operation, her behaviour was noticeably subdued. Freeman and Watts elaborated:

> ... from the day after operation (and we demonstrated this repeatedly to the timorous ward personnel) we could playfully grab Oretha by the throat, twist her arm, tickle her in the ribs and slap her behind without eliciting anything more than a wide grin or a hoarse chuckle. (pp. 406–407)

The frequently arbitrary character of the criteria used to define a surgical outcome as intimating improvement is nowhere better illustrated than in the following amusing reminiscence by the Scottish psychiatrist R. D. Laing (1967):

> Jimmy McKenzie was a bloody pest at the mental hospital because he went around shouting back at his voices. We could only hear one end of the conversation of course, but the other end could be inferred in general terms at least from: "Away tae fuck, ye filthy minded bastards . . . !" It was decided at one and the same time to alleviate his distress and ours, by giving him the benefit of leucotomy. An improvement in his condition was noted. After the operation he went around no longer shouting abuse at his voices, but: "Whats that? Say that again! Speak up ye buggers, I cannae hear ye!" (p. 146)

Arbitrary and unsophisticated criteria of postoperative improvement are less likely where a thorough assessment of an individual's preoperative condition and adaptation has been undertaken, targets have been formally determined and a systematic and wide-ranging postoperative evaluation has been performed. A within-subject controlled design most readily facilitates this type of analysis, since assessment must be sensitive to preoperative individual variation. However, few of the studies claiming experimental control present within-subject analyses, preferring group designs that offer only aggregate data. Optimal control and sensitivity would seem realizable by grafting within-subject analyses on to between-group designs. Consider, for example, Moore's arguments on the effects of psychosurgery on emotional behaviour:

> In a patient who has always been over-sensitive, too self-critical, too much lacking in confidence, too introspective, this change to extraversion may, on balance, make him more efficient and a more useful

citizen, better adapted to cope with life's problems. In a patient who is already too complacent, too casual, too prone to project his failings on to his environment, this change may be a higher price than he can afford to pay. (pp. 126–127)

Nuances of this sort may be obscured by looking only at group averages. A similar point can be made with regard to adverse sequelae. Thus, optimal studies would present individual analyses as well as aggregate group data.

In summary, a detailed examination of some 50 or so psychosurgical studies in this chapter reveals that they are pitifully poor in terms of design. The data offered must therefore be treated with a measure of suspicion and the inferences drawn from them tempered accordingly. Even the so-called "controlled studies" suffer from several major weaknesses. As indicated in Chapter 4, difficulties include biases in selection and allocation to groups, failure to control important subject variables, biases in aspects of the subject's treatment other than whether psychosurgery is or is not conducted, differences in postoperative treatment, unsophisticated and questionable assessment procedures and insufficient follow-ups.

Table 7.29 summarizes the general design features of the most cited of these controlled studies; inspection of this table merely reinforces our evaluation in Chapter 4. First of all, it should be appreciated that most of the more recent enterprises are retrospective. Second, only two of the studies listed, Jenkins *et al.* (1954) and Marks *et al.* (1966), bothered with the essential safeguard of blind assessment. Third, no effort has been made to control for the non-specific effects of psychosurgical intervention. The studies listed in Table 7.29 have without exception no treatment-control designs; none of

Table 7.29 Design features of most widely cited "controlled" studies

Study	*Prospective*	*Retrospective*	*Single blind*	*Double blind*	*Ordinary/ no-treatment control*	*Placebo control*	*Other treatment control*	*Within-subject control*
Friedman *et al.* (1951)	√	–	–	–	√	–	–	–
Jenkins *et al.* (1954)	√	–	√	–	√	–	–	–
Freeman *et al.* (1954)	√	–	–	–	√	–	–	–
Medina *et al.* (1954)	√	–	–	–	√	–	–	√
Baharal (1958)	√	–	–	–	√	–	–	–
Robin (1958a)	–	√	–	–	√	–	–	–
Robin (1958b)	–	√	–	–	√	–	–	–
McKenzie and Kaczanowski (1964)	–	√	–	–	√	–	–	–
Marks *et al.* (1966)	–	√	√	–	√	–	–	√

these have formally compared psychosurgery with alternative treatment modes, and none have attempted any proper placebo control. As such, they afford a less than rigorous test of psychosurgery's specific efficacy.

Table 7.29 describes the techniques used for allocating patients to the treatment and no-treatment condition in these studies. There are no instances of random allocation to groups and in several studies the control group comprises patients for whom permission for surgery was not forthcoming. As indicated in Chapter 4, there are good grounds for suspecting that such patients constitute a less than ideal comparison group. A control group comprising patients considered less likely to benefit from psychosurgery is even more problematic. While several of these studies have at least attempted to match treatment and control patients on various prognostic indicators, the techniques and criteria used for matching and allocation have frequently been rudimentary and unsophisticated. Further, as pointed out in Chapter 4, it is generally the case that the more rigorous the procedure and the better the match, the less the results flatter psychosurgery (cf. Robin, 1958a, b).

Table 7.30 Method of assignment of patients to "experimental" and "control" groups

		Matched		*Alternate*			*Risk*	
Study	*Random*	*Group*	*Individual*	*Group*	*Individual*	*Refusal*	*Poor*	*Good*
Friedman *et al.* (1951)	–	√	–	–	–	√	?[1]	
Jenkins *et al.* (1954)	–	√	–	–	–	–	–	–
Freeman *et al.* (1954)	–	–	–	–	–	√	–	–
Medina *et al.* (1954)	–	–	√	–	–	√	–	–
Baharal (1958)	–	?[2]	–	–	–	–	–	–
Robin (1958a)	–	–	√	–	–	–	–	–
Robin (1958b)	–	–	√	–	–	–	–	–
McKenzie and Kaczanowski (1964)	–	√[3]	–	–	–	?[4]	–	–
Marks *et al.* (1966)	–	–	√	–	–	–	–	–

[1] Patients were selected for the surgery group on a "therapeutic basis"
[2] Patients were considered "comparable" to the operation series
[3] Patients were deemed to be "similar"
[4] The control group included some "refusals"

Clearly, caution must again be exercised when drawing conclusions from reports designated as "controlled studies".

We have insisted previously that it is up to psychosurgeons to provide an unequivocal case for psychosurgery's efficacy. We can but conclude from our analysis of matters pertaining to design and assessment that this case has not been satisfactorily made. As such, our conclusion is at odds with Culliton's (1976) comment based on a preview of the assessment of the National Commission for the Protection of Human Subjects of Biomedical and Behavioural Research (Mirsky and Orzak, 1977). Culliton asserted that "psychosurgery can be good for one's mental health" (p. 301). Interestingly enough, of the three studies commissioned for the National Commission, both the empirical studies offer little comfort to psychosurgery. Disregarding the 11 patients treated primarily for chronic pain (which does not count as psychosurgery under our definition), Teuber *et al.*'s (1977) data indicate that only about a third of the remaining 34 patients displayed lasting clinical improvement after cingulectomy. In the other study, Mirsky and Orzak (1977) reported that only just over half of their 27 patients could be described as presenting a "very favourable outcome" (i.e. "very much improved" or "cured" – p. 17). While neither study offers conclusive evidence of efficacy, they do appear to indicate a lower risk of adverse sequelae relative to that which attended the older procedures. Indeed, Valenstein (1977) in the review that comprised the third of the National Commission's studies, was careful to distinguish between clinical efficacy and adverse sequelae. He concluded that contemporary psychosurgery seemed to attract a low incidence of side effects and commented that this "... finding stands in sharp contrast to the results from older lobotomy operations" (p. 96). Our own assessment is largely in line with the conclusion that modern psychosurgical operations cannot boast substantially higher clinical improvement rates than their predecessors, although they might very well entail a lower risk of adverse sequelae. However, such a result may well reflect improved surgical techniques (and more limited surgical ablations) rather than intimate the emergence of more valid and theoretically justified procedures. The theoretical basis of psychosurgery is the subject of the next chapter.

8

Theoretical basis of psychosurgery

When assessing the validity of any therapeutic procedure, two areas of information require close examination. The first relates to the practical effectiveness of the therapy. Here the questions are essentially empirical. Does the therapy work? The last five chapters dealt with the empirical justification for psychosurgical procedures. The second area for scrutiny concerns the theoretical underpinnings of the therapy. Is the therapy based on an adequate scientific rationale? In this chapter we shall examine the theoretical rationales offered for psychosurgery. To what extent do they constitute a secure base from which to embark on surgical excursions into the brain for the purpose of adjusting behaviour? Are the rationales offered consistent with current knowledge about brain functional organization?

At the outset it is important to appreciate that the manner in which the brain controls our behaviour continues to belie easy comprehension. Nevertheless, important clues to the workings of the brain continue to emerge from a wide variety of sources: neurophysiology and neuropsychology, the experimental psychology of humans and other animals, psychiatry.

Before delving into the rationales offered for psychosurgery, it might be profitable to chart the progress and development of ideas about the functional organization of the brain. This should provide a general context within which to consider psychosurgical theory.

The brain was first credited the role of orchestrating our perceptions, thoughts and actions some 25 centuries ago by Alcmaeon of Croton. In addition, Alcmaeon argued that the brain was far from undifferentiated with regard to psychological functions. Each sense modality was considered to have its own territory or localization within the brain. Thus, since the brain was first implicated in the control of behaviour, the idea of specificity or localization of function, i.e. that different brain regions housed different psychological functions, was prevalent. Clearly, any systematic account of brain functional organization would have to address itself to the question of specificity.

The first account of specificity to gain widespread acceptance was the theory of ventricular localization. Here, the psychological functions of memory, imagination, etc. were sited in the brain's ventricular spaces. It was with Gregor Reich at the end of the fifteenth century that ventricular theory received its first comprehensive description. His depiction of functional localization within the brain (Figure 8.1) indicates that the ventricles were suitably enlarged to accommodate their new status. The theory of ventricular localization held sway throughout the sixteenth and seventeenth centuries. However, the theory was without a shred of empirical support.

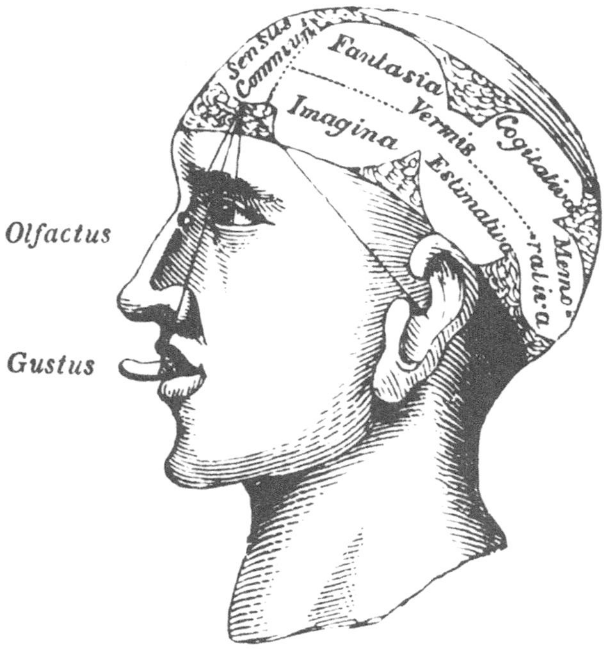

Figure 8.1 Ventricular localization depicted by Gregor Reich

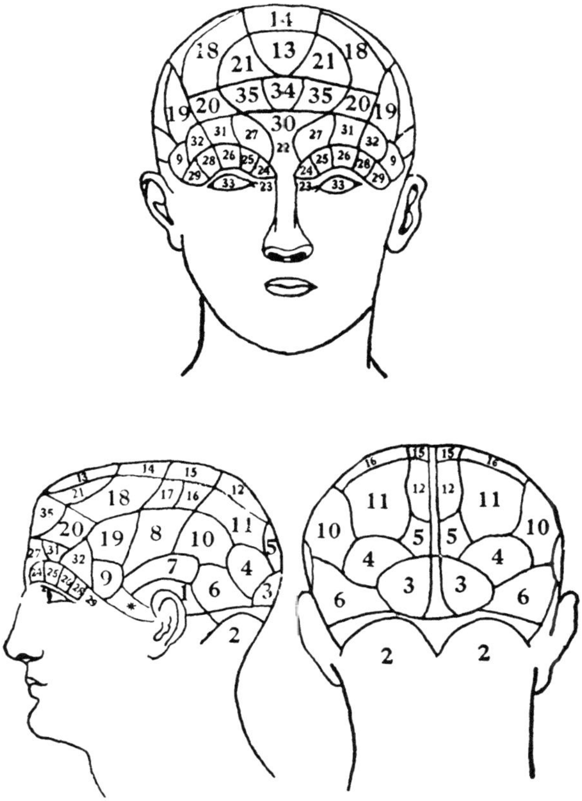

AFFECTIVE FACULTIES

PROPENSITIES

? Desire to live
* Alimentiveness
1 Destructiveness
2 Amativeness
3 Philoprogenitiveness
4 Adhesiveness
5 Inhabitiveness
6 Combativeness
7 Secretiveness
8 Acquisitiveness
9 Constructiveness

SENTIMENTS

10 Cautiousness
11 Approbativeness
12 Self-Esteem
13 Benevolence
14 Reverence
15 Firmness
16 Conscientiousness
17 Hope
18 Marvelousness
19 Ideality
20 Mirthfulness
21 Imitation

INTELLECTUAL FACULTIES

PERCEPTIVE

22 Individuality
23 Configuration
24 Size
25 Weight and Resistance
26 Coloring
27 Locality
28 Order
29 Calculation
30 Eventuality
31 Time
32 Tune
33 Language

REFLECTIVE

34 Comparison
35 Causality

Figure 8.2 Phrenological localization of function

Its roots lay not in science and direct empirical observation but in mysticism and magic.

Two centuries elapsed before empiricism was brought to bear on the question of brain localization. The anatomist Franz Joseph Gall provided a major impetus. The young Gall had been struck by the marked individual differences displayed by his classmates. In particular, he noted that those with efficient and reliable memories (Gall's mnemonic abilities were modest) were frequently characterized by protruding eyes. Subsequent inspection, first of the skulls of prisoners and lunatics and later of his friends, complemented by examination of plaster casts of the heads of the famous, led Gall to elaborate his schoolboy observations into a thesis that argued a precise relationship between cranial characteristics and psychological functions. Initially, Gall localized 27 functions in this manner. His collaborator Spurzheim extended and redefined Gall's scheme, providing a completed localization system that accounted for some 35 or 36 functions. Elaborate skull maps depicted the location of these functions (Figure 8.2). Spurzheim dignified the new discipline as "phrenology".

The phrenological system of localization had evolved through correlational analysis. While subsequent neurological and neuropsychological investigations adopted an analogous methodology, the procedures of Gall were far from adequate. His style of correlational analysis lacked the necessary rigour, system and objectivity demanded of science.

The essence of phrenology can be distilled as four basic propositions. First, it proposed that consciousness can be neatly compartmentalized into discrete functions or faculties. Nineteenth-century philosophy was much opposed to this attack on our psychological unity. The phrenological classification of faculties was clearly arbitrary, intuitive and invalid. Phrenology's second proposition asserted that faculties or functions so delineated have specific locations within the brain. While Gall and Spurzheim's localization maps are patently preposterous, their inadequate methodology and fanciful scheme of faculties did not permit a realistic test of this as a general proposition. Thirdly, phrenology assumed that conformation of the exterior of the skull mirrored the conformation of the interior and the topography of the brain. This assumption does not survive close inspection. The thickness of the skull varies greatly, idiosyncratically and adventitiously. Phrenology's final proposition, that an excess of any faculty is reflected in an enlargement of a corresponding brain region, is also correctly regarded as myth.

While it is easy in hindsight to dismiss phrenology as pseudoscience, its historical impact should not be underplayed. As Fulton (1955) attested, phrenology was embraced "by some of the best intellects of the age" (p. 3). The journal of phrenology was born in Edinburgh in 1823 and, although passing through a series of transformations, survived until as recently as 1911. Phrenology had persisted for almost a century. Further, phrenologists were never reticent in proclaiming the social benefits that could accrue from their new science. As Chorover (1976) recently pointed out:

> ... like the popularizers of psychology and psychiatry in our own times, the phrenologists of the nineteenth century told their contemporaries how to be happy, how to solve personal problems, how to choose a mate, how to raise children and how to succeed in business. (p. 742)

Phrenologists also expounded on the important social issues of their day. Coombs, an early and respected convert to the phrenological cause, submitted that phrenological evidence confirmed racial differences in intellect. Intellectual capacity was viewed as located in the frontal areas of the brain and revealed by the topography of the forehead. The Negro forehead was observed to be somewhat narrower than the Caucasian "highbrow". Thus, the relative social stations of the races could be explained on phrenological grounds. Phrenological considerations were also brought to bear on crime and insanity. If social and mental excellence could be accounted for in terms of the brain's geography, so too could social and mental shortcomings.

The history of phrenology is not without comedy. Phrenology had nurtured an interest in brain size as well as cranial prominences. Prevailing wisdom had it that brain size mirrored intellectual evolution. Consequently, the skulls of great men were studied after their death. Byron's skull is purported to have housed a brain of some 2000 grams, an organ much larger than the average 1360 grams. Gall's skull was an obvious candidate for close scrutiny. However, although he was a man of considerable gifts, his brain was much smaller than average, weighing in at only 1100 grams. Further, inspection of Gall's cranial geography revealed that "combativeness", "destructiveness" and "secretiveness" were all well developed.

Nevertheless, his phrenology made its mark in more subtle ways; it had created a climate highly receptive to the idea of precise functional localization. It was in this climate that more direct neurological and neuropsychological investigations were launched.

However, not everyone was convinced of the correctness of a highly differentiated brain. Pierre Flourens expressed alternative opinion with the clearest voice. During the first half of the nineteenth century he conducted a meticulous series of experiments selectively extirpating parts of the central nervous system in pigeons and noting the behavioural consequences. On the basis of his observations that large portions of the pigeon's brain could be removed without impairing any specific functions independently, Flourens contested the highly specific localization of functions. Instead, he asserted the functional unity of the nervous system.

It was not long, though, before Flourens' doctrine of the unity of the brain was challenged. In 1861, Paul Broca described the case of a patient with a severe disturbance of expressive speech. This was apparently the man's sole defect; he communicated intelligently by signs. An autopsy revealed a lesion in the interior frontal gyrus of the patient's left cerebral hemisphere. Drawing on subsequent cases, Broca postulated that the posterior third of the left interior frontal gyrus is the centre for motor images of the world, i.e. the centre for language expression. The loss of expressive speech apparent with damage in this area was termed "aphasia" by Broca, a label that has endured admirably.

Broca's conclusion was received with unprecedented enthusiasm. It clearly derived from direct empirical observation. While both Broca and Gall relied on correlational analysis, the objects of Broca's analysis pertained much more directly to the matter of brain functional organization. Consequently, Broca was able to reassert the phrenological principle of specificity on acceptably scientific grounds.

It is difficult to understate the impact of Broca's investigation. It provided both the conceptual framework and the clinical methodology of mainstream neurological and neuropyschological study for the next 80 years or so. A mere decade saw its influence realized. In 1873, Carl Wernicke described a sample of patients with lesions in the posterior third of the left superior temporal gyrus. While expressive speech was relatively unaffected in these patients, they demonstrated a marked inability to comprehend spoken language. Wernicke concluded that this region marked the centre for the understanding of speech.

Specific sensory and motor centres were soon grafted on to the emerging scheme. In 1870, Fritsch and Hitzig announced the experimental discovery of motor functions in the cerebral cortex. Applying electrical stimulation to the cerebral cortex of a dog, they found that in certain anterior portions, movement consistently accompanied stimulation. In 1876, Sir David Ferrier confirmed and extended these observations in monkeys and extrapolated his findings to the human brain. The localization of sensory functions quickly followed.

Sensory and motor localization was soon complemented by the allocation of complex mental processes to narrowly restricted areas of the brain. Broca's clinical methodology was enthusiastically brought to bear on a wide variety of human activities. By the beginning of this century, elaborate functional maps started to appear. Although these differed in topographical detail from early phrenological charts, the conceptual similarities were striking. In fact, Franz (1912) was prompted to parody these new efforts at exact localization as "the new phrenology". The most detailed of the "narrow localization" charts were produced by Kleist (1934), following clinical scrutiny of an extensive sample of World War I veterans. Kleist delineated centres in the brain for such functions as "falling reaction", "singing", "gazing downward" and "gazing upward" (Figure 8.3). The "personal and social ego" attracted its own unique and separate compartment. In the same vein, Nielson (1946) described a circumscribed area of the brain as the "centre for the perception

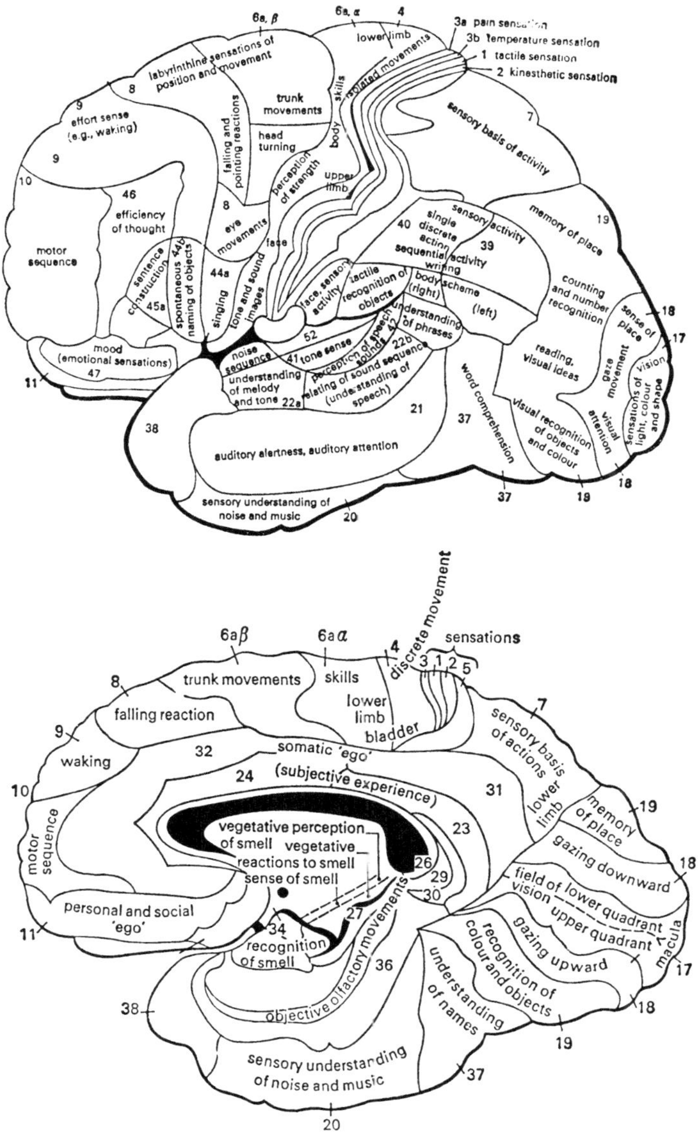

Figure 8.3 Kleist's localization map

of living objects", distinguishing it from an area concerned with the perception of inanimate objects.

While the narrow localization view certainly dominated thinking in these matters, in would be wrong to suppose that it developed unchallenged. Criticism focused on several issues. The proponents of narrow localization relied heavily for their data on experiments performed by nature, namely on brains violated by disease or accident. Surgery (neurosurgery and later psychosurgery) has provided additional material for study. Precise functional localization clearly demands a precise specification of the anatomical extent of the lesion. However, this is no easy matter. Even with lesions that result from surgical intent rather than mishap, exact specification of the boundaries of tissue removal is often impossible. Surgical accuracy has been discussed already.

Other problems exist. For example, space-occupying lesions such as tumours produce pressure inside the skull. This can drastically distort the shape of the brain, detrimentally affecting tissue at some distance from the site of primary disruption. Apart from transfer of intracranial pressure, contiguous cerebral oedema and the disruption of neural connections between regions can each induce marked alterations in distant parts of the brain. In addition, pathologically affected tissue may interfere physiologically with the normal cerebral functioning of neighbouring neurons. In some circumstances chemical changes in pathological cells may adversely affect the chemical integrity of neighbouring cells or even the rest of the brain. Finally, it should be noted that the presence of diseased tissue is not necessarily associated with the same behavioural symptoms as comparable tissue absence or removal. Such considerations substantially weaken the narrow localization case. The brain lesion studies were not sufficiently delineated to justify the neat cerebral arrangements that were advocated. In addition, the strict specificity of Kleist is difficult to reconcile with observations of gross individual differences in lesion effects. As early as 1933, Dandy informed us that lesions that are apparently similar in most respects can result in quite different disturbances in different individuals. The behavioural assessment procedures used by narrow localizationists have also attracted criticism. The psychology of the period was, as Luria (1973) had indicated, "very imperfect". In many of the clinical studies, it was wielded with little insight or practical skill. In conceptual sophistication it resembled closely the "faculty psychology" of the phrenologists.

Finally, the basic reasoning applied to the clinical data by narrow localizationists has been seriously challenged. They argued that a function could be considered localized when its permanent loss followed damage to some circumscribed area of the brain. To illustrate how such an inference can be misleading, critics have generally resorted to simple physical analogies. For example, if the fuel tank of an automobile were removed, we would not be surprised to find the automobile incapable of movement. However, few of us would entertain the conclusion, based on this clinical fact, that the function of a fuel tank is to propel an automobile. While simple mechanical analogies are generally to be mistrusted in any debate on complex neural processes (a point to which we shall return), they nevertheless illustrate the need for caution in drawing conclusions from clinical neuropsychological observations. Jackson's (1932) pronouncement on the cerebral localization of speech continues to be pertinent here: "To locate damage which destroys speech and to localize speech are two different things" (p. 130).

The proponents of narrow localization also drew support from research on the effects of stimulating the cortex electrically. Early examples of such research have already been cited. The work of Penfield and his associates (Penfield and Rasmussen, 1950) presents us with the most dramatic recent illustration of the tradition. They demonstrated with human subjects under local anaesthetic that parts of the precentral and postcentral gyri are related to different parts of the body. In addition, they found that stimulation in parts of the occipital lobes produced sensations of lights, flashes, visual movements and colours. With stimulation in the temporal regions, auditory sensations were reported by subjects. However, difficulties similar to those surrounding the lesion studies attend inferences of specificity drawn from brain stimulation effects.

In addition, the electrical stimulation technique has attracted several specific criticisms. First of all, stimulation elicits psychological effects in some areas, i.e. the primary and secondary motor areas, but not in the electrically "silent" areas, which lie anterior to the precentral gyrus and in the extensive posterior parietal regions. Consequently, cortical stimulation tells us little about these "silent" regions and their significance for higher mental functions. Second, such stimulation is necessarily artificial. A single cortical "spot" cannot be stimulated without affecting adjoining areas (Fulton, 1947). Third, neural tissue is highly sensitive to variations in the nature of the electrical stimulus – its frequency, intensity, duration and waveform. Finally, restimulation of the same "spot" with the same electrical stimulus frequently produces dissimilar effects, i.e. a different sensation or movement. The more recent observations with electrical stimulation in subcortical structures again belie a narrow localization account of brain organization. As Valenstein (1973a) indicated:

> The experimental data clearly indicate that electrodes that seem to be in the same brain locus in different animals often evoke different behavior, and electrodes located at very different brain sites may evoke the same behavior in a given animal. (p. 89)

The question of what the behavioural effects of brain damage and stimulation imply for brain functional organization is complicated still further by observations that stimulation and destruction of the same neural tissue are not necessarily associated with reciprocal effects (e.g. Ellison and Flynn, 1968).

In summary, the obvious problems that surround the stimulation and lesion data and the inferences that can be legitimately drawn from them would seem to make the narrow localization thesis untenable. As Meyer (1960) remarked:

> ... there is lability or plasticity inherent in cerebral tissue that prevents the attempt to localize functions at specific points. (p. 531)

Valenstein (1973a) was similarly explicit:

> ... there are few areas of the brain that are concerned with the regulation of one and only one behavior and there is no single area in the brain that has complete control over any behavior. (p. 122)

The inadequacies of the view that functions are narrowly localized tempted some critics back to Flourens' doctrine of unity. The most prominent of these was Karl Lashley who (Lashley, 1929) emphasized the patterning of neural activity rather than the locus. The primary empirical impetus for his assertion of unity or equipotentiality was provided by a series of experiments on the effects of brain lesions on maze learning in rats. Errors in maze learning and retention were plotted against the amount and location of cortical tissue destroyed. Lashley concluded that decrements in performance were independent of the location of tissue damage. Instead, disruption depended on the extent of the cortical lesion.

While the thrust of Lashley's ideas continue to have more than archival interest, it is clear that the notion of complete equipotentiality save for primary motor and sensory areas, is no more acceptable than that of strict localization. A sample of the criticisms specifically directed at Lashley's work illustrate this contention. First of all, the validity of generalizing from rats, or for that matter from any non-human subject, to humans, has been seriously questioned. Meyer (1960), for example, strongly objected to the practice:

> The findings of animal studies are of little value in determining cerebral functions and their localization in man, because of the general trends of neural development towards encephalization. In lower animals the higher cortical centres display more generalized functions, and, as they gradually evolve phylogenetically from a relatively undifferentiated structure of tissue (pallium), they become gradually structurally differentiated, more complex and increasingly specialized with regard to function which they take over from lower centres. (p. 534)

Further, Luria (1973) has argued cogently that the distinctive human reliance on complex and dynamic symbolic systems intimates distinctive neural arrangements. In addition, it has been suggested that the equipotentiality observed by Lashley could have been an artifact of the maze task used. According to Hunter (1930), all sensory modalities contribute almost equally to the control of behaviour in the maze. Consequently, a lesion in any sensory projection area should disrupt performance to approximately the same extent, giving merely the appearance of equipotentiality. Pickett (1952) provided some experimental support for this interpretation. He used a maze that could be run only on the basis of tactile and kinaesthetic cues. The results did not favour equipotentiality.

Clearly, neither precise compartmentalization nor complete equipotentiality offer an adequate account of behavioural processes and their organization within the brain.

A compromise solution to the problem lay in the idea of "regional equipotentiality," i.e. the theory that while a behavioural function may be localized in a particular area of the brain, within that area all parts contribute equally to maintaining the function. While regional equipotentiality has some attraction, it has yet to receive serious elaboration.

A recent treatment, which embodies some of the character of regional equipotentiality and is at the same time sufficiently elaborated, is Luria's (1973) systems approach. Luria prefaced his account with a re-examination of the basic concepts of "function" and "localization". He noted that the term "function" has been used in two quite distinct ways. On the one hand, "function" has been used to refer to the specialized activities of particular tissue, e.g. the function of the pancreatic tissue to secrete insulin or the function of the giant pyramidal cells of Betz to generate motor impulses. On the other hand, "function" has also been used to denote complex physiological and psychological activities, such as digestion and perception. In this usage, a function cannot be considered as the prerogative of a given small unit of tissue.

Such complex activities are more appropriately understood as "complex functional systems", a term that emphasizes their dependence upon a whole series of simple tissue functions. Luria surmised that many of the difficulties attending the study of the cerebral organization of psychological functions stem from treating them as simple functions. While simple tissue functions can, by definition, have precise locations, complex functional systems can in no way be limited to circumscribed areas of the brain. According to Luria, two distinguishing features of complex functional systems preclude this: the complex composition of a functional system, which always includes both afferent and efferent components, and the interchangeable character of many of the components in a functional system.

In summary, Luria replaced the competing notions of isolated faculties and psychic unity with the concept of complex functional systems. Narrow localization and equipotentiality have been supplanted by the idea that complex functional systems are organized in systems of concertedly working zones, each of which performs its role in the complex functional system. These concertedly working zones may be distributed in geographically diverse areas of the brain. Thus, Luria's scheme states that each complex behavioural function depends on a variety of brain areas and that each brain area contributes to a variety of complex functions. As such, it represents a major conceptual advance over earlier representations.

Having plotted the development of ideas about brain functional organization, let us now consider the timing of psychosurgery in this historical scheme and the theoretical accounts that marked its progress. At the outset, however, it should be emphasized that such accounts are notable primarily by their meagreness and infrequency. Psychosurgeons have always relied more on practical and empirical arguments. The atheoretical flavour of early psychosurgical activities was clearly conveyed in Fulton's (1951) monograph:

> In 1935–36, when the lobotomy operation was first proposed, knowledge of frontal lobe function both in man and in animals was limited, and the procedure which gained wide acceptance was in large measure empirical and paid little heed to the broader problem of functional localization in the human brain. (p. 100)

Willet (1960) indicated that little had changed in the intervening decade, a decade that witnessed the emergence of many new operative procedures:

> ... surgeons appear to have been prompted by hunches and empirical experience rather than by clearly formulated hypotheses when proposing their various modifications. (p. 569)

As recently as 1977, Valenstein was asserting the same point. Comparing the empirical and physiological rationales forwarded for psychosurgery, he commented:

> The physiological rationale for psychosurgery is based on much more indirect, heterogenous and often tortured sets of arguments. (pp. 9–10)

It is difficult to attribute such persistent dissatisfaction to chance.

In the opening chapter, we credited Burckhardt, at the end of the nineteenth century, with the first published account of psychosurgery. At that time, Flourens' doctrine of unity was still competing vigorously with the emerging system of narrow localization. Burckhardt's own account acknowledged the dispute but clearly expressed his sympathies in the matter:

> Whoever sees in psychoses only diffuse illness of the cortex ... for him there would naturally be no point in excising relatively small portions of the cortex in the hope of influencing a psychosis favourably by it.
>
> One, therefore, has to be, as I am, of a different opinion, namely that our psychological existence is also made up of single elements, which are localized in separate areas of the brain and keep their places for life. (p. 544)

Thus it was Burckhardt's commitment to the narrow localization view that provided the main impetus for his surgical explorations.

Burckhardt's initiative was critically received. His call to colleagues to "tread the path of cortical extirpation with even better and more satisfactory results" yielded no immediate recruits. The prevailing climate of ideas was unfavourable. Some fifty years later, when Moniz reported the results of frontal lobe surgery, it was noticeably better; by the 1930s the concept of cerebral specificity was widely respected.

The concept of narrow localization, then, featured strikingly in the emergence of psychosurgery. If this theory constituted the sole rationale for modern surgical efforts, the whole enterprise could be readily dismissed, simply as a "phrenological mistake" (Chorover, 1976, p. 764). However, it is apparent from even their earliest pronouncements that many psychosurgeons did not and do not explicitly subscribe to a highly compartmentalized view of the brain and instead have sought justification for their activities elsewhere. Reminiscing in 1956, Moniz revealed his reasons for focusing on the frontal areas:

> Inasmuch as I was convinced of the importance of the prefrontal lobes in mental activity, I chose this region for the experiments. (p. 136)

Moniz's conception of the workings of the prefrontal region was undeniably vague. However, he considered it a much less differentiated structure than did many of his contemporaries. In fact, Moniz's major physiological rationale for frontal lobe surgery did not lie in structural organization but instead stemmed from considerations at the neuronal level. Here, Moniz relied heavily on the then prevalent notion that fixed connections occurred between nerve cells during learning. He proposed that in psychoses such fixed neural connections have become abnormally stabilized. Thus, the recurrent anxieties and morbid fantasies of psychotic patients were viewed as reflecting the abnormal stabilization of neural connections. Surgery was undertaken to destroy these stabilized connections and the compulsive thought patterns they embodied. Moniz (1948) elaborated:

> ... to cure these patients we must destroy the more or less fixed arrangements of cellular connections that must exist in the brain, and particularly those which are linked to the frontal lobes. (p. 46)

These early and tentative ideas of Moniz have themselves shown remarkable durability. The notion of abnormally fixed, closed neural circuits in the frontal areas has constituted the major rationale throughout most of psychosurgery's evolution. Minor embellishments have been added to Moniz's orginal version. Freeman and Watts (1950) exemplify:

> Fixation of ideas, according to the Moniz hypothesis, is the functional expression of pathologically stabilized synaptic connections of various

> cells groups. It would seem likely, therefore, that fantasy becomes to a certain extent irreversible. ... One may express this psychologically as a complex, or physiologically as a closed neural circuit. This circuit or this complex is highly endowed with emotional tone. (p. 561)

Freeman and Watts considered that such emotional tone derived from the thalamus.

As recently as 1971, Freeman was reiterating this same general theme:

> The most tenable theory would seem to be that the fibres severed in transorbital lobotomy are collaterals of the thalamofrontal projection. It would further seem that these collaterals are highly unstable and thus unimportant in mental health, but that during the course of a functional mental disorder they become stabilized in their synaptic connections and thus serve to perpetuate the stereotyped thinking disorder and emotional reaction that underlie the psychosis. *Thus the original hypothesis of Egas Moniz appears more probable than ever*. (p. 622, italics in original)

It should be emphasized here that this sort of formulation is purely metaphorical. Neither Moniz nor those who followed his initiative had concrete evidence of the existence of any "fixed arrangements of cellular connections". Similarly, the corollary that psychological compulsions and complexes reflected the operation of closed neural circuits around which impulses incessantly reverberated owed more to analogy than to neurophysiological observation. Frequently, however, theoretical presentations in psychosurgery do not make explicit the metaphorical character of their arguments.

The use of such analogies to explain brain mechanisms is an activity of some precedent. Every age seems to have deployed its own technological achievements in developing neurobehavioural metaphors. For example, Descartes' formulations owed much to the marvels of seventeenth-century French plumbing and the elaborate fountains fashionable at the time.

In this century, we have seen the brain likened to a giant telephone exchange and, more recently, to computers. The former represents the neurophysiological corollary of the narrow localization position. Essentially, exponents of the telephone exchange theory proposed that precise and fixed connections are forged during learning between cells or cell systems in the sensory areas of the brain and cells in the motor areas, in a fashion akin to the connection of two telephones by wires through a series of exchanges. It is this analogy which characterizes Moniz's rationale for lobotomy and underlies many subsequent psychosurgical perspectives. Scoville (1949) illustrates:

> Let us compare the frontal lobes and their thalamic connexions to a telephone switchboard with its connecting cable to various telephones.

> Pool with his topectomy actually cuts out sections of the switchboard proper. Smith, Dax and Reitman with their superior and orbital leucotomies have cut parts of the telephone cable. Wycis and Spiegel with their thalamotomy have cut out a considerable number of the telephones and the speaker with his selective under-cutting has stepped behind the switchboard and cut the wires connecting various portions of it to the cable. (pp. 4–5)

It has long been obvious, however, that the telephone exchange metaphor is totally unsatisfactory. Lashley's work (Lashley, 1952) exemplified some of the shortcomings of such accounts at the behavioural level. His research demonstrated that rats retained the ability to run mazes in spite of being deprived of large areas of cortex after their initial learning experiences. Either Lashley's extirpations uncannily avoided the pertinent neural connections (an unlikely proposition) or the brain just does not operate like a telephone exchange.

Contemporary physical analogies are decidedly more complex. In computers we have devices that behave in ways that can be considered intelligent. Like our brains, computers recognize patterns, receive and store information, solve problems, play complicated games and so on. Accordingly, it is not surprising to find such clever machines, together with sophisticated mathematical techniques, pressed into the service of modelling brain mechanisms. On the whole, however, psychosurgical theory has paid little heed to such developments. Rather, it has tended to persist with earlier and simpler metaphors. Where computer technology has been invoked, its application has been idiosyncratic and glib. The rationale presented recently by Sano and his colleagues (Sano *et al.*, 1972) for posterior hypothalamic surgery can be regarded as typical:

> The human brain is often compared with the computer. The limbic system and the brain stem including the diencephalon are the elaborate "hardware." Major parts of the neocortex are also the "hardware" more elaborate than the former. The frontal association areas which are the most conspicuously developed in Homo sapiens, may be compared, however, with the "software." Here is the seat of the higher intellectual functions which put the "hardware" to good use.
>
> Personally we are rather reluctant to operate on the "software" as are many contemporary psychiatrists. It may, however, be permissible to operate upon the "hardware", if the operation does not cause serious side effects. This is our principal attitude towards psychosurgery. (p. 57)

Sano would do well to consider Somerhoff's (1974) treatment of brain–computer comparisons. Somerhoff clearly harbours serious misgivings:

> Comparisons between brains and computers can mislead in a number of ways. They can mislead not only by suggesting analogies where

> none in fact exist, but also because in applying computer concepts to the brain we may unwittingly commit ourselves to tacit assumptions which are valid enough in engineering but have no valid foundation in biology. (p. 12)

Sano's rather naïve venture into this idiom would seem a case in point.

Sano's attitude, however, that the appropriate sites for psychosurgery comprise limbic and brain-stem structures, is now widely shared. There are exceptions. Scoville (1971), for example, expressed serious doubts about the efficacy of limbic-system operations in psychosis.

Nevertheless, there has been a marked shift in surgical focus from the frontal to the frontolimbic and limbic areas; this has been discussed previously. However, it is important to stress that even in the early development of psychosurgical theory, medial brain structures were attributed more than nominal status. So far in this chapter, we have discussed only those aspects of Freeman's formulations that parallel the theme initiated by Moniz. However, Freeman and Watts elaborated several additional and separate hypotheses. In essence, they suggested that frontal operations did not disrupt the fixed ideational patterns *per se* but rather eliminated the emotional impact of the ideas.

In addition, Freeman and Watts (1947b) firmly implicated the thalamus in this emotional blunting. Frontal lobotomy, they insisted, worked "to divorce ideation and affect by subtotal section of the anterior thalamic radiation" (p. 658). Freeman and Watts' thesis strongly commended the restriction of surgery to medial frontal areas. In 1950, they argued:

> ... it should be possible to limit the incisions in the frontal lobe so that only the medial nucleus would be affected and only enough to bring about the desired reduction of affectively charged psychotic behaviour with preservation of the rest of the personality as intact as possible. (pp. 290–293)

Livingston (1969) outlined the subsequent development of this theme, expressing the now popular view that where benefit accrued from the older frontal operations, it did so because of the alteration of limbic system functioning. Aside from prompting more circumscribed operations addressed specifically to those portions of the frontal regions with limbic system connections, this emphasis also pointed to selective ablation of limbic structures, such as the thalamus, cingulum and amygdala.

Finally, in addition to the shifts in the site and extent of surgical interventions, prevailing opinions regarding the sorts of patients considered appropriate for surgery have undergone revision. This change has been detailed previously.

Are these newer, more circumscribed procedures maintained by a more sophisticated theoretical framework than the older, frontal operations?

Willet's (1960) assessment, cited previously, would suggest not. Other authorities seem to concur; Valenstein (1973a) for example, was strikingly disapproving:

> The theory that accompanied these selective or "fractional" psychosurgical procedures has remained at a very speculative and tenuous level. The functions of the particular brain areas selected for ablation are still not understood, and for the most part theoretical statements simply paraphrase what is believed to be the more striking postoperative changes. (p. 275)

The arguments used by Crow to justify restricted interior frontal lesions illustrate this sort of speculation:

> ... the cells of the inferior third of the frontal lobes are contained in a system, the functions of which are to produce fear sensation. When the neuronal system is only slightly active, we may call the sensation "apprehension" and when it is very active we may call the sensation "terror." It can be plausibly argued that such a fear system is favourable, and possibly necessary, for survival among higher animals including man. I have also speculated that an essential component of what we call happiness is a suppression of the general level of activity of this hypothetical fear-system. In other words, happiness is the absence of fear at a time when we have in our consciousness a set of concepts which we have learned to consider attractive. I have come to consider that these particular patients were ill because they had inherited or through environmental influences in some way developed fear-systems which had become chronically overactive with intermittent paroxysms of severe overactivity .... (Quoted in Valenstein, 1973a, pp. 275–276)

More recently, Heath and Cox (1976) elaborated a similarly styled rationale, applying it to most of the usual psychosurgical procedures. They postulated the existence of two separate but interacting systems of emotion in the brain: an adversive system and a pleasure system.

Examination of the theoretical statements that adorn the practice of cingulotomy provide validation of Valenstein's unfavourable assessment. Yakolev (1965), for example, presented the following account:

> The cingulum is a bundle strategically situated to mediate activities of the limbic cortex to the entire forebrain. On general grounds one might speculate that these activities have something to do with the outward expression of the visceral, i.e. of the internal states or "emotions." Its interruption in cingulotomy modifies in some way the behavioural expression of the distraught internal states. (p. 269)

A decade later, Ballantine *et al.* (1977) were no less vague:

> If one assumes that in some way cingulotomy favorably affects patients with intractable disorders of affect, the improvement could be attributed to anatomic disruption, to the neurochemical after-effects of such disruption, or to a combination of the two. (p. 350)

In the same volume, Teuber *et al.* (1977) provided no additional insight:

> In attempting a physiological interpretation, one can only speculate that the therapeutic effects ... might be the result of the induction of some change in chemically specific pathways, possibly at some remove from the area directly approached. (p. 361)

More critical to psychosurgery than the analogies provided by technological developments have been those derived from animal experimentation. Valenstein (1973a) recorded this influence: "Almost every new development in psychosurgery has been directly inspired by animal experimentation" (p. 326). Before assessing the contribution of particular animal researches, two points must be emphasized. First of all, great care should always be exercised when projecting the results of brain lesions in the experimental animal to humans. The reasons for caution here have been rehearsed earlier in this chapter. Second, the risk of errors in generalizing from animals to humans is substantially aggravated when the appraisal of animal lesion effects is highly selective. It is unfortunate that psychosurgeons have frequently been guilty of gross selective perception in this respect.

While some doubt surrounds Moniz's motivation, it is apparent that the conference paper presented by Fulton and Jacobsen on the behavioural changes that followed bilateral frontal lesions in chimpanzees is generally regarded as a key factor. Certainly, Fulton (1951) was convinced of its influence.

Fulton and Jacobsen's observations have been summarized in Chapter 1. Nevertheless, it is important to emphasize here that the main burden of their paper was that serious intellectual deficits followed frontal ablations in chimpanzees. What apparently caught Moniz's attention, however, was their aside that one of the animals displayed a marked postoperative reduction in the frustration or experimental neuroses generated by the primary experimental exercise, the delayed response task. According to Freeman and Watts' (1950) account:

> He (*Moniz*) compared in his own mind the querulous, the deluded, the agitated and the obsessed with these apes of Fulton and Jacobsen. (p. xvi)

Jacobsen, however, was at some pains to point out that the rather restricted phenomenon of "experimental neuroses" should be carefully distinguished from the equivalent label applied in a psychiatric setting.

The development of cingulotomy also owes much to the somewhat selective appraisal of particular animal studies. Fulton's Withering Lectures in 1948 are considered crucial. Fulton (1951) took up the story:

> In my Withering Lectures I raised the question of whether a lesion in the cingulate area might not be chiefly responsible for the behavioral changes which occur in man after radical frontal lobotomy. This suggestion was based largely on behavioral changes reported in monkeys by Wilbur Smith and Arthur Ward. (pp. 82–83)

Smith and Ward both reported that following cingulotomy, their animals appeared much tamer towards both their cagemates and their human handlers. It was this increased tameness that impressed psychosurgeons. However, there is more to the behaviour of cingulotomized monkeys than simple pacificity. Ward's (1948) account patently illustrates that "tameness" provides an utterly inadequate description of the behaviour of operated animals. The complex character of disturbances produced by cingulate surgery can be intimated by recounting some of Ward's description. The cingulotomized monkey showed "no grooming behaviour, no acts of affection towards its companions" and seemed "as though it had lost its social conscience". With regard to its cagemates, the operated animal "treats them as inanimate objects and will walk on them, bump into them if they happen to be in the way, and will sit on them", and "will openly eat food in the hand of a companion without being prepared to do battle and appears surprised when rebuffed", and "never shows actual hostility to its fellows". Ward concluded by asserting that such monkeys "lose the ability to accurately forecast the social repercussions of their own actions".

More recent psychosurgical procedures have also leaned heavily for justification on the results of animal experiments. The research prompted by Klüver and Bucy's initiative was markedly influential. Klüver and Bucy (1938) reported a syndrome of behaviour changes in monkeys following bilateral temporal lobotomy. These have been detailed in the opening chapter. They are similar in many respects to the changes observed by Smith and Ward to follow anterior cingulate lesions. Subsequent research revealed that this Klüver–Bucy syndrome could be produced by lesions restricted to the amygdaloid nuclei. As in the case of cingulate lesions, it was primarily the taming effects of amygdala surgery that attracted the interest of psychosurgeons.

Narabayashi (cf. Narabayashi *et al.*, 1963; Narabayashi and Uno, 1966) was a pioneer with stereotactic amygdalotomy in 1958, and the number of individuals subjected to the operation has been increasing slowly but continuously ever since. The usual behavioural indications for surgical referral are behaviours designated as "aggressive", "violent" and "uncontrollably" explosive.

Some practitioners have advocated limiting amygdalotomies to aggressive and violent patients with symptoms of temporal lobe epilepsy (e.g. Mark and Ordia, 1976; Vaernet, 1972). This could be considered as elevating the operation to the status of neurosurgery, given that neuropathological indices of epilepsy provided the grounds for surgery. However, it is difficult to discern the primary surgical indications with such patients. Opponents of amygdala surgery contend that even with epileptic patients, the main impetus for surgery is aggressive behaviour. This interpretation is not without foundation. For example, Mark *et al.* (1972) stated:

> When present, interictal episodes of uncontrolled violent behavior are usually a more disabling symptom to the victims of temporal lobe epilepsy than the seizures themselves. Thus the treatment of this aspect of the disorder is of prime importance. (p. 140)

In addition, while an orderly relationship between episodic aggressive behaviour and temporal lobe epilepsy has been postulated (cf. Mark and Ordia, 1976; Mark and Sweet, 1974), many authorities remain unconvinced (cf. Goldstein, 1974; Rodin, 1973).

For psychosurgeons like Narabayashi, though, such considerations would appear to be largely cosmetic, since stereotactic destruction of the amygdala is conducted explicitly for the control of violent behaviour. Here the complexities of temporal lobe epilepsy are not permitted to cloud the metaphor provided by Klüver and Bucy's monkeys.

As we have indicated already, the psychosurgical treatment of animal brain research is frequently cavalier. The highly selective evaluation of the animal amygdala research is exemplary. Fortunately, in the case of the amygdala, many of the major deficits that characterize the Klüver–Bucy syndrome in animals, such as hypersexuality and compulsive orality, rarely result from human surgery (Mark *et al.*, 1972; Narabayashi, 1972). A literal application of the early animal research would have predicted otherwise. In a sense, the absence of some of the Klüver–Bucy deficits following human amygdalotomies serves to re-emphasize the general problems of simple animal analogies. Further, psychosurgeons operating on the human amygdala had no independent grounds for suspecting only fractional Klüver–Bucy effects.

More recent research on the effects of amygdala lesions on monkeys in non-laboratory, free-ranging settings is exceptionally revealing. It clearly demonstrates the crucial influence that postoperative social context has on the behavioural effects observed to follow ablations. The implications of this result have not, as yet, been explicitly represented in psychosurgical theory. Some hint of the importance of social context for lesion effects was provided in an early experiment by Rosvold *et al.* (1954). They noted that the effects of bilateral amygdalotomies on rhesus monkeys reflected the prevailing social dynamics within the group of monkeys to which the operatee belonged.

Kling and his colleagues have substantially expanded this style of experiment. Amygdalotomies were performed on monkeys selected from large free-ranging and semi-free-ranging colonies. The preoperative behaviour of these animals was subject to careful observation. They were then isolated from the colony, lesioned and, following a short period of postoperative recovery and laboratory-based observation, returned to the colony, where their behaviour was again closely scrutinized. Kling's results are of major significance. First, they throw some light on the absence of hypersexuality and increased orality in human amygdalotomized patients. These components of the Klüver–Bucy syndrome were observed by Kling to be present only in a restricted postoperative environment.

More importantly perhaps, Kling's research reveals a dramatic pattern of postoperative deficits in social behaviour apparent only when the monkeys rejoin the colony. Nothing in the usual postoperative laboratory behaviour directly intimated such striking social maladjustment. Essentially, amygdalotomized animals in the monkey colony seemed no longer to comprehend the established social norms. They failed to respond appropriately to social communications and continuously appeared confused and fearful. Frequently, when approached by a monkey in a non-threatening way, they would respond by cowering or fleeing. Alternatively, operated animals would, on occasion, react provocatively when threatened by a dominant colony member. A severe beating was the price of such social incompetence. In adult monkeys, the failure to resocialize postoperatively was total. Complete social isolation was invariably followed by death from starvation or from attacks by predators.

Kling (1972) offered an explanation for these effects, distilling what seemed like a primary deficit:

> It may be, then, that one of the effects of amygdalotomy is a reduction of control over visual input resulting in a "depersonalized-like" state in which the subject is hyperattentive, distractable and confused resulting in withdrawal from those communications which cannot be sorted out. As the environmental complexity is reduced, the operated subject would show increased attention and responsiveness to those limited objects in its visual world permitting the expression of the characteristic hyperorality, hypersexuality and approach behavior toward normally avoided objects and man. (p. 529)

Incidentally, recent observations suggest that a similar lack of resocialization follows cingulate lesions (Meyers and Swett, 1970, cited by Kling, 1972).

Kling's observations and conclusions offer little encouragement to those committed to surgical experiments on the human amygdala. To the prospect of taming aggressive behaviours, gleaned from the early animal research, it is necessary to graft on the likelihood of doing untold damage to complex social behaviour, as revealed by subsequent animal research.

Finally, the rationale offered by Roeder and his colleagues (Roeder and Müller, 1969; Roeder *et al.*, 1972) for ventromedial hypothalamic surgery as a treatment for paedophilic homosexuality provides perhaps the most striking recent instance of the selective perception of animal research results. A film of Schreiner and Kling's animal experiments provided the main impetus. We can do no better than allow those psychosurgeons to speak for themselves:

> The experimental animals (cats), which had exhibited the hypersexuality typical of the post amygdalectomy syndrome, lost it after supplemental destructions of the hypothalamic ventromedial nuclei, but with the appearance of aggressivity.
>
> This film, exhibited by Schreiner and Kling at the International Neurologic Congress in Brussels (1957), was a mine of information for human sexual pathology. Without going into more specific details, much of what was observed in the behavior of male cats after lesions in the region of the amygdaloid nucleus resembles human perversions. Already this film convinced us that there were solid reasons for undertaking a therapeutic stereotaxic procedure. (pp. 87–88)

Several important points should be made here. First of all, as indicated previously, hypersexuality appears as a consequence of amygdalotomy only in confined postoperative environments. Consequently, its validity as a metaphor for human sexual perversions would seem questionable. Second, there is evidence to implicate the ventromedial hypothalamus in a wide range of behavioural and biological functions in addition to sex (cf. Valenstein, 1973a, b). Third, Roeder and his colleagues derived support from the assertion of Dörner and his associates of separate male and female sex centres in the brains of their laboratory rats. In the usual cerebral arrangement, one of these centres is considered to dominate, depending on the sex of the animal. The destruction of one centre results in a change of dominance. Thus, if the female sex centre (localized in the ventromedial hypothalamus) is destroyed, male sexual behaviour should dominate and any male homosexual tendencies would be abolished. Dörner's views are not shared by most of the mainstream scholars of sexual biology. Few consider that single and separate sex centres regulating the behaviour of each sex represents an acceptable characterization of available evidence. Finally, there is a compelling body of argument to commend the view that, while structural and hormonal influences may dominate with regard to the intensity of sexual interest, in higher animals, especially humans, learning plays the crucial role in the mode of expression of that interest, i.e. its direction (cf. Zuckerman, 1972).

In summary, we can only lament with previous reviewers that the rationales for psychosurgery lack both substance and consistency. Psychosurgeons have tended to resort to rather loose and tenuous allegories as a substitute for direct and sophisticated physiological theory. Further, the general perspectives of brain organization that have traditionally governed their activities are no longer tenable.

As indicated earlier, the concept of narrow localization, with its complementary representation of neural processes as operating like a telephone exchange, was much in evidence in early psychosurgical discourse. Such an outlook on cerebral functioning did much to foster and sustain the development of psychosurgery. Theoretical commitments are never recklessly discarded. Hence, it should be no surprise to find the notion of a highly specific brain persisting in current psychosurgery. Admittedly, its influence is less explicit. Nevertheless, as recently as 1977, Dagi couched the logic for psychosurgery in the following simple terms:

> A syllogism may be proposed:
> I. All function has some anatomical basis
> II. Behavior is a function
> III. Therefore, behavior has some anatomical basis.
> When this syllogism is followed with two possible corrolaries, complexity is gained:
> IIIa. All behavior has a specific locus; therefore, pathological behavior has some specific locus; or
> IIIb. Pathological behavior has a specifically pathological locus.
> It is on these bases that one obtains philosophical justification for the ablation of focal areas. (pp. 518–519)

In addition, the contemporary statements of many psychosurgeons betray a continued allegiance to precise cerebral specificity. Roeder's insistence on a "female sex centre" located in the ventromedial hypothalamus and the treatment of the amygdala as a centre for aggressive behaviour (cf. Hitchcock *et al.*, 1972) serve as examples. Finally, advocacy of narrow localization can be discerned in the ongoing debate about psychiatric disorders and specific brain structures.

Many psychosurgeons have argued vigorously that different psychiatric disorders necessitate different, specifically localized lesions. Cox and Brown (1977) illustrate this view:

> Knowledge of brain function and of neuroanatomical localization of emotion has progressed to the point that specific targets can now be selected for the treatment of certain psychiatric syndromes. Psychosurgery is not a non-specific procedure. (p. 477)

It is difficult to seriously sustain arguments of specificity, however, when it is apparent that identical behavioural disorders often attract radically different surgery. For example, while Sano and his colleagues choose posteromedial hypothalamotomy as the preferred "sedative" for aggressive behaviour, others, such as Balasubramaniam and Narabayashi, treat aggressive behaviour with amygdalotomy.

Some psychosurgeons, in fact, deny that different psychiatric disorders require differently located lesions. Scoville has consistently advocated equipotentiality. As recently as 1972, Scoville wrote:

> Different types of mental disease probably do not require different areas of ablation. The author at variance with some surgeons, believes there is no need to vary the location of operation for neuroses, depressions, schizophrenia, or psychic pain. (p. 18)

The question of specificity in psychosurgery has remained unsolved throughout the history of the practice. Peraita and Lopez de Lerma (1977) recently commented on the lack of consensus attending the practice of traditional frontal lobe surgery:

> Some supported the idea of a quantitative mechanism of action and a close relationship between postoperative deficits and therapeutic result, others attributed more importance to the selectivity of the lesion. (p. 211)

There is no greater agreement today. Valenstein (1977) has commented that such disunion characterizes the level of understanding of basic physiological mechanisms.

Finally, there is little to suggest that settling this dispute would substantially elevate the theoretical status of psychosurgery. Any solution to the specificity question must explicitly acknowledge that the behavioural targets of psychosurgery are complex psychological processes, maintained by intricate arrangements of events in the environment and serviced by a system of cerebral structures working in a concerted and dynamic fashion. Further, any one structure in such a system will contribute to other functional systems in the brain. If this analysis is even marginally accurate, it would seem unreasonable to suppose that psychosurgery can ever aspire to specific effects.

9

Ethical implications of psychosurgery

Several important ethical issues are raised by the practice of psychosurgery; in the present chapter we shall examine these. At the outset, however, it should be appreciated that it is difficult, in the context of psychosurgery, to disengage a discussion of ethics from several recent legal and legislative deliberations. Nevertheless, separation will be attempted, since it should simplify matter of organization. Consequently, Chapter 10 will deal specifically with the legal prescriptions pertaining to psychosurgery. In the present chapter the treatment of the ethical issues will be essentially non-prescriptive. Discussion will centre around the brain's inviolability, the irreversibility of psychosurgery, the moral implications of psychosurgery's scientific status and the problems surrounding consent.

While psychosurgery is presently at the forefront of biomedical ethics, it is important to emphasize that many of the ethical issues stimulated by the practice could be justifiably raised in connection with many contemporary psychiatric and psychological procedures. In fact, in many ways, psychosurgery represents a curious focus for ethical debate. As Brown *et al.* (1975) reflected

> Although psychosurgery is a powerful means of changing behavior, the ethical problems posed by the modification of behavior with drugs or psychotherapy are probably of greater import because these means of control are available to a much wider range of potential "abusers" than are the techniques of psychosurgery. (p. 232)

In a similar vein, Shuman (1977) has urged that drug therapy constitutes a far more urgent subject for ethical consideration. Comparing the scope of behaviour control by drugs and surgery, Shuman commented:

> Even if we leave aside behavior modification drugs dispensed by physicians untrained in psychiatry, prescribed for young children by so-called child psychiatrists, and prescribed by pediatricians, it is clear that the number reachable by drugs is enormously greater than the number reachable by surgery. (p. 96)

Further, techniques that rely on external environmental manipulations should be included in any comprehensive moral discourse. In fact, most forms of behaviour control concentrate on manipulating the external rather than the internal environment. The therapies derived from classical and operant conditioning usually spring to mind in this context. However, such practices seem merely to represent highly streamlined versions of the processes that conventionally regulate human socialization and development, that govern behavioural control via the media and via formal education and that operate more or less casually in everyday social encounters.

This would seem to imply that it is in the phenomenon of behaviour control *per se* that demands careful scrutiny rather than any particular style of control. However, the very omnipresence of this phenomenon necessarily prohibits fruitful ethical debate. In essence, behaviour control is an ethically vacuous topic. Begelman (1973) pinpointed the difficulty:

> Ethical issues arising over behavioral control are not – nor can they ever sensibly be said to be – issues over whether behavioral control is morally legitimate. This is because the concept of behavioral control itself is too wide or generic to permit meaningful moral questions to be raised concerning it. Such questions can only arise in connection with undertaking specific types of behavioral control in particular circumstances. (p. 413)

Begelman's argument, that for ethical questions to be meaningful they must be asked in the context of specific techniques of behaviour control, is persuasive. However, he does not tackle the issue of why moral questions are far more commonly posed in conjunction with some techniques, such as psychosurgery, than others. Why should psychosurgery constitute a primary focus for contemporary debate? Two major factors might be considered.

First of all, there is the fairly widespread opinion that the human brain is inviolable. Neville's (1975) commentary indicates the contention that the human brain demands unique respect:

> Whereas his environment, perhaps even his hair and fingernails,

legitimately might be alienated from him for good social reasons, his body, especially the irreplaceable brain and nervous systems, are more nearly inviolable in a moral sense. (p. 88)

Some proponents of the inviolability thesis point to the utter complexity of the brain compared to other surgical targets and the commensurate ignorance that attends its workings. They submit that incomplete knowledge precludes surgical interventions. Two sorts of opposing argument have been voiced. The first asserts that substantial ignorance is usually a temporary condition; the second that all knowledge is incomplete anyway. Certainly, these arguments temper the case for inviolability based on complexity. By citing precedent, i.e. seeming complexity did not preclude surgical innovations on other organs, and asserting that the present ignorance will subside as brain science advances, they suggest that an inviolability thesis, can only, at best, be maintained temporarily. However, these two arguments should not escape comment. First of all, while the biological rationale for psychosurgery is no more inadequate than that governing other drastic techniques of behaviour control (electroconvulsive shock therapy is a case in point), the conceptual ignorance surrounding psychosurgical operations far exceeds that associated with other major surgical enterprises. Secondly, future advances in brain science seem just as likely to condemn psychosurgery as they are to commend it.

It is more usual to find the inviolability thesis relying not on cerebral complexity but on the psychological or even spiritual significance of the brain. Here, the brain is variously cited as "the seat of the soul", "the spiritual self", "the most intimate environment of the person himself" or "the executive apparatus of the individual" (cf. Shuman, 1977) in order to convey its sanctity. Such status is presumed to exempt the brain from psychosurgical interference. Some psychosurgeons have been decidedly unimpressed by this sort of advocacy. Ballantine (1972) exemplifies: "The brain is no longer a sacred organ, excluded from surgical therapy because it houses the human soul" (p. 30).

While it is possible that psychological events might be mediated by cerebral processes yet somehow transcend them, the neurosciences assume not. Behaviour is viewed as stemming from the concerted working of neural systems. However, asserting that the behaviour of man depends on systems of neurons does not in itself license surgical tampering as Ballantine seems to presume. As indicated in the previous chapter, the manner in which neural systems regulate behaviour is a crucial consideration.

It is fairly apparent that, in its usual expression, the inviolability thesis does not possess the necessary precision and objectivity to satisfy scientific discourse. However, what it lacks in rigour and clarity, it certainly makes up for in affective tone. This tone has been accurately captured by Gaylin (1975):

> We all have a healthy revulsion against penetration of our innards, and surgically messing around with the brain has its own built-in controls in the aversive effect the very images present. (p. 21)

Delgado (1969) is undoubtedly correct in asserting that the notion of inviolability of the brain is simply a social construct, like nudity. However, it is a peculiarly academic conceit which insists that as such it should not impinge on therapeutic conduct. Widely and intensely held feelings in such matters should never be summarily dismissed, even though they may lack any obvious rational basis.

One final aspect of the inviolability thesis deserves mention. Its proponents usually reserve submissions of inviolability for psychosurgical procedures. Neurosurgical operations embarking from clear indications of organic pathology are exempted. This implies that feelings regarding inviolability are mediated to a large extent by concern at the destruction of healthy tissue. The intentional destruction of healthy tissue certainly warrants discussion. Those defending the practice in psychosurgery point out that it is a usual feature in surgical interventions. One of Gaylin's (1975) numerous examples illustrates his general proposition:

> An individual with a peptic ulcer in his duodenum may have his healthy stomach removed because of the functions of the stomach in secreting hydrochloric acid (due to conditions unknown but often psychologically aggravated) encourage ulceration of the duodenal wall. (p. 16)

Moving to the brain, an example is afforded by the corpus callosectomies conducted by Vogel in California. These were undertaken to limit severe epileptic discharges. Here again the surgical target was noticeably displaced from any pathological focus; the tissue excised was healthy. These ablations and, in particular, their cognitive and perceptual sequelae occasioned mild curiosity rather than widespread disquiet. Such precedents seem to undermine any general "healthy tissue" principle. However, it should be stressed that, although healthy tissue was excised in each of the cases above, surgery was undertaken in the interests of alleviating an explicit organic pathology. In psychosurgery there are no firm organic indications to give comfort to the surgeon. Surgical indications are solely behavioural. Thus, a somewhat qualified "healthy tissue" principle would seem to distinguish psychosurgery from most other surgical endeavours.

The disappearing practice of bilateral hand amputation to curb kleptomania, where there is nothing to implicate physical pathology might also be fitted into this modified "healthy tissue" model. Breggin (1973a) was certainly impressed by the similarities:

> ... psychosurgical operations are best compared to the still more ancient practices of cutting off a limb or poking out the eyes of accused criminals. (p. 13)

The second major issue that has undoubtedly focused ethical attention on psychosurgery is the matter of irreversibility. Its critical role in ethical deliberations has been recognized by several authorities. The primary concerns regarding irreversibility seem to stem from the presumed permanence of the behavioural changes engineered through psychosurgery and not from the fact of permanent anatomical damage. It is argued that this permanence distinguishes psychosurgery from other means of behavioural control. In contrast to psychosurgery, behavioural changes achieved through manipulation of the external environment are considered reversible, as are alterations produced by many pharmaceuticals.

There is good cause, however, to question the adequacy of this dichotomy. First of all, while permanent behavioural change may be a likely result of permanent neural interference, it is not a necessary or certain outcome of such disruption. Behaviour functions frequently show remarkable resistance in the face of gross neural insults. Brain lesions frequently cause far less disruption to behavioural capacity than might be immediately expected from the volume of tissue destroyed.

Further, the systems model of brain functional organization, described in the preceding chapter, stresses cerebral flexibility and plasticity. Luria (1973), it will be remembered, contended that psychological functions are best conceived not as simple functions with narrow cerebral locations but as complex functional systems having correspondingly complex structural foundations. A major characteristic of complex functional systems according to Luria, is the interchangeability of their components. Thus, in contrast to a narrow localization telephone exchange perspective on brain organization, a systems approach clearly allows for substantial functional reorganization following a brain lesion.

It is interesting to note that critics relying on the irreversibility argument frequently assume what seems like a narrow localization perspective. For example, Phyllis Breggin (1974) argued:

> Psychosurgery is an irreversible process; damaged brain cells deteriorate rather than regenerate. A victim of such an operation can never recover the loss of a portion of his brain and his related capacities to create, to learn, to choose, in essence, to be a free person. Certain choices and responses have been irrevocably taken away from him. (p. 21)

Although the acknowledgement of cerebral plasticity in no way justifies contemporary psychosurgery, it does, however, diminish opposition based exclusively on the notion of irreversibility.

A second aspect of the irreversibility case concerns the notion that other modes of behavioural control are reversible. Control based on manipulation of the external environment is usually cited as the clearest example. However, while behavioural changes so based are in theory reversible, in practice they frequently defy easy subsequent amendment. The intransigence of well-learned habits has been extensively documented.

In addition, it now seems quite likely that, with prolonged exposure, other organic therapies eventually disrupt cerebral integrity as much as psychosurgery. Electroconvulsive shock therapy provides us with a good example. As Scoville (1973) commented:

> ... it is to be remembered that any extensive or long continued shock therapy may well be more destructive to brain function than are the new limited surgical operations. (p. 7)

Behavioural control by drugs has also been credited with irreversible tissue disruption. Thus, it would seem that, if permanent destruction of neural tissue in psychosurgery is to attract ethical scrutiny, the other organic therapies should not escape notice.

In conclusion, irreversibility would seem a rather weak base from which to mount scientific opposition to psychosurgery. First of all, as we stressed earlier, irreversible neural disruption does not necessarily imply irrevocable changes in functional capacity. Second, there is little reason to suspect that, in practice, non-surgical behavioural influences, including environmentally based effects, produce changes that are phenomenally less permanent than those produced by surgery. Finally, and most importantly, it is the ambition of all behavioural interventions to fashion reliable alterations in behaviour. Consequently, it is not on the reversibility of a behavioural change that our critical focus should be trained, but on its desirability. (Desirability is an issue to which we shall return.)

We have now considered aspects of psychosurgery that have been cited as accounting for its prominence in current ethical discussions. However, it has proved difficult to isolate scientifically-reliable grounds for distinguishing psychosurgery from other behavioural control procedures and/or surgical practice. The qualified "healthy tissue" principle elaborated previously seems to provide the most tenable rational basis for according psychosurgery special status. Submissions based on irreversibility are not totally compelling. In addition, the conspicuousness of psychosurgery seems to stem in part from beliefs that although widely shared, do not readily permit logical analysis. Some of the expressions of the inviolability thesis provide examples here. Such opinion obviously constitutes a legitimate part of moral and social discourse. However, any expressedly rational treatment of psychosurgery should be more usefully served by concentrating on those issues which are accessible to analysis.

Ultimately, the ethical status of psychosurgery interacts intimately with its scientific status. Questions of inviolability and irreversibility necessarily defer to questions of validity and efficacy.

As Shuman (1977) stated:

> Only when there is adequate scientific reason to believe that a change will probably be desirable ... should surgical intervention be considered as a potentially proper treatment. (p. 103)

However, it should be stressed that decisions regarding desirability are mediated to an extent by social and political considerations. They are not simply a matter of science. As Winkler (1977) commented, "Desirability depends on who and where you are in a society" (p. 92). Nevertheless, questions of scientific justification remain important. In Chapter 11, we shall examine some of the dynamics of social influence. For the moment though, let us consider the importance of psychosurgery's scientific status in ethical matters.

The ethical issues that attend a scientifically valid and efficacious procedure are invariably different from those surrounding an invalid and ineffective one. We are not suggesting here that ample validity somehow discharges behavioural manipulations from the moral arena. As Begelman (1973) advised, "Therapeutic practice without exception is inextricably bound up with values, in both subtle and complex ways" (p. 414).

Several enthusiastic advocates of psychosurgery apparently believe otherwise. Debating the ethics of psychosurgical approaches to a wide range of behavioural and social problems, Rollin (1973) offered the following dismissive comments:

> I have often been dismayed by the pontification of those who oppose such approaches to these problems; the overriding needs of the sufferer are then lost in sterile debate. (p. 594)

Begelman (1973) dealt harshly with such myopia:

> Proponents of the amorality of using certain techniques of behavior change do not belong in therapy, because they do not belong anywhere. (pp. 418–419)

Certain ethical issues seem to transcend, at least to an extent, the scientific status of a therapeutic enterprise. Questions regarding consent feature among these and will be considered later in this chapter. Problems surrounding the concepts of mental health and abnormality will be dealt with in Chapter 11. However, many of the moral implications of psychosurgery are plainly shaped by considerations of its validity.

It is clear from our previous discussion that opinions differ markedly regarding the scientific status of psychosurgery. In order to acquire the stamp of scientific approval, it is usual for a prospective therapy to fulfil two main conditions. First of all, there must be sound empirical evidence that the therapy achieves its stated aims. Second, the therapy must be supported by a consistent and adequate theoretical infrastructure. When a therapy is relatively more intrusive, assaultive and hazardous, we might reasonably insist on a further condition: that it is relatively more effective than less risky procedures.

What, then, is the scientific status of psychosurgery, and what ethical dilemmas does it consequently present? It is clear that, in spite of protestations to the contrary, psychosurgery is still without a reliable and substantial biological rationale. However, clinical practice has invariably placed greater emphasis on empirical evidence of effectiveness. Here the superficial indications at least are more favourable. However, a more critical examination of the empirical evidence relating to psychosurgical procedures tends to dispel overconfidence. Glaring weaknesses in experimental design and clinical assessment, persistent problems with surgical accuracy and the ever-present shadow of adverse sequelae combine to substantially undermine the empirical case for psychosurgery.

Is psychosurgery, then, to be accorded merely experimental status? Our assessment of the theoretical and empirical indications for psychosurgical procedures would hardly commend the thesis that they possess adequate scientific credentials.

If we consider that "experimental" constitutes an appropriate designation, questions of degree arise, such as how experimental is psychosurgery? At one end of the continuum of clinical experimentation can be located purely experimental research. Here therapeutic aspirations and pretensions are minimal. Psychosurgery as a purely experimental exercise is clearly deplorable. Even the most committed of psychosurgeons assure us of their disapproval.

By consistently invoking therapeutic aims, psychosurgeons have circumvented much of the moral indignation that would attend purely experimental cerebral ablations. Bailey *et al.* (1977) illustrate this commitment to the therapeutic perspective:

> ... the operator proceeds on the basis that he expects and strives to do good, to relieve suffering, pain, or deformity to the best of his professional skills as required by the current state of the art. (p. 501)

Thus, if psychosurgery is to be viewed as experimental, the model preferred by psychosurgeons would be that of therapeutic research. The ideal therapeutic experiment should be appropriately placed at the other end of the clinical research continuum, to pure scientific research. Andy (1977) characterized it as follows:

> Therapeutic research is therapy that has not been clinically established and proven, but there have been sufficient clinical experience and scientific knowledge to justify its use and to expect the individual to benefit from the procedure. Therapeutic research in psychosurgery

> should not be based on scientific data obtained only from animal experimentation. It should be based principally on a critical retrospective analysis of clinical observations and experience. (p. 506)

It is clear that a wide range of psychosurgical procedures do not meet Andy's criteria of ideal therapeutic research. Roeder and his associates, for example, embarked on ventromedial hypothalamic surgery solely on the basis of animal experimentation. From our discussion in the previous chapter, it is clear that a similar dependence on animal research characterized the development of other operations. In fact, some commentators have speculated that the whole modern practice of psychosurgery would never have emerged but for that placid chimpanzee Becky.

It may be reasoned that the ethical obstacles presented by hazardous experiments on human subjects increase markedly as one moves along the experimental continuum from ideal therapeutic research to pure experimental activities. In this respect, it should be stressed that to qualify as ideal, therapeutic research must be based on substantial retrospective clinical data. The definition of ideal is not a matter of the vigour of the surgeon's protestations regarding patient benefits. The psychosurgeons undertaking the experiments mentioned above uniformly insisted on the primacy of patient interests. However, it is readily apparent that from the extensive frontal incisions of the past to the more restricted variations of the present, psychosurgical experiments have rarely had the support of even the most modest retrospective clinical data.

In summary, psychosurgery has frequently failed to conform to even the most lenient interpretation of what constitutes ideal therapeutic research. In spite of benevolent declarations of therapeutic intent, many procedures would seem more appropriately located at some distance from the therapeutic experimental end of the continuum.

Psychosurgery's precise experimental status has important implications for recent discussions about a prospective controlled trial. There seem to be three opinions in this matter.

First of all, it has been argued that with a therapy of such proven accuracy a controlled trial is redundant. From this perspective several other ethical issues emerge. Brown *et al.* (1975) indicated the basis dilemma:

> While good clinical practice demands that the individual always be a patient first, scientific studies often demand the witholding of an experimental treatment from some patients while providing it to others in order to compare the effectiveness of the new treatment with older treatments or with no treatment. However, there are those who dispute the right to withhold treatment of potential value from anyone under any conditions. (p. 233)

This "right to treatment" thesis in its widest context represents a general reaction against those critics of contemporary psychiatric practice, such as Szasz (1961), who advocate the deinstitutionalization and deprofessionalization of mental health care. This is a matter to which we shall return in Chapter 11. Let us for the moment consider the right to treatment in the specific context of a proposed prospective controlled trial of psychosurgery. Clearly, the right to treatment here is difficult to defend on rational grounds. Without previous satisfactory controlled trials, statements according to psychosurgery "potential value" have minimal scientific status.

A second class of opinion also opposes a controlled trial, but on the grounds that psychosurgery lacks acceptable theoretical support and the sort of ratio of positive to negative empirical indications that favour further research. A controlled trial, it is argued, would simply expose patients to ill-founded and potentially dangerous procedures. Our overall assessment of psychosurgery certainly commends this argument more than the previous one.

A third body of opinion holds that a prospective controlled trial is long overdue and should help settle much of the controversy that surrounds contemporary psychosurgery. The Report of the Research Committee of the Royal College of Psychiatrists (1977) illustrated:

> Psychosurgery has never been subjected to a prospective controlled trial, which contemporary scientific opinion regards as essential for the assessment of new treatment. (p. 176)

Two major considerations favour a prospective controlled trial. First mainstream opposition to psychosurgery seems fairly receptive to a scientifically sound proposal. Although some commentators base their criticism very much on the spectacular abuse, studied opposition to psychosurgery is more usually founded on errors of omission rather than commission. It is argued that psychosurgical experiments fail to meet the usual demands of scientific objectivity. A prospective controlled trial would seem a natural corollary of the contention that the superficial indications of success from uncontrolled studies should not be trusted. While the impoverished theoretical foundation of psychosurgery constitutes a contraindication, it can again be countered that theory frequently lags behind therapeutic practice. The urgency of clinical demands rarely permits otherwise. However, it must be interjected here that only a few of the many psychosurgical procedures can boast even superficial indications of success.

The second argument for a controlled trial is decidedly more cynical. Psychosurgery is almost certain to continue in the foreseeable future, albeit in a more regulated milieu. It would seem markedly preferable to embed future operations in a prospective controlled trial than to carry on in the present informal and uncontrolled manner. In concluding this discussion, we can do no better than direct the reader to Strauss's (1973) apt remarks. Strauss posed the following question:

> The question I wish to raise is whether it is ever ethical to employ a new therapy except under such conditions that valid conclusions regarding its value can be drawn. (p. 1183)

Strauss's answer was unequivocal:

> Let me now answer my original question by stating that no experimental method of treatment may be ethically employed except under such conditions that valid conclusions may be drawn. "Informed consent" of the patient is not enough, and committees on human experimentation should carefully consider experimental design as well as risk. (p. 1183)

The preceding discussion has been conducted on the premise that psychosurgical procedures are still experimental. While our analysis clearly indicates this perspective, let us for the moment abandon scientific purism and give greater credence than previously to superficial indications of success – the results of uncontrolled studies and the informal testimonials of experienced clinicians that psychosurgery works. A question of some moral significance immediately arises. In what manner does psychosurgery work? Has a cure been effected, or is the operation simply a palliative measure?

Curative measures are depicted as directly attacking a pathology at its source. Palliative therapies, on the other hand, may alleviate symptoms, but this is achieved indirectly, i.e. through mediating processes. However, mediation is an elusive matter. It is rarely possible to distinguish a direct from a mediated effect with any measure of confidence. A more tangible distinction between curative and palliative measures might be based on the related issue of specificity. "Cure" would here be reserved for the specific elimination of specific target symptoms, with "palliative" denoting instances of non-specific, generalized outcomes and/or non-specific behavioural aims. In palliative surgery, the incidence of a specific target symptom may be attenuated but only because the change with regard to the target symptom is subsumed in a fairly general constellation of operative effects. The change in the target symptom arises from its correlation with other more general processes disrupted by the operation. Alternatively, the procedure may be explicitly acknowledged as palliative, i.e. only general behavioural aims were entertained.

Given the validity of this distinction, there are several reasons for regarding psychosurgery as an essentially palliative measure. First of all, the systems model of brain functional organization advocated earlier postulates that even the most localized lesions will give rise to a constellation or syndrome of effects rather than to changes in some specific symptom or other. Second, the early psychosurgical operations can be considered palliative. While the behavioural aim of these procedures was to eliminate the compulsions and obsessions of disturbed psychotic patients, any resultant symptomatic relief was embedded in a range of emotional and behavioural changes.

Although the newer psychosurgical procedures are more circumscribed in terms of tissue destruction, there is little reason to suspect that their essential character has altered. In fact, the language of many modern psychosurgeons clearly betrays the palliative nature of their activities. "Behavioural management" increasingly replaces more specific symptomatic objectives, while "sedative neurosurgery" readily conveys a palliative intent. Even where more specific curative aims are invoked, it is extremely doubtful that cures are, in fact, being effected. Roeder and his associates (e.g. Roeder *et al.*, 1972) exemplify. The symptoms of male paedophilic homosexuality, it will be recalled, comprise Roeder's specific surgical target. The ventromedial hypothalamus is accordingly ablated. While Roeder insists that a specific cure is affected, Valenstein's (1973a) assessment is probably more accurate:

> ... the evidence presented makes it clear that the major effect of surgery is to produce a general lowering of sexual drive. (p. 323)

The manner in which psychosurgery works, cure or palliative, has an important ethical consequence. Although there is nothing intrinsically repugnant about palliative measures, they should be more susceptible to the constraints of "risk" than curative procedures; i.e. while risky curative procedures are ethically permissible, risky palliative procedures are not. Given our ignorance of cerebral processes, psychosurgery could easily be regarded as risky. Certainly, it is decidedly more risky than alternative, less assaultive, psychotherapeutic palliatives.

Psychosurgery continues to provide a necessary focus for several wide-ranging ethical issues. For the remainder of this chapter we shall consider the most consistently controversial of these – the issue of consent.

Ideally, the requirement for consent should guarantee a patient's active involvement in decisions affecting him. McCaughey (1977) illustrated:

> Consent must not be thought of simply as a legal protection for the doctor. It is an essential way of involving others in the responsible decision of the surgeon. (p. 106)

However, even the most casual perusal of pronouncements on psychiatric decision making reveals little consensus on the matter of how the burden of decision making should be distributed. Andy (1977), for example, strongly advocated the primacy of the doctor and the institution employing him. Patient consultation was presented as discretionary rather than mandatory.

In defending their relative primacy in the matter, doctors frequently argue that the patient's very act of coming to hospital constitutes a delegation of decision making to the doctor. As Crow (1977) insisted:

> A patient comes to me and says he is suffering and he asks for help. I give it if I can, I do not go out and offer treatment to people ...

> Patients ask for treatment, they are not sought out by psychiatrists and surgeons ... (p. 120)

Neville (1975), however, indicated the shortcomings of this argument:

> It is doubtful, however ... that the consequences of hospital admission can ever be predicted with sufficient clarity for this argument to hold. Therefore consent rests with the patient or his proxy. (p. 108)

Clearly, treatment without patient consent is morally pernicious. There is a fairly general consensus on this matter. However, merely obtaining mechanical consent is insufficient. Where patient participation in therapeutic decision making is simply a platitudinous exercise, consent amounts to no more than a surety for doctors and their immediate employers.

In order to ensure patient control over psychosurgical procedures, the consent facility must embody certain crucial attributes. Consent should be informed, it should be rational and it should be voluntary. Let us consider each of these in turn.

Several commentators have emphasized that proper consent must be informed. For consent to be classed as informed, the patient must receive a reasonable explanation of the proposed procedures. This explanation must identify those aspects of the procedure which are experimental; the most conservative model of what comprises an experimental procedure should apply here. Not only should potential benefits be described but also attendant risks and discomforts. Possible alternatives to the proposed therapy must be rehearsed, and the patient should be encouraged at all times to ask questions.

Neville (1975) examined the circumstances that counteract optimally informed consent. First of all, the procedure for which consent is required may have unpredictable consequences. Neville surveyed the implications of unpredictability:

> Procedures that are "experimental" are those for which it is problematic that informed consent can be given. It is dubious that informed consent is possible when the doctors can say only that possible results fall within a wide range of alternatives. In these cases no one would be in a position to give or to withhold consent, and the procedure should not be employed. (p. 109)

It is perhaps unnecessary to recount that our previous analysis is not inconsistent with the view that contemporary psychosurgery comprises just such "experimental" procedures. However, Neville permitted an exception to the usual prohibitions consequent on unpredictability. This occurs when one of the wide range of possible outcomes would be as undesirable as refraining from the procedure or employing an alternative procedure.

However, psychosurgery can hardly be regarded as a critical intervention, i.e. as an emergency treatment. Psychosurgery is not a response to sudden infirmity; invariably the pertinent behavioural symptoms have been available for inspection and treatment for some time. Further, as indicated previously, alternative, less assaultive therapies rarely wield the same potential for catastrophe as psychosurgery. In defence, psychosurgeons usually protest that surgery was considered only after less assaultive therapies had been tried and found unsuccessful. While such protestations have been effective in the past, they are now treated with due scepticism (cf. Valenstein, 1973a).

Informed consent can also be limited by the doctor's failure to provide the patient with available information. The requirement for full disclosure, it can be argued, should be waived under certain exceptional circumstances, such as emergency treatment. The range of exceptions are usually subsumed under the general rubric of "therapeutic privilege". In its most frequently encountered form, "therapeutic privilege" attests that if it can be reasonably assumed that a patient's condition would be worsened by full disclosure, then disclosure is not required. However, as Shuman (1977) was quick to point out, such privilege is readily open to abuse:

> The therapeutic privilege is easily abused because treating physicians can so readily manipulate patients and situations to create an environment in which fuller disclosure plausibly would have "worsened the patient's 'condition'." The therapeutic privilege thus becomes a mechanism by which a sincere but authoritarian physician, convinced that the patient's medical condition cannot be improved except by a proposed therapy, can insure the receipt of informed consent by defending the nondisclosure of relevant risks. (p. 147)

In the specific milieu of psychosurgical operations, "therapeutic privilege" would seem a morally pernicious practice. With psychosurgery, we can see no alternative to properly informed consent.

To be meaningful, consent should not only be informed but also rational. Neville (1975) indicated what is implied by "rational" in this context:

> This means that the decision maker must not only be apprised of the consequences of the alternatives, he must also be able to approach the decision in a normal frame of mind, enabling him to act with maximum sensitivity to the real values involved. (p. 109)

The frequently encountered assertions that psychosurgery should not be permitted on young children, mental retardates or involuntarily institutionalized individuals is to some extent founded on the belief that such individuals cannot give rational consent.

However, decisions regarding an individual's rationality are notoriously difficult. They should not be the exclusive responsibility of the treating physician since, as in the case of "therapeutic privilege", abuses would be inevitable in such circumstances.

Where rationality cannot be assumed, the conventional practice is to revert to proxy consent. This immediately poses the question of who would best act as proxy consenter. Various possibilities suggest themselves – the treating physician, next of kin, an independent committee and so on. A case has been made in the past for the treating physician (cf. de Lange, 1973). However, the doctor as proxy consenter would undermine the whole consent requirement. Simply by labelling a patient's opinions as pathologically derived, the treating physician can circumvent the consent procedure. Neville (1975) clearly favoured the next of kin. The legitimacy of the next of kin in matters of proxy consent is widely approved.

While the next of kin model might be satisfactory in most cases, specific problems can be readily envisaged. The next of kin must be maximally sensitive and rational. In some instances, this will be in doubt, and the validity of proxy consent will be compromised accordingly. Neville (1975) provided an example:

> We would be disinclined, for instance, to allow a mother suffering from severe postpartum depression to make decisions concerning procedures to sustain the life of a deformed child. (pp. 109–110)

Clearly, superordinate decisions have to be.made regarding the suitability of the next of kin as a proxy consenter. It is here that an independent committee would be useful. The same committee could reasonably preside over questions regarding the patient's fitness to consent or dissent. It could also be enjoined to consider the other conditions of consent, i.e. to ensure that consent was informed and voluntary. Thus the committee's usual role would be that of a referee, policing the general circumstances of consent and ascertaining the competence of the patient and his personal proxy. However, where neither the patient nor his personal proxy were deemed to meet acceptable standards of sensitivity and rationality, the committee should assume powers of proxy. The general role of such an independent committee in psychosurgery will be explored more fully in the next chapter. For the moment, it is sufficient to indicate here that the committee must be broad-based and fully informed.

In developing protocols for ideal consent procedures it is usual to insist that consent should not only be informed and rational but also voluntary, i.e. the consenter should be free from coercion. Much of the controversy that has recently surrounded psychosurgery stems from its use in essentially coercive environments. Our discussion here will focus exclusively on involuntarily institutionalized mental patients. Considerations relating to individuals confined for reasons of criminal behaviour and/or sociopolitical deviance will be waived until the next chapter.

One body of opinion holds that voluntary consent is impossible for patients in an involuntary, institutional milieu. It is possible to discern two propositions in arguments of this sort. The first submits that the actions of voluntary and involuntary patients are governed by qualitatively different dynamics. Consequently, these two groups of patients should be regarded as different for purposes of consent. The second proposition is dependent of the first: namely, that the involuntary patient's singularly vulnerable status in fact disqualifies him from the consent process. This has been referred to as the "no consent doctrine" (Shuman, 1977). Let us consider these in turn.

First of all, are voluntary and involuntary patients phenomenally different and do they merit separate consideration as regards consent? Many psychosurgeons appear to attach little significance to the now well-documented case that, within a total institution, the distribution of power is markedly uneven and the vulnerability of inmates is considerable. Andy (1977) illustrates:

> The guidelines for psychosurgical therapeutic experimentation upon institutionalized patients should be the same as those established for the non-institutionalized. (p. 509)

Here, equivalence regarding consent is advocated from a rather narrow perspective that makes light of the coercive aspects of institutional existence.

The argument that voluntary and involuntary patients should be treated alike is more persuasively based on the thesis that coercion is not a consequence of an involuntary status but constitutes a general feature of physician–patient interactions. As Gaylin (1975) perceptively inquired, "Isn't there always a coercive aspect inherent in the authoritarian position of the physician?" (p. 12)

The social pressures that motivate the voluntary patient are both subtle and pervasive. Winkler (1977) commented:

> People defining themselves as ill are reflecting the institutional structures in the society in which they live, and people requesting treatment may well be reflecting the social pressures to define themselves in certain sorts of ways. It takes a strong will to resist these pressures. (p. 120)

Thus, it would seem difficult to defend an absolute or even qualitative distinction between voluntary and involuntary patients; both groups are subject to coercion. However, there is every reason to suspect that a quantitative distinction exists; the involuntary patient is subject to a much more single-minded and compelling regime. While this analysis certainly commends vigilance in matters of consent with regard to the involuntarily institutionalized, it does not inevitably imply that separate consent criteria be established for voluntary and involuntary patients.

According to the second proposition, involuntary patients are necessarily incapable of voluntary consent. A range of options immediately present themselves:

1. Consent is not needed with involuntary patients; treatment can proceed without it.

2. Since they cannot give adequate consent, involuntary patients should be exempt from certain procedures; it is with this option in mind that the proposition is usually voiced.

3. Proxy consent is the appropriate practice with involuntarily institutionalized individuals.

At the outset, it is important to stress again that treatment without consent remains a morally precarious undertaking. The second option has little more to commend it. Exempting or disqualifying involuntary patients from particular procedures on the basis of consent is hard to justify on any grounds. How can consent criteria be established that permit some procedures and prohibit others for involuntary patients while, at the same time, allowing voluntary patients access to both? In addition, it can be argued that the selective prohibition of treatments for involuntarily institutionalized individuals constitutes a further encroachment on their already eroded civil liberties. Rather than affording inmates protection from institutional coercion, prohibitions of this nature simply compound the circumstances of coercion. Finally, while proxy consent might provide an adequate solution in many cases, it should not be regarded as a general answer to the problem of consent with respect to involuntarily institutionalization.

Whenever feasible, consent should rest with the patient. As indicated previously, ideal consent procedures distribute the burden of medical decision making more equitably and, in particular, ensure the active participation of the patient in decisions that intimately affect him. Sentiments that serve merely to isolate further the involuntarily institutionalized individual by minimizing his access to medical decisions seem decidedly misplaced.

Our consent committee might usefully assume responsibility for scrutinizing the conduct of consent procedures in involuntary patients. Working from the brief implied by the analysis above, that involuntary institutionalization *per se* does not preclude consent, the committee would be charged with assessing whether the involuntary status of a particular patient in a particular setting undermined the other requirements of consent (i.e. that consent must be informed and rational). If the patient's status was deemed to mitigate rationality, the power of consent would be delegated to an acceptable proxy. If the usual proxy (next of kin) proved unacceptable, the committee, as indicated previously, should assume the role. In the absence of full disclosure, whether from negligence or insensitivity on the part of the institution or from the unpredictability of the proposed therapy, the committee would not allow treatment to proceed.

In this chapter we have examined the ethical issues that attend psychosurgery. In doing so, we have outlined a format for policing the requirement for consent. In the next chapter we shall consider the various models for policing and regulating the practice of psychosurgery.

10

The regulation of psychosurgery

In the preceding chapter we considered the ethical issues surrounding psychosurgery. However, our treatment of these issues was, for the most part, divorced from the matter of regulation. Accordingly, in the present chapter, we shall focus specifically on the various prescriptions that have been offered for policing and controlling the practice of psychosurgery.

At the outset, it is important to indicate that clinical practice has rarely been subject to formal external regulation (Bromberger, 1977). Certainly, the first wave of psychosurgical operations encountered no formal regulatory obstacles. Addressing the problems involved in drafting a statute to police the use of lobotomy, the Stanford Law Review (1949) concluded:

> ... the greater good will be achieved by avoiding legislative fetters and relying for protection on the high standards of the medical profession and the individuals who compose it. (p. 474)

This laissez faire ethic prevailed for the next two decades. As Annas and Glantz (1974) commented, "throughout the 1950s and 1960s, psychosurgery was ignored by the legal community" (p. 251). It is an arrangement that continues to attract wide support from the medical profession. In an editorial of *Biological Psychiatry*, Wortis (1972) contested the wisdom of legislating against contemporary psychosurgery. His comments are reminiscent of the 1949 submission:

> There is room in our society for some mandatory laws for health and sanitation, but they should be few and cautious. It is simply not possible to settle our scientific differences through legislation, or to insure good medical practice of judgment by laws. (p. 100)

In the face of such persistent opposition within the medical profession, are there persuasive arguments in favour of regulation? There are, in fact, several good reasons for submitting that psychosurgery warrants regulatory attention.

First of all, our present analysis indicates that psychosurgery still lacks an adequate scientific rationale and possesses only superficial and precarious empirical support. Given that the efficacy and validity of psychosurgery are still in doubt, regulation is appropriate. Second, only in a regulated milieu will it be possible to insist on the experimental control and assessment procedures necessary to properly evaluate the therapeutic status and utility of psychosurgery.

Third, there is now substantial public concern and even alarm about psychosurgery, particularly in the United States. Admittedly, much of this is based on the perhaps unlikely proposition that psychosurgery offers the potential for unlimited social control and the somewhat metaphysical construct that the brain is inviolable. Nevertheless, widespread and intensely held views, whether grounded in logic or not, demand formal recognition; the regulation of psychosurgery would seem the appropriate response.

Finally, in spite of protestations to the contrary, psychosurgery is not simply a medical concern. It is, as we have indicated in the previous chapter, a matter of social ethics. In fact, it is difficult to contest the case that all medical treatment and experimentation embodies issues of morality. This is emphatically so when the treatment or experiment is aimed specifically at altering behaviour. (The failure of some psychosurgeons to even recognize the existence of fundamental ethical problems is, in itself, a powerful argument for external regulation.) When confronted with far-reaching ethical questions, the matter of consent, for example, it has usually proved propitious to formulate regulations for the purpose of guidance and arbitration.

Having established that external control is warranted – to protect patients exposed to experimental procedures, to improve the conduct of psychosurgery, to reflect the public concern, and to provide clarification on complex ethical issues – let us consider what style of regulation would be appropriate. Several models have been put forward.

The least radical and intrusive model for regulation involves the scrutiny of proposals for psychosurgery by peer review committees. As Offir (1974) wryly commented, these are "the physician's peers, not the patient's" (p. 59). Since 1966, such committees have been an integral part of federally funded American hospitals. Further, some legislation has placed great emphasis on peer review committees. For example, in Australia, the New

South Wales Mental Health Act of 1959 (cf. Maddison, 1977) made provisions for the establishment of a leucotomy committee to deal with proposals for psychosurgery on involuntarily committed patients. The committee, currently consisting of three psychiatrists and a neurosurgeon, presents its recommendations to the Director of State Psychiatric Services for approval and the notification of the next of kin for proxy consent. If the proxy disapproves, and the Director considers this disapproval unreasonable, the matter is put before the Master of Protective Jurisdiction of the Supreme Court for determination. Several Australian commentators have been critical of this review system. Winkler (1977), for example, contended that, since most psychosurgery in Australia is conducted in private practice, any review procedure should be widened to include voluntary patients.

The legislation recently enacted in California does, in fact, make this sort of provision for voluntary patients. This legislation has been effective since 1977 and is directed specifically at voluntary patients, whether institutionalized or not. Separate legislation has been enacted for individuals within the criminal justice system, and this will be considered later. The California review committee comprises three physicians. They are charged with reviewing both the patient's consent and the merits of the operation; in particular, the committee must be satisfied that all alternative, less drastic treatments have been exhausted before granting approval for psychosurgery.

The rationale underlying the peer review system is straightforward. Edgar (1975) elaborated:

> The theory is that the professional deals with issues and utilizes techniques requiring special expertise, and that only those blessed with expertise can assess his (*the psychosurgeon's*) skill. (pp. 130–131)

Edgar clearly harboured doubts concerning this thesis:

> The argument may be grounded more on monopoly than in reason. (p. 131)

Several other commentators have voiced similar concern about peer review systems (cf. Valenstein, 1973a).

Winkler (1977) cited a case (Tom) to illustrate the inadequacies of the Australian peer review system:

> Although Tom's case was initially considered by the State Government appointed Leucotomy Committee, serious errors of management were evident. In 1968 permission was obtained from the relatives with almost no attempt to inform them of the reason for operation and its possible effects and side-effects. Relatives who were readily available and interested were not consulted by the Committee either in 1968 or 1973. The operation in 1973 was done without a further investigation by the Committee, the approval 5 years earlier being considered adequate

> for the purpose. In 1973 the permission for operation was obtained from the relatives at the last minute as an afterthought. The law considers such permission unnecessary for involuntary patients; the relatives did not know the patient was involuntary. There are serious grounds for questioning whether the operation in 1973 should have been performed. These events almost culminated in Tom's death from a suicide attempt, with little, if any, positive gain from one half-completed and a second completed surgical intervention. (p. 98)

Winkler concluded that membership of the Australian Leucotomy Committee should be broadened to provide a properly independent review which would apply to both voluntary and involuntary patients.

Winkler's proposal for a mandatory review by a committee comprising both physicians and non-physicians and would seem to overcome some of the problems associated with peer reviews. Many American hospitals already possess broad-based review bodies of this sort. In fact, in October 1973, the Department of Health, Education and Welfare in the United States proposed that all institutional review committees should consist of individuals of varying backgrounds and should contain at least five persons in all.

The first comprehensive American state legislation specifically aimed at psychosurgery gives the onus for decision making to a broad-based review board. The Oregon statute was enacted in 1973 and reflected the initiative of two neuroscientists (a neurologist and a neurophysiologist). The statute provides that psychosurgery may be performed only with the approval of at least six members of a nine-member review board. The review board operates on a statewide basis, and its nine members are appointed by the Governor of Oregon from specified medical, psychological, neuroscientific and lay backgrounds.

The function of the Oregon board is twofold. First of all, it is charged with determining, according to statutory guidelines, whether the consent of the patient or his proxy is properly informed and voluntary. For this purpose a consent hearing is arranged by the board for the patient or his proxy and, where desired, a legal representative. Second, having satisfied itself about consent, the board has to decide whether the operation has clinical merit and is an appropriate treatment for the patient. In making its determination, the review board is encouraged to consult physicians knowledgeable in the field. It must also be satisfied that all other viable alternative methods of treatment have been tried and have failed to produce satisfactory results.

In England, the Government White Paper (September, 1978), reviewing the Mental Health Act of 1959, places similar emphasis on review by a broad-based committee or panel. In its recommendations it argued of certain treatments, which included psychosurgery:

> Treatment which is irreversible, hazardous or not fully established should not be imposed without the patient's consent (except to save life), and, even if the patient (whether informal or detained) does give consent treatment should not be administered without a concurring second opinion. (pp. 141–142)

Three modes of second opinion were considered by the White Paper: an independent psychiatrist's opinion, a committee in each hospital charged with oversight of the rights and responsibilities of staff and patients (essentially, a peer review committee), and/or a multidisciplinary panel especially established for the purpose. The British Government at that time clearly favoured the final alternative:

> There was a good deal of support for the multidisciplinary panel on the grounds that this would add a new and important safeguard in relation to contentious treatments. Much, but not all, medical opinion was against the introduction of multidisciplinary panels, but it is hoped that, in the light of the widespread support for them, the medical profession will feel able to go along with this proposal. (p. 135)

While it is clear that such committees are likely to afford the patient much more protection from equivocal treatments than a peer review arrangement, the systems outlined above have attracted criticisms. Annas and Glantz (1974) pointed to what they regarded as weaknesses with the Oregon legislation:

> At least a majority and as many as seven members of the nine-member board may be physicians. Only one need be an attorney and only one is designated as a "member of the general public". The board is thus heavily biased toward the scientific research community and may approve the performance of psychosurgery even against the dissent of the "lay" members. (p. 263)

The British White Paper did not offer much guidance regarding committee membership. However, it is clear that here only one lay member was envisaged.

Annas and Glantz were also critical of the Oregon consent hearing. They indicated that the hearing, as presently structured, could permit surgery against a patient's wishes:

> If the patient has a legal guardian, the board is required to review only the consent of the guardian and the appropriateness of the proposed procedure. The patient himself need not testify, and the board may approve the procedure even if the prospective patient specifically opposes it. (pp. 263–264)

Let us consider these two criticisms in turn. First of all, while lay membership of such committees might reasonably be strengthened, minority lay opinion is always likely to bow to majority professional opinion. For example, one of the lay members of the consent committee in the celebrated Detroit psychosurgery case (reviewed later) declared his own lack of competence and explicitly acknowledged the heavy reliance he placed on the good intentions and technical competence of the medical assessors. Annas and Glantz seem to imply that lay domination in review committees is required to provide optimal patient protection. However, there is no reason for believing that lay members possess better judgement and greater moral integrity than their professional co-members. The present authors submit that it is not the exact composition of the panel that is crucial, save that it must be broad-based, but its independence.

The second problem cited by Annas and Glantz stems to a large extent from Oregon's failure to distinguish between legal competence and the capacity to give informed consent. This is an issue we considered in the previous chapter. It is perhaps sufficient here to recount our submission that involuntary status should not in itself render a patient incompetent to consent to or dissent from psychosurgery. It is noteworthy in this conext that the California legislation recognizes that an individual judged to be legally incompetent as a general matter may nevertheless retain the specific capacity for informed consent to psychosurgery.

Ervin (1977) indicated what is perhaps a more fundamental difficulty with the Oregon statue. It is a problem Oregon shares with other prescriptions relating to psychosurgery:

> The one thing that the committee has not established – and I hope it will – is a mechanism for systematized pre-operative plus post-operative clinical and psychological evaluation. (p. 126)

Edgar (1975) also stressed the importance of regulating not simply whether or not an operation is performed in a particular case but also the manner in which psychosurgical experiments are generally conducted.

Several commentators have proposed a two-tier committee system; usually a peer review followed by a broader-based assessment. For example, Ervin (1977) strongly recommended this system to the Australians:

> In regard to all research in both mental hospitals and prisons in Australia I would make a strong recommendation for the establishment of a two-level committee. One, a "peer review committee" which would review the research design and would include people from outside the particular speciality – a lawyer and so on. The second level committee primarily would be a "community committee". For example in a prison three out of five members could be prisoners selected by the prisoners themselves, whilst the outside people could include attorneys. The first committee would deal with the scientific aspects and the second commit-

tee would examine the human and social consequences of the research. (p. 127)

The Massachusetts Task Force Report (Stone, 1975) also advocated the two-tier approach in hospitals considering psychosurgery:

> The evaluation system must include a two-tier review at the hospital: first, appropriate peer review; and second, review by the human studies committee at the hospital, a group which must include non-physicians. Both peer review and human studies committee must endorse the investigation or experimentation. (p. 28)

Further, unless a hospital's submitted protocol satisfies the Department of Mental Health that it possesses such facilities, psychosurgery would not be permitted there.

The majority report proposed that peer review should comprise at least two physicians plus an outside psychiatrist appointed by the Department of Mental Health. The minority report strongly opposed this latter proposal. However, both minority and majority factions stressed the importance of appropriate pre- and post-operative assessment and acceptable experimental design. A central state registry was proposed to enable the collation of data from past and future psychosurgical exercises so that the effectiveness of the procedures could be accurately evaluated.

The recent report, from the United States, of the National Commission for the Protection of Biomedical and Behavioral Research in 1977 also advocated a central monitoring agency for psychosurgical procedures. This agency, the National Psychosurgery Board, would compile and assess information on the nature, extent and outcomes of psychosurgical procedures performed in America, the indications for the procedures, and the types of patients on which they are performed. In a novel version of the two-tier system, the National Commission indicated that peer review would only be instituted following a favourable determination by the Psychosurgery Advisory Board that a particular psychosurgical procedure is of demonstrable benefit to a particular sort of patient. Other matters relating to the operation would be left up to a mandatory peer review board in the referring institution. The peer review board would include a neurosurgeon, a psychiatrist, a neurologist and a psychologist and would preside over matters such as the competence of the surgeon; whether it is appropriate, based on sufficient assessment of the patient, to perform the procedure; whether pre- or post-operative assessment would be adequate; and the validity of the patient's consent.

While the two-tier system has gained wide acceptance in the United States, in general it would seem to offer little, if any, advantage over a single broad-based committee, especially where the membership of one of the two tiers has close and pervasive links with the physicians proposing the treatment. In addition, it is questionable logic that separates the issues surrounding psychosurgery, as some proposals do, into scientific/medical and ethical/social, where the former are deemed the prerogative of a peer review and the latter the concern of a "community" committee. These concerns are, as we indicated in the previous chapter, intimately interwoven. In determining the scientific status of a proposal for psychosurgery, a peer review body necessarily establishes the framework for subsequent ethical deliberations in the community committee. Finally, committees are somewhat cumbersome and unwieldy instruments; given that no sources of information are lost, one is always better than two.

With regard to the National Commission recommendations, the establishment of a national apparatus for the ongoing evaluation of psychosurgical procedures would seem a genuine advance. However, the role proposed for the National Psychosurgery Advisory Board might be usefully expanded. In addition to evaluating data from psychosurgical studies, the board should also establish firm guidelines that optimize and standardize the quality of the data available; i.e. crucial matters of experimental design and assessment should be regulated centrally and not left to the discretion of local peer review committees. In fact, the main weakness of the National Commission's submission is that it places too much reliance on local, institutional peer review. As we indicated previously, there are strong precedents for doubting the appropriateness of peer reviews in matters of patient protection. Further, given that the National Psychosurgery Advisory Board also amounts to peer review, the whole regulatory system appears somewhat "incestuous".

Court review offers an alternative to peer review or review by a broad-based committee. An example of this alternative is provided by California's penal legislation. Enacted in 1976 and addressed to involuntary institutionalized individuals (pursuant to California penal code), the California statute provides for mandatory court review of any proposed psychosurgery. The confining institution is required to petition for a court order authorizing the operation. Before issuing an order, the court, having appointed both an independent medical expert and a public defender for the indigent, must be satisfied that the patient has the capacity for informed consent and has, in fact, consented, and that the operation has clinical merit. Here the court must determine that the psychosurgery proposed is beneficial; that there is compelling evidence justifying the operation; that there are no less onerous alternatives available; that the operation is in accordance with sound medical and psychiatric practice.

A similar provision for involuntary patients has been recommended by the National Commission; that in addition to the assessment of the Psychosurgery Advisory Board and institutional peer review, proposals for psychosurgery on involuntary patients should satisfy court review. According to the Commission, proposals for psychosurgery on children would be subject to the same sort of regulation.

It is important to note at the outset that these schemes make no distinction between involuntarily institutionalized psychiatric patients, where the grounds for confinement are psychiatric (this class of detainees would generally encompass what are conventionally understood as the criminal insane*) and prisoners (criminals, social and political deviants), where the motives for confinement are social rather than psychiatric. However, it is submitted that these two classes of involuntarily institutionalized individuals merit independent consideration. We shall return to this matter later and, in particular, the thesis that psychosurgery on prisoners should be prohibited.

For the moment, though, let us focus on the appropriateness of court review for involuntarily institutionalized mental patients. We have already indicated in the previous chapter that the grounds for treating involuntary and voluntary patients in a qualitatively different manner are rather weak. Either the nature of psychosurgical procedures necessitates close control of these procedures or it does not. The manner of regulation should be determined by the status of the treatment and not by the status of the patient. It is a point emphasized by King (1977) in her dissenting statement in the National Commission's report. King clearly viewed the Commission's judgement in this matter as groundless.

Further, the National Commission's recommendations and the California legislature embody noticeable inconsistencies in their approach to involuntarily institutionalized patients. While both submissions take care to distinguish between the legal status (voluntary or involuntary) and the psychological status of an individual in the matter of capacity to give informed consent, legal status is deemed of major significance in establishing the clinical merit of a psychosurgical procedure, by prescribing the manner in which such a determination is made. However, clinical merit would seem markedly less likely to interact with the legal status of the patient than the capacity to consent.

One solution here is to require all proposals for psychosurgery, whether aimed at voluntary or involuntary patients, to be subject to court review. However, we are not convinced that this is the optimal means of affording patient protection. There seems little reason for trusting that a lay judge and jury, exposed to fairly limited expert testimony, are capable of better judgement than a broad-based committee, serviced by centrally collated data,

* It is clear that particular individuals traditionally subsumed under the rubric of criminal insanity present us with substantial classification problems. In particular, difficulties surround the criminal psychopath category. Most psychiatrists and psychologists would not view the psychopath as psychiatrically disturbed or ill in the same way as the psychotic. Few would agree on the attributes that define the psychopathic condition, and many would deny that any such condition exists. This latter position is starting to attract official support. Given these definitional difficulties and the marked absence of a consensus, no distinction will be made here between the criminal and what some psychiatrists and courts label the criminal psychopath; i.e. the criminal psychopath will be considered subject to the same regulations that govern psychosurgery on criminals.

evaluations and guidelines. The judgements of courts in matters relating to psychosurgery have not, to date, been noticeably consistent. Further, court review as a matter of course for all psychosurgery proposals is likely to prove an awkward and protracted business.

Finally, several critics have called for a ban on psychosurgery. Breggin's has undoubtedly been the most insistent and uncompromising voice. In his submission in the *Congressional Record*, Breggin (1972a) unequivocally stated, "... I believe that all forms of psychosurgery should be outlawed in America as they were in Russia" (p. 5576). (Psychosurgery has been prohibited in the Soviet Union since 1951.)

Few serious students of psychosurgery share Breggin's commitment to total abolition.

It is more usual to find the abolition case expressed in terms of partial or selective, rather than total, prohibition. Psychosurgery would be allowed but only, for example, in specific classes of institution or psychiatric facility; or, alternatively, psychosurgery might be permitted only for certain categories of patient; or, finally, only certain psychosurgical procedures might be allowed.

Undoubtedly the most far-reaching and prohibitive proposal for institutional regulation was drafted by United States Representative Louis Stokes in 1973. Stokes' bill would have outlawed psychosurgery in federally connected health-care facilities. The practice of psychosurgery in violation of this bill would result in institutions and/or individual physicians being barred from federal government support. Further, the bill envisaged fines of up to \$10 000 per operation. A watchdog committee would be established to investigate whether psychosurgery was taking place and what penalties should be levied against those practising it. In addition, the bill would have opened the district courts to civil actions by patients.

There are, however, two major weaknesses with the Stokes bill. First of all, the parameters of the bill were not allied in any systematic manner to the scientific, clinical and social status of psychosurgery. As Meister (1975) pointed out:

> ... the mechanisms and rationale of the Stokes bill are not made functions of the therapeutic usefulness or social liabilities of psychosurgery at all. (p. 182)

Second, if psychosurgery is to be performed anywhere, it should be in the most sophisticated and accountable facilities (cf. National Commission Report, 1977). The Stokes Bill would have undoubtedly had the opposite effect.

Various authorities have proposed outlawing psychosurgery for particular classes of patients (e.g. Annas and Glantz, 1974; Chorover, 1974). Usually, it is argued that psychosurgery should not be permitted for involuntarily institutionalized individuals. By far the most influential advocacy for this style of selective ban arises from the ruling of the Wayne County court in the *Kaimowitz v. the Department of Mental Health* case (Gass, 1975; Gaylin *et al.*, 1975, Appendix). While the decision of a lower court in the United States establishes only weak precedent, the ruling of the three judges in Wayne County is of some consequence. As Annas and Glantz (1974) testify:

> Although this lower court opinion has no binding precedential effect in Michigan or any other jurisdiction, it is likely to influence future judicial and legislative activity if only because it is the first judicial pronouncement in this area. (p. 261)

For a detailed and critical account of the case and its implications, the reader is referred to Shuman's (1977) scholarly account. The present treatment will be necessarily brief.

The case arose from an application by Doctors Robin and Gottlieb to examine the comparative efficacy of amygdalotomy and the drug cyproterome acetate in controlling violent and aggressive behaviour. The scientific and ethical validity of the study was approved by a scientific review committee and a multidisciplinary human rights committee, respectively. Initially, it had been hoped that 24 subjects would be recruited, but only one person was deemed suitable. This candidate had been confined for 17 years in a Michigan state hospital as a criminal sexual psychopath. Following the acquisition of consent (both from the subject and his parents), the subject was scheduled for electrode implantation as a diagnostic preliminary to surgery. The proposal sparked off intense controversy, and before the researchers could in fact proceed, Gabe Kaimowitz, a senior attorney for the Michigan Medical Committee for Human Rights, brought suit to prevent the experiment. Although the subject subsequently recanted his consent and was discharged from hospital, and the Department of Health withdrew its approval for the project, the Wayne County court considered that the case raised questions of permanent significance.

Consequently, the three judges heard testimony from a variety of expert witnesses and set themselves the task of determining whether involuntarily confined patients could, in fact, legally consent to participate in this sort of experiment.

The court ruled that psychosurgery for the amelioration of aggressive behaviour should be regarded as highly experimental. Having established the status of the operation, the court then ruled on the matter of consent and, citing the whole text of the Nuremberg Code of 1947, concluded that the inherently coercive atmosphere of lengthy institutionalization reduces the involuntarily confined individual's independence and hence competence to give rational and voluntary consent to a highly experimental venture. The experimental status of the procedure was viewed as undermining the knowledgeability requirement of consent.

It is important to appreciate that in the court's determination, it is the combined or interactive effects of institutionalization and a highly experimental procedure that mitigated adequate consent. The court noted that its ruling did not prevent involuntarily confined individuals from giving adequate consent to neurological procedures or even to amygdalotomy should it become an accepted, non-experimental treatment. This ruling that patient status and treatment status interact in the matter of consent has clearly puzzled a number of commentators: Shuman (1977) was particularly critical of the court's ruling.

> What reason is there to believe that a committed patient who enjoys sufficient competence and equality of "bargaining power" to give "truly" informed consent for such complex but nonexperimental surgery as a portal-caval shunt for cirrhosis, an internal mammary artery myocardial implant, or even an ileostomy for ulcerative colitis, suddenly loses that competence and equality because the procedure is experimental psychosurgery? (p. 153)

There would seem to be a great deal of merit in the contention that a procedure is either sufficiently unpredictable and risky to suggest prohibition or it is not. The status of the patient would not seem to interact with this. Further, if consent is deemed a requirement for a particular treatment (emergency treatments may be exempted from the consent requirement), either the patient's status prevents adequate consent or it does not. The scientific status of the procedure does not logically impinge on the patient's rationality or voluntariness. In addition, as we argued earlier, it is important to distinguish between the patient's legal status as involuntary and his incompetence to consent. The two are not inevitably dependent. Rada (1974) indicated the reactionary nature of the Kaimowitz ruling in this respect:

> ... the progressive trend in mental health law has been to refute the concept of legal incompetence based solely on mental patient status (voluntary or involuntary), but the logical extension of the Kaimowitz ruling runs counter to that progressive trend. (p. 98)

It is an ironic aspect of the Kaimowitz case that when the constitutionality of the subject's detention was challenged, he was released on the basis of expert testimony that he was competent to return to society. Thus the patient was ruled competent to leave hospital by one court while judged incompetent to give consent by another.

The Wayne County court also ruled that proxy consent was legally inadequate in the matter of amygdalotomy. While it considered that proxy consent may be legally adequate when arising out of traditional therapeutic circumstances, it is legally ineffective in the case of psychosurgery. Stated simply, the court ruled that a proxy cannot do what the patient is legally unable to do.

The Kaimowitz ruling would seem fraught with difficulties. If a procedure mitigates adequate knowledgeability, it is difficult to see how the matter of proxy consent arises anyway. It should only arise when, given knowledgeability, the patient's circumstances mitigate rationality, either through his intrinsic incapacities or through the coercive character of his surroundings. It is important to re-emphasize however, that an adequately informed and sensitive proxy consent should never be permitted to overrule patient dissent in instances where the patient's competence is compromised by a coercive environment.

The Wayne County court also presented constitutional reasons for not permitting the subject's consent. The court argued that the First Amendment of the United States Constitution, which guarantees freedom of speech, necessarily protects freedom of thought and mental processes and that psychosurgery, by interfering with mental processes, infringes on this constitutional freedom. The subject's consent was therefore seen as unacceptable. The constitutional barriers to consent established by the Kaimowitz case have been treated with notable scepticism (see Shuman, 1977, for a detailed discussion).

In summary, this "no consent" ruling would seem an unfortunate further infringement on those already poorly endowed with civil liberties.

As we indicated previously, it is important to distinguish between involuntarily confined mental patients and individuals institutionalized for other reasons, i.e. prisoners. While psychosurgery can be considered a "legitimate" part of the treatment package available to involuntary patients, it would seem entirely inappropriate for criminal, social or political "deviance". Several psychosurgeons have, in fact, registered their disapproval of psychosurgery in these areas. Scoville (1973) has undoubtedly been the most persistently explicit:

> I am alarmed by the present trend of questions asked us by both politicians and news reporters as to whether mental surgery will benefit criminals, rebels and social misfits. Mental surgery will never restore social conscience, character defects or infantile sexual arrest. (p. 35)

Let us consider the case against psychosurgery on prisoners. First of all, it is important to recall that psychosurgery is sustained by the assumption that some concealed cerebral dysfunction underlies particular patterns of disturbed behaviour. While inferences of cerebral pathology would seem to constitute legitimate speculation when dealing with grossly disturbed psychotic behaviour, they are entirely unjustified in the area of criminal behaviour, where there now exists a convincing body of evidence demonstrating the overriding importance of complex social learning processes and the pervasive influence of social and cultural context (cf. Feldman, 1977).

Second, there is now a large backlog of experience (negative as well as positive) in the area of treating mental patients with psychosurgery. Substantial data have been gathered over the years. While much of these are suspect, they at least offer clues to effectiveness and risk. The use of psychosurgery on prison inmates can boast no such tradition. It possesses no data base to intimate effectiveness and risk. In addition, issues regarding experimental control and design and evaluation have at least received occasional rehearsal in the context of traditional psychosurgery. No such discussion has attended the matter of psychosurgery on prisoners.

In conclusion, these two considerations, the existence of contrary theoretical indications and the absence of pertinent empirical data, reveal that psychosurgical operations on prisoners represent a highly experimental activity. We have already indicated in Chapter 9 our strong opposition to purely experimental psychosurgery. Prohibition would appear the appropriate recourse. It is important to appreciate that, in contrast to the Wayne County ruling, prohibition would be based solely on the highly experimental nature of procedures as they relate to this class of individual, i.e. prisoners. It is not premised on the issue of coercion. As such, our present submission is without implications regarding the matter of consent.

In view of current alarm, one particular subgroup of prisoners deserves special mention. These are political "deviants" (revolutionaries and "terrorists" are subsumed here). Given the prevailing political climates in countries such as the United States and Britain, this subgroup would at present appear an unlikely target for psychosurgical intervention. However, practices in the Soviet Union (discussed in the next chapter) demonstrate how readily psychiatric diagnosis and treatment can become instruments of political repression. The activities of Societ psychiatrists should caution us against complacency. It was clearly with sociopolitical abuse in mind that the National Commission (1977) stated:

> The Commission affirms that the use of psychosurgery for any purpose other than to provide treatment to individual patients would be inappropriate and should be prohibited. (p. 58)

The difficulty with this sort of pronouncement is that it affords the political dissident only marginal protection and does not, in fact, counter the more pernicious Soviet-style practices. By simply attributing politically inspired deviant behaviour to individual psychiatric pathology, treatment, including psychosurgery, is rendered acceptable. A more explicit formulation, prohibiting psychiatric intervention in cases of political deviance, would seem appropriate.

Children comprise another class of patient frequently deemed appropriate for special protection. Both Chorover (1974) and Older (1974), for example, have advocated that psychosurgery on children should be outlawed. While few formal submissions have explicitly addressed the issue of psychosurgery and children, the National Commission (1977) argued that patients under the legal age of consent be subject to analogous regulations as those proposed for involuntary patients, i.e. psychosurgery may be performed but only after a favourable determination by the National Psychosurgery Advisory Board, a recommendation by an Institutional Review Board, and the approval of a court in which the patient had legal representation. The informed consent of both parents was considered necessary.

However, the Commission conceded that it did not, in fact, review data relating to psychosurgery and children. This certainly moderates their submission that psychosurgery should be permitted on children.

Had the Commission undertaken such a study, it might have uncovered two fairly persuasive arguments in favour of prohibiting psychosurgery on children. The first relates to differences in neural organization between children and adults, the second to behavioural differences.

As we detailed in Chapter 8, the functional organization of the brain is not static, but dynamic. In particular, neural organization changes dramatically during the course of development. The effect of brain damage on psychological processes is demonstrably dependent on the age of the brain damaged. Luria (1973) presented impressive evidence that the disruption of the same cerebral structures in children and adults has markedly different consequences. For example, while damage to primary sensory areas in adults has fairly circumscribed consequences for sensory processes, damage in the same regions in children can result in the failure to elaborate the higher intellectual capacities that depend for their evolution on the early integrity of these primary processes.

The general implications are clear enough. Because of the changing significance of cerebral structures during development, identical surgical lesions in adults and children can have markedly different consequences. As we have already seen, the behavioural effects of psychosurgical interventions in adults are far from perfectly predictable. The dynamic character of cerebral organization makes prediction even more difficult for children. In addition, the nature of the interdependence of cerebral structures in children intimates the very real possibility of stifling later higher development through psychosurgery, by excising its anatomical prerequisites.

The second argument against psychosurgery in the case of children concerns behavioural rather than neural fluidity. Stated simply, children have a far greater capacity for behavioural change and recovery than adults in the areas of emotional instability and social malajustment. Highly disruptive children frequently emerge as competent and responsible adults, with no or only minimal formal therapeutic intervention. The distribution of "hyperactivity" in children attests to this. "Hyperactivity" is disproportionately frequent before the age of eight, becomes less frequent thereafter and is almost totally absent in children during their middle teens. Yet "hyperactivity" is one of the main behavioural indications for psychosurgery in children.

In summary, there appears to be a strong case for excluding children from psychosurgery.

The final style of partial ban mentioned involves the selective prohibition of particular psychosurgical procedures. Thus, some psychosurgical procedures would be permitted, while others would be banned. Overall, this approach has much to commend it. It embodies an acknowledgement that psychosurgery comprises a collection of procedures of varying scientific status. It is a point missed by most of the prescriptions for regulating psychosurgery. The National Commission (1977) proposal, however, is a noteworthy exception. Here, a National Psychosurgery Advisory Board would be charged with determining whether any "specific psychosurgical procedure has demonstrable benefit for the treatment of an individual with the psychiatric symptom of disorder of the patient" (p. 62). It is clearly implied that the Advisory Board might find some procedures acceptable, i.e. having demonstrable benefit, and others not. A list of those not, at present, meeting even the least stringent requirements is likely to include, for example, amygdalotomy for aggression, in the absence of firm signs of temporal lobe dysfunction irrevocably connected with the patient's behavioural difficulties.

In conclusion, our present analysis strongly favours the vigilant and assiduous regulation of psychosurgery. Of the models considered, a broad-based review committee, servicing a group of hospitals rather than anchored at one institution, would seem to provide maximum patient protection without unduly hampering essential clinical research. The committee would deliberate on both the ethical and scientific merits of any psychosurgical proposal, as well as examining consent protocols. However, by itself, in the absence of backup in the form of firm and unambiguous guidelines, a broad-based committee is likely to prove inadequate. Thus, some additional and superordinate regulatory medium is required.

The prior provision of criteria to the review committee would seem preferable to *post hoc* monitoring. Two mechanisms suggest themselves here. First of all, legislation could be enacted to curtail certain practices. Psychosurgery on children and prisoners would seem appropriate areas for legislative prohibition. Similarly, psychosurgery could be prohibited where there is no facility for broad-based review.

A national Psychosurgery Advisory Board offers a second mechanism for guiding the deliberations of broad-based review committees. Elaborating the National Commission's proposal, an Advisory Board would concern itself with the following: collating and evaluating data from psychosurgical studies; advising review committees on the theoretical and empirical status of any particular psychosurgical procedure; providing pertinent research summaries and bibliographies; indicating the types of alternative treatments available; establishing firm guidelines regarding the conduct of proposed psychosurgery (particularly in matters of design and pre- and postoperative assessment), in order to maximize the quality of the Advisory Board's data base. This final matter should be nationally directed and not, as the National Commission proposes, left to local wisdom. Thus, the status of psychosurgical procedures would attract continuous and co-ordinated review, and guidelines would be modified accordingly. The facility for ongoing amendment embodied in this mechanism is not readily available with formal legislative control. It should be stressed that a national Psychosurgery Advisory Board would not determine the merits of individual proposals. The onus for such decision making would rest with the broad-based review committees.

Finally, broad-based review would also, as indicated previously, be charged with establishing the validity of consent. Again it should proceed from explicit guidelines. Here, however, a national Psychosurgery Advisory Board would seem an inappropriate mechanism, since the issues surrounding consent are of general significance and not simply matters pertaining to psychosurgery. A special commission to establish principles governing consent would seem worthwhile, given that there is little existing consensus.

Our previous discussion affirmed that consent must be both informed and rational. It would be for the review committee to determine the knowledgeability and rationality of consent. If it is deemed irrational, then a proxy should be appointed. Proxy would conventionally be invested in the patient's next of kin. Involuntarily committed patients should not be denied access to consent on prima facie grounds, i.e. simply on the basis of their involuntary legal status. It would be up to the review committee to determine, in a particular case, whether the patient's environment was sufficiently coercive to mitigate rationality. In the event of such a determination, proxy consent would again seem the appropriate recourse. However, in cases of this sort, therapy should never proceed against the patient's wishes, i.e. proxy consent should not be allowed to overrule patient dissent.

11

Sociopolitical aspects

It has become increasingly evident in recent years that the issues attending therapeutic practice extend beyond the boundaries of conventional medical deliberation to embrace matters of wider, sociopolitical significance. The controversy that surrounds contemporary psychosurgery clearly reflects this growing "social awareness"; the sociopolitical status of psychosurgery attracts as much attention as its medical status. In fact it is possible to discern two distinct styles of opposition to psychosurgery; while some opponents have directed their criticism at the clinical and scientific status of psychosurgery, others have focussed on its implications as an instrument for social and political control. It is to this latter aspect, i.e. the sociopolitical role of psychosurgery, that we shall address the present chapter.

At the outset, it should be noted that there are two senses in which psychosurgical intervention have been deemed political (cf. Meister, 1975). First of all, it has been argued that psychosurgery is overtly and explicitly political. Hence, the surgeon's knife is regarded as an instrument for extirpating political opposition. Second, psychosurgery can be regarded as political in the wider and more implicit sense that all therapeutic interventions are concerned with values, a matter considered briefly in Chapter 9. Let us consider each of these aspects of psychosurgery in turn.

Several commentators have contended that psychosurgery, along with other contemporary psychotechnologies, is being exploited for explicitly political ends (cf. Breggin, 1972a; Chorover, 1976). It is certainly possible to point to instances where psychiatric diagnosis and treatment have been pressed into the service of political repression. Recently well-publicized practices in the Soviet Union provide the clearest illustrations. Since our present account will be necessarily brief, the reader is referred to Lader (1977) and Wing (1978) for more detailed discussions of psychiatry and political dissidence in the Soviet Union.

There is now well-documented evidence that Soviet psychiatrists have consistently and systematically facilitated political repression by offering diagnosis of mental illness in cases where no disorder existed. Individuals have accordingly been confined to mental hospitals when, in fact, their only "disorder" was political dissent, i.e. expressing their disagreement with official Soviet policy.

Let us consider the fairly typical case of Leonid Plyushch, an apparently sane man diagnosed insane and confined to a "special" psychiatric hospital. Plyushch's first dissident act occurred in 1964, when, while employed as a mathematician in the Cybernetics Institute of the Ukranian SSR Academy of Sciences, he wrote a letter to the Central Committee of the Communist Party, outlining ideas for the democratization of the Soviet Union. His letter reached the KGB, and he was formally cautioned not to engage in such correspondence for a period of two years. Two years later, in 1966, Plyushch began to contribute to the underground *Samizdat* (self-published) literature, advocating the gradual development of democracy. In the spring of 1968, in an open letter to the editors of *Komsomalskaya Pravda*, he condemned the current wave of political trials. He was subsequently dismissed from his post at the Cybernetics Institute. Other letters and declarations followed, culminating in Plyushch co-founding the Moscow-based Initiative Group for the Defence of Human Rights in the USSR. As a consequence of the latter enterprise, he lost his temporary job as a bookbinder. Plyushch was finally arrested in Kiev in 1972; the charge was anti-Soviet agitation and propaganda. Following his arrest, Plyushch was permitted to write one letter from prison to his wife. Wing (1978) has examined this letter and concluded of it:

> . . . shows no evidence of thought disorder or other impairment. Not only does it demonstrate his intellectual clarity but it is full of feeling for his family and is totally free from self-pity. (p. 182)

A year after his arrest, Plyushch appeared before two psychiatric commissions for assessment. Both diagnosed him as a "sluggish schizophrenic". Neither Plyushch nor his wife, Tatyana, were present during the assessment, and he was not permitted access to the evidence pertaining to his case. His wife's subsequent letter to the chairperson of one of these commissions (from Serbsky), testifying to her husband's normality, was not apparently considered material.

From 1973 to 1976, Plyushch was confined in the Dniepropetrovsk "special" mental hospital. Both he and his wife have subsequently presented detailed accounts of his treatment and condition there. He was "treated" primarily with haloperidol, a major tranquillizer. Until then, Plyushch had retained a high level of intellectual functioning. However, with haloperidol his condition markedly deteriorated. Plyushch indicated that his interest in political issues disappeared, along with scientific curiosity and his concern about his family. His speech became jerky and broken, his gait awkward and his memory impaired. Tatyana, visiting the hospital in 1973, was hardly able to recognize her husband. Lader (1977) had this to say about Plyushch's state:

> This state is due to the neurological side-effects of the major tranquillizer. It can be ameliorated by giving medication (antiparkinsonism drugs), but this was allegedly withheld. General lassitude and torpor are other side-effects, which can only be treated by lowering the dose of the tranquillizer. (p. 133)

Plyushch was released from hospital in 1976, following mounting pressure from the West. The French Communist Party is considered particularly instrumental in this respect.

Those Western psychiatrists who have had access to the official evidence relating to Plyushch's psychiatric condition have been decidedly unimpressed by the Soviet diagnosis. Three Senior Fellows of the Royal College of Psychiatrists informally examined Plyushch and found no signs of schizophrenia or any other mental disorder.

While there would appear to be nothing in contemporary American and British psychosurgical endeavours to match the conscious subversion of psychiatry to sociopolitical expediency apparent in the Soviet system, many observers have contended that it is not the actual political abuse of psychosurgery that prompts their concern, but its potential for such abuse (Kolb, 1973; Ukena and Nichols, 1972). Contentions of this sort have not gone unchallenged. Snodgrass (1973), for example, questions the logistics of psychosurgery as a means of mass sociopolitical control:

> There are approximately 3000 neurosurgeons in the United States. Taking things to the ultimate absurdity, if each did nothing but psychosurgery and each did two procedures a day, six days a week, the total would be 1.9 million a year. Actually, however, neurosurgeons usually operate in teams and 95% of their work is totally unrelated to anything psychosurgical. Complete concentration on psychosurgery would mean there would be no one available to operate for head injuries, brain tumors, slipped discs, and many other conditions. (p. 915)

While Snodgrass's mathematics are undoubtedly accurate, his argument is clearly fallacious. The fallacy lies in the assumption that in order to achieve sociopolitical control, large numbers of operations would be required. As Older (1974) correctly pointed out:

> In fact, there is no need for mass surgery to keep a populace tame and obedient. One only need tame the popular leaders and the occasional malcontent to keep the masses in order. Historical examples of cowing the people through destruction of leadership abound. A few well-publicised operations would do the job ... (p. 671)

Psychosurgery could indeed be subject to political abuse, and its practitioners should guard against complacency.

It is important to emphasize that the activities of scientists and technologists, including psychiatrists, generally reflect the political systems that envelop them. In line with democratic political arrangements, American and British psychiatry indulges diverse opinions and approaches. In contrast, political power in the Soviet Union is narrowly concentrated and services a single ideology. Soviet psychiatry is characterized by a similarly monolithic perspective. It is this single-mindedness that facilitates the subjugation of science to dogma and the deployment of psychiatry for political repression.

Psychiatrists and psychosurgeons in the West should beware, however, of taking too much comfort from this analysis. Gross inequalities in social power exist, and science and technology are always more likely to service those who have power at the expense of those who do not. The likelihood that psychosurgery or similar psychiatric technologies will be enlisted for politically odious purposes grows in proportion to the extent that power is monopolized by any single interest.

In addition to these general concerns about political abuse, two specific charges have been levelled at psychosurgery: first, that it is "racist"; second, that it is "sexist". Let us consider each of these in turn.

Several commentators have either implied or asserted that psychosurgery is "racist" (Breggin, 1972a, b; Mason, 1973); that it is being selectively applied to stifle racial minorities. Mark *et al.*'s (1967) letter to the *Journal of the American Medical Association*, in which they hypothesized a possible neuropathological basis for America's racial riots, has undoubtedly done much to foster this impression. Psychosurgeons have occasionally demonstrated a lamentable insensitivty in the area of race relations. Freeman and Watts' (1950) assertion, echoed by Greenblatt *et al.* (1950), that Negroes comprised the most suitable candidates for lobotomy, provides the best quoted example. However, by far the most extreme sentiments in the context of psychosurgery have been expressed by the English physician J. C. Carothers. Drawing from observations in colonial Kenya, Carothers (1951) submitted that the descriptions of postoperative behaviour following lobotomy characterized the usual behaviour of East Africans.

> The writer has, indeed, often been struck by the fact that words and phrases used with reference to leucotomized patients were equally

> applicable to most East Africans. It seems also not without significance that at least one of the few Europeans leucotomized in Kenya has, since his operation, consorted much more happily with Africans than Europeans, in marked distinction from his previous behaviour, and to the great embarrassment of his relations. (pp. 37–38)

Many observers have regarded Mark, Sweet and Ervin's letter as simply one more outburst in this unsavoury tradition. Let us consider their letter in detail. They begin by asserting that while the environmental causes of urban violence have been well rehearsed, other factors, such as brain dysfunction, have been ignored:

> That poverty, unemployment, slum housing and inadequate education underlies the nation's urban riots is well known, but the obviousness of these causes may have blinded us to the more subtle role of other possible factors, including brain dysfunction in the rioters who engaged in arson, sniping and physical assault. (p. 217)

Having noted that rioting is a minority pursuit they then pose the following question:

> ... if slum conditions alone determined and initiated riots, why are the vast majority of slum dwellers able to resist the temptations of unrestrained violence? Is there something peculiar about the violent slum dweller that differentiates him from his peaceful neighbour? (p. 217)

Mark, Sweet and Ervin go on to acknowledge in passing that the urban rioter has no monopoly on violence and finish by advocating what seems to be large-scale diagnostic screening.

> The goal of such studies would be to pinpoint diagnose and treat those people with low violence thresholds before they contribute to further tragedies. (p 217)

Several questions immediately arise.

First of all, given limited state budgets and the acknowledged social causes of mass violence, why deflect already patently inadequate resources from social welfare into medical screening? Both scientific reason and socially deprived communities would seem much better served if resources were concentrated at combating the "well-known" social causes of urban disquiet.

Second, on which sectors of the population would screening focus? Countering the charge of racism, Mark (1973) contended that a theory that stresses the role of brain disease in violence does not imply selective attention to one particular race. If this is the case, then why raise the issue in connection with violence in black ghettos? Given that it would be impossible (irrespective of whether it is warranted) to subject the entire population of the United States or any other country to protracted neurological and psychiatric scrutiny, the suspicion remains that screening would focus on particular racial and ethnic groups, in most cases adding further insult to a history of degradation.

Third, given the acknowledged social preconditions for violence, why specify the rioter as the likely source of pathology rather than his docile and uncomplaining neighbour? In the face of massive deprivation (the existence of which Marks and his associates readily admit), surely docility would seem a far from adaptive response. In this context, it is interesting to note that, following a review of empirical studies dealing with the attributes of black protesters, Caplan (1970) concluded:

> ... militants are no more socially or personally deviant than their non-militant counterparts. In fact, there is good reason to believe that they are outstanding on some important measures of socioeconomic achievement. (p. 60)

Finally, it can be argued that because change is a difficult process for many social institutions, theories that attribute pathological motives to protesting forces function to minimize the impact of their opposition and perpetuate the social conditions that prompted their protest.

By way of defence, Mark (1973) insisted that neurosurgical interest lay only in those violent individuals whose violence was clearly the outcome of organic brain disease or dysfunction:

> It is one thing to advocate neurosurgical procedures for certain kinds of violent behaviour caused by organic brain disease or dysfunction. It is quite another to advocate them as general methods of behavior control. My own belief is that no form of conditioning, drug therapy, or surgery is necessary or desirable to control normal-brained members of our society, no matter what their political views are or how they express them. (p. 3)

It is important to note, however, that for some surgeons (e.g. Narabayashi) interested in the amygdala and aggression, signs of organic pathology appear largely superfluous. While Mark's sentiments are entirely laudable, they again prompt the question of why the issue of brain disease and treatment (by implication, surgical) was raised in the context of the ghetto riots, especially when we find that the main thrust of the authors' thesis is aimed at personal aggression rather than mass social violence (cf. Mark, 1973; Mark and Ervin, 1970). As various authorities testify (cf. Billig, 1976, for a scholarly analysis), the latter cannot be usefully understood in terms of the former.

In conclusion, Mark, Sweet and Ervin's letter would seem, in both content and timing, a remarkably insensitive document. Since its contribution to the understanding of large-scale displays of violent behaviour is negligible, the impropriety is compounded.

Thus, it is easy to see how accusations that psychosurgery is "racist" arise.

However, to what extent are such charges justified in terms of the racial and ethnic identities of contemporary psychosurgical candidates? Is there, in fact, a predominance of operatees from racial minorities?

While it is difficult to obtain hard data, Valenstein's (1977) analysis of the responses of America's most active psychosurgeons suggests that black minorities are not over represented. The National Commission (1977) provided the following summary:

> Minorities account for very few of the psychosurgical patients. In fact, based upon correspondence with some of the most active psychosurgeons in the country, Valenstein reports that in a combined total of 600 patients, one was black, two were Oriental Americans, and six were Hispanic Americans. (p. 30)

Nevertheless, a "racist" potential still exists in particular social settings. As Mark and Neville (1973) admitted:

> ... there is the grave social danger that certain state institutions, in which blacks might have a disproportionately large representation (for instance, state mental hospitals or even some prisons), might present their inmates as candidate for psychiatric neurosurgery out of custodial or even punitive motives, not strictly for therapeutic motives. (p. 769)

Clearly, this is a situation that warrants continued vigilance.

Let us now examine the second claim, that psychosurgery is "sexist". Again this charge was undoubtedly nurtured by the insistence of early practitioners that women comprised the preferred candidates for psychosurgery. While there is no firm evidence of a racial bias, demographic analyses do reveal that more women are subjected to psychosurgery than men.

This sex bias (approximately three women receive operations for every two men) seems to be both consistent across time (surveys published in 1947 and 1977 reveal the same inequities) and across countries (it is a feature of American and British practices). However, it is important to emphasize that the order of this difference closely mirrors the magnitude of sex difference apparent in the general psychiatric population and, in particular, in the diagnostic categories that attract psychosurgical treatment. Consequently, it would seem it is not selection for psychosurgery *per se* that requires our immediate attention, but general biases in diagnosis (Dohrenwend and Dohrenwend, 1976) and the social processes that result in more women than men coming to the notice of psychiatric agencies (Gove and Tudor, 1973).

Nevertheless, it is not difficult to find instances of sexual bias in psychosurgical practice. The lower social status accorded women in Western society would seem to make them particularly vulnerable in the context of psychosurgery (Barahal, 1958). Specific examples will be elaborated later in this chapter.

Let us now turn to the second, less explicit manner in which psychosurgery can be considered political. As we indicated previously, therapeutic interventions are ultimately bound up with values. In this broad sense, then, all therapy is political. Breggin (1975) stated the case:

> Therapy is applied politics. From hospitalizing a patient to offering psychoanalytic insight, a therapist's every action reflect his own attitudes toward political issues, including individual freedom vs. state control, or capitalism versus socialism. (p. 369)

However, it is not simply that individual therapists, wittingly or unwittingly, permit their values to colour what they recommend as appropriate therapeutic goals. More importantly perhaps, ideological factors are considered to pervade the theoretical perspectives that underlie fairly general modes of therapeutic conduct. What is defined as a problem and the style and focus of subsequent analysis/treatment are both seen as reflecting sociopolitical interest as well as scientific judgement.

The theoretical perspective that underlies a great deal of contemporary psychiatric practices, including psychosurgery, is the "medical model". Strange and distressing patterns of behaviour are here regarded as illnesses and are assumed liable to those concepts and instruments of biology that have proved so conspicuously effective in countering physical illness.

However, allegiance to the "medical model" in such matters is far from unanimous. Thomas Szasz undoubtedly ranks as one of the most vociferous critics. He has persistently maintained that mental illness and physical illness are phenomenally different; mental illnesses are regarded as metaphorical diseases, standing in the same sort of relationship to literal or physical diseases as disapproved-of television programmes stand to defective television receivers. In short, mental illness is viewed as a "myth".

Szasz's distinction between physical illness and mental illness has been echoed by others. Brown and Harris (1978) summarized this style of criticism as follows:

> There is a difference between physical illness and mental illness. The former is more objective because it involves physiological symptomatology and aetiology; mental illness is a matter of subjective opinion and value-judgement made about deviation from normal behaviour. (p. 41)

They continued:

> Mental illness is more vaguely defined involving definitions that are more subject to social values. (pp. 41–42)

If this distinction is valid, the sociopolitical character of the "medical model" in such circumstances is immediately apparent. The diagnosis of mental illness is a matter of social attribution – a function of dominant social values.

However, Szasz's dichotomy is somewhat unsophisticated. As Shuman (1977) noted:

> ... it overestimates the biological component of nonmental diseases and underestimates that component in mental disease. (p. 177)

In countering Szasz, Wing (1978) indicated that all diseases represent inferences or theories:

> Szasz says that we cannot demonstrate schizophrenia in the dead body of someone who is supposed to have had the condition during his lifetime, in the way that he thinks that pneumonia, say, can be demonstrated. But *no* disease can be "seen" in this way. The pneumonic consolidation is a theory put forward to explain a particular pattern of events, many of them psychological in nature and available only because the patient has described his subjective experience. (p. 32)

Here, physiological pathology is viewed as simply part of the pattern of data pertinent to the inference of disease. While the confirmation of gross pathology will no doubt increase validity, it is not a prerequisite for the formulation of a disease theory. This analysis clearly stresses the usefulness and consistency of a disease theory, rather than the presence or absence of observable physiological pathology. It also attests that in both mental and physical illness, judgement is influenced by social forces. However, Wing stresses that in both cases, the greater the social component in the data used to infer a disease, the less useful a disease theory is likely to be.

It is possible that much of the controversy surrounding "mental illness" stems from the two quite different connotations of the term "illness".Wing (1978) described these distinct usages:

> In one usage, someone is regarded as sick (or regards himself or herself as sick), because of some experience or behaviour that departs from a standard of health generally accepted in that community. Such standards vary widely. In one society, multi-coloured spots on the skin indicate health, in another they indicate illness. Moreover, the norms of health are vague and shifting so there can be a good deal of latitude as to what is regarded as unhealthy ... In the second usage, for which we are reserving the term "disease" a limited and relatively specific theory about some aspect of mental or bodily functioning is put forward because it is thought to be relevant to the reduction of some recognizable impairment. (p. 140)

We shall follow Wing's nomenclature, reserving "illness" for the first usage and "disease" for the second.

This distinction between "illness' and "disease" is important. The two terms reflect substantially different versions of the "medical model". "Illness" is clearly a social concept, since it denotes a departure from the socially defined ideal – "health". Likewise, "mental health" and "mental illness" are socially derived – a function of prevailing social forces. This "illness" style of "medical model" has been widely championed. In 1974, the World Health Organization added its endorsement, when it announced that "health" signified a state of complete physical, mental and social well-being and not merely the absence of disease.

In contrast to "illness", "disease" denotes much more circumscribed and socially detached phenomena. Wing elaborated on the requirements of a disease theory:

> The first requirement of a disease theory is the recognition of a cluster of undesirable traits or characteristics that tend to occur together; solidity is given to such a cluster if it can be shown to have a degree of stability over time as well ... the third characteristic of clusters for which a disease theory might usefully be put forward (is) that the constituent characteristics can be defined without recourse to social phenomena. (p. 22)

Wing continued:

> The second essential element in any disease theory is the hypothesis that the cluster of traits is "symptomatic" of some underlying biological disturbance. The more the symptoms making up this syndrome are definable in non-social terms, the more likely are we to be able to suggest the nature of the underlying disorder. (p. 22)

Two implications of this dichotomy are immediately apparent. First of all, the criticism that a diagnosis of "mental" illness primarily represents sociopolitical rather than scientific judgement would seem more readily applicable in the "illness" rather than in the "disease" version of the "medical model". Second, while the "disease" model restricts psychiatric intervention to those fairly circumscribed aspects of human behaviour that can be usefully subsumed by a disease theory, the illness model offers psychiatry unlimited licence. With regard to the World Health Organization's assertion of the "illness" approach, for example, Lader (1977) noted:

> ... this is *reductio ad absurdum*: psychiatrists could use it to claim that anybody not healthy is ill, and since nobody is ever in "a state of complete physical, mental and social well-being", then everybody is sick. (p. 195)

While psychiatry has indeed expanded into all manner of human activities, it is in the area of social deviance that psychiatrists have mounted their most concerted attack. Wing (1978) described the phenomenon:

> Departures from normal are regarded as pathological, i.e. medical terminology is taken over to describe what are mainly social deviations. (p. 33)

Shuman (1977) identified such psychiatric intervention in matters of deviance as "medical role fascism" (the attribution of neutrality to value-loaded activities) and indicated its origins in the subjugation of the "disease" model by the "illness" model.

> It is hardly surprising that in deviance labelling one encounters the most insidious role of fascism. The pernicious belief that disease and illness are the same ... generates a nearly incontrovertible justification for doctors, psychiatrists and other health field specialists to regard themselves as appropriate and exclusive labellers of deviance. (p. 177)

In summary, the value-laden character of many psychiatric diagnostic practices, the expansion of the psychiatric prerogative, and medical role fascism have all been primarily precipitated by the "illness" version of the medical model. A "disease" model that demands the elaboration of a clinical syndrome with a limited social component, requires an adequately reasoned hypothesis of underlying biological disturbance and appreciates the theoretical character of the "disease" would seem to avoid many of these problems. It is perhaps not surprising, then, that some psychiatrists have recently demanded a more circumscribed "disease" orientation. As Lader (1977) advised:

> Many people need help but not necessarily of a medical or psychiatric nature. The treatment of definable mental disease is the province of the psychiatrist; the promotion of well being is his concern but not his responsibility. (p. 195)

Two other sociopolitical aspects of the "medical model" have been stressed by its critics. First of all, the "medical model" is regarded as extremely individualistic, i.e. it firmly locates the cause of a problem within the individual; social conditions external to the individual are likely to attract little systematic attention. As Coleman (1974) indicated:

> The stamp of medical expertise and benevolence simultaneously focuses attention on sick individuals while diverting attention from ailing social and political institutions. (p. 675)

Thus, the "medical model" generally emphasizes individualistic repair rather than social reform. This would appear to be an orientation markedly congenial to the status quo. Unfortunately, psychiatrists have often failed to address themselves to this feature of the "medical model". As Halleck (1971) pointed out:

> There is a strange and unfortunate tendency among psychiatrists to believe that professional activities designed to change the status quo are political and activities tending to strengthen the status quo are medical or neutral. (p. 36)

Psychosurgeons, in particular, have frequently been guilty of excluding the immediate and wider social context from their analysis. The search for causes and the application of treatment in such cases extends no further than the individual expressing the "problem symptoms". Some examples will serve to illustrate this myopia. Knight (1973) provides the first:

> A woman of 38 suffered from tension and anxiety since childhood. Following marriage to a sadist she developed multiple jerks and sweating, so severe that she had to change her clothes several times a day, and obsessional tidiness and depression. The effort to tidy her wardrobe was exhausting. (p. 101)

Following psychosurgery the woman was reported to have recovered.

Clare (1976) rightly deplored Knight's total failure to examine the marital environment and wryly commented that, if psychosurgery was at all the appropriate recourse here, the sadistic husband would seem the more suitable candidate. Sargant and Slater (1972) described a very similar, although hypothetical, case:

> Another type of depressive illness that may be helped by leucotomy is the reactive depression in which environmental factors of an irremediable kind are involved. A depressed woman, for instance, may owe her illness to a psychopathic husband who cannot change and will not accept treatment. Separation might be the answer but is ruled out by other ties such as children, by the patient's financial or emotional dependence or by her religious views. Patients of this type are often helped by antidepressant drugs. But in the occasional cases where they do not work, we have seen patients enabled by a leucotomy to return to the difficult environment and cope with it in a way which had hitherto been impossible. (pp. 105–106)

In both of these cases the operations are advocated to enable a distressed wife to accommodate a disturbed and recalcitrant husband – a husband who was, in both cases, clearly the primary instrument of the woman's malaise. Not only do the rationales offered for psychosurgery here reflect a total failure to appreciate the dynamics of these particular marital environments, they also betray a view of marriage and women's status that is patently "sexist". As such, they not only belie protests of sociopolitical neutrality, but also reinforce accusations of sex bias in psychosurgery.

The well-publicised case of "Thomas R" provides us with another example where presurgical analysis of the individual's behaviour lacks a reasonable appreciation of the significance of his social and marital environment. A patient in the Boston violence project, Thomas R was introduced by Mark and Ervin (1970) as a talented and inventive engineer in his mid-30s. His manner was described as quiet and reserved, courteous and sympathetic. Thomas's chief problem was identified as outbursts of violent rage, sometimes directed at his coworkers and friends, but usually at his wife and children. He was reported to harbour the paranoid belief that his wife no longer cared for him and was, in fact, "carrying on" with a neighbour; he nursed grudges and brooded incessantly over his delusion. Her denials evidently provoked a frenzied response and Thomas would attack her, even picking her up when she was pregnant and throwing her against the wall. Electroencephalographic evidence of temporal lobe epilepsy is offered, along with the assertion that other brain abnormalities existed. As various authorities attest, this evidence is not wholly convincing (Chorover, 1974; Coleman, 1974). At any rate, any connection with Thomas's violent outbursts is nowhere unequivocably demonstrated.

Thomas was reported to have been enraged by the initial overtures concerning surgery, but he eventually consented to bilateral amygdalectomy. In *Violence and the Brain*, Mark and Ervin (1970) concluded:

> Four years have passed since the operation, during which time Thomas has not had a single episode of rage. He continues, however, to have an occasional epileptic seizure with periods of confusion and disordered thinking. (pp. 96–97)

However, other versions of Thomas's postoperative adjustment do not bear out Mark and Ervin's suggestion of success (Breggin, 1973b; Chorover, 1974; Scheflin and Opton, 1978). In addition, Mark and Ervin's report failed to mention one crucial detail in the Thomas R case. Scheflin and Opton (1978) elaborated:

> . . . Mark and Ervin's reports omit an important detail here: namely, that while Thomas was in the hospital undergoing brain stimulation studies through eighty implanted electrodes, his wife sued him for divorce, served the documents upon him in the hospital ward, and married the man who was the object of Thomas's suspicions. (p. 300)

Clearly, Thomas's concern over his wife was not wholly unfounded, and his outbursts were undoubtedly triggered by something more tangible than delusions. This turn of events again illustrates the importance of closely examining the social context in which behaviour occurs.

What, then, of Thomas's postoperative behaviour? Scheflin and Opton (1978) provided the following summary:

> After seven months, Dr. Mark removed the electrodes and released Thomas in the custody of his mother. She found him "sickly, pale and weak." His life subsequently has been a phantasmagoria of confusion, violence, delusion and incarceration. He never worked again, but drifted back and forth between police lock-ups and mental hospitals. The Veterans Administration declared him "totally disabled" on October 26,

> 1968, although his surgeons were still citing him as a success much later. (p. 300)

It is obvious, however, that certain conditions will only yield to individual intervention. The conventional dysfunctions attracting neurosurgery provide us with a case in point. No amount of social intervention or political reform will suffice here. The only effective and rational way of dealing with some cerebral disorders is by means of a direct surgical assault on the brain. Political neutrality can hardly be challenged in these circumstances. Clearly, then, accusations of reinforcing the status quo are valid only when individualistic repairs are undertaken on the basis of inappropriate inferences of medical/biological causation. Consequently, it is with the "illness" version of the "medical model" that concern should focus. Whereas the "disease" model, as indicated previously, imposes strict preconditions on a theory of disease, the "illness" model allows unbridled and unsupported attribution of medical causation.

We do not mean to imply here that the application of a "disease" model somehow extricates psychiatrists from considering the wider social context – quite the reverse! In order to formulate a useful disease theory, the psychiatrist must confront the possible influence of social and cultural systems. Finally, there is nothing in the "disease" approach that inherently opposes social reform.

The second additional feature of the "medical model" that has attracted criticism concerns the subtle social functions served by medical language. It has been widely argued that the application of a psychiatric label of diagnosis to patterns of unusual or distressing behaviour generates particular role expectancies for the individual so diagnosed. Reiss (1972) characterized the argument as follows:

> ... the label "mentally ill" attributes to the person so labeled a particular social role. The role is the sick role – a role of helplessness and debilitation. (p. 73)

Thus, the ascription of the term "illness" to certain patterns of behaviour is considered to be a signal to the individual that he is irresponsible, ineffective and no longer in control of his behaviour. Since the sick role is relatively well defined, it is argued that others with access to the individual's diagnosis conspire to reinforce the impact of the label. They, too, are governed by similar expectancies and regard subsequent modes of behaviour as confirming the validity of the label.

The ease with which diagnostic labels are acquired, and the subsequent social impact they have, are admirably illustrated by Rosenhan's (1973) study. Eight experimental subjects gained admission to a variety (12 in all) of American psychiatric hospitals simply by complaining of "voices". When questioned, the subjects responded that the voices were unclear but seemed to be saying "empty", "hollow" and "thud". No other symptoms were presented. In all bar one case the admitting diagnosis was schizophrenia. Once hospitalized, the subjects recorded that their every action was interpreted by the staff as reflecting their "illness". Thus, rather than normal behaviour on the ward prompting a revision of the diagnosis, the converse occurred. The subject's behaviour and past history were distorted by staff observers to conform with a popular theory of the dynamics of the schizophrenic reaction.

Two distinct forms of the style of criticism can be discerned. The first recognizes the existence of some primary problem or disability that brings the individual into contact with diagnostic agencies. The acquisition of a diagnosis and related societal reactions serve to compound the primary disability by selectively refining and stereotyping the individual's social role. The second form asserts that either there is no primary problem or, if there is, it is a relatively trivial one; disability only exists after a formal diagnosis has been made.

Wing (1978) indicated that empirical evidence favoured the first form of critique. However, the Rosenhan study cautions that the more pervasive and casual the application of diagnostic labels, the more trivial and illusory the problems subjected to diagnostic stigmatization. Wherever diagnosis services an all-consuming "illness" model, inappropriate aspects of human behaviour are likely to be diagnosed as "mental illness". In contrast, applied on the basis of a circumscribed and carefully elaborated disease theory, diagnosis should highlight the nature of some primary disability. In short, while a "disease" version of the "medical model" is unlikely to precipitate secondary "labelling" effects in the absence of a clear primary disability, this is not the case with the "illness" model. Further, it can be argued that the social processes induced by a diagnostic label depend on the nature and, in particular, the specificity of the label. A diagnostic label intimating some specific and circumscribed disease is likely to have quite different implications from one announcing some vague deviation from the approved social and behavioural ideal. While the thesis that diagnostic labels serve social as well as medical functions is generally compelling, it is reasonable to presume that the non-medical consequences recede as the specificity of the diagnostic referants increase. Consequently, the secondary social effects of a diagnostic label are likely to be far less when diagnostic practice conforms with the "disease" rather than the "illness" model.

We have now examined several of the criticisms that have been levelled at the "medical model" underlying most psychiatric (including psychosurgical) practice. All proclaim its subtle sociopolitical character. Faced with such challenge to the "medical model", psychiatrists and psychosurgeons have been quick to respond. Unfortunately, much of their reaction has been off-target and protectionist. The critics (collectively diagnosed as "antipsychiatrists"), they argue, list only problems; rarely are remedies intimated. Mark (1974) illustrates:

> Up to this point, the antipsychiatrist arguments have consisted only of criticism. It is time for them to disclose a positive program, if they have one. (p. 86)

However, it should be appreciated that the failure to offer solutions in no way mitigates the validity of criticism.

A more extreme reaction posits that the criticism of the "medical model" reflects some devilish conspiracy to deprive mentally ill patients of effective treatment in order to highlight gross social and economic inequalities. Thus, criticisms of traditional psychiatry can be parried as a threat to the individual's "right to treatment". While the more exuberant presentations of psychiatry's critics are clearly open to interpretations of this sort, polemic and counterpolemic must not obscure the accuracy and importance of many of the charges made against mainstream psychiatric theory and practice. Pronouncements about the "right to treatment" are no substitute for careful reflection and resynthesis in the face of valid criticism. Incidentally, a "right to treatment" would seem a somewhat imperialistic and ill-considered ethic. If individuals are to be formally accorded "rights" in such matters (and there is good reason to believe that they should), what they require is the "right to *valid* treatment *being available*". The additions are important; individuals must be protected from treatment that has no scientific merit or is of unproven scientific merit, i.e. they have a "right to the right treatment". In addition, individuals must also retain the capacity to refuse a particular treatment.

In conclusion, psychiatrists should aspire to a more considered analysis of the criticisms attracted by the "medical model". Our present analysis, it is hoped, is less hysterical than most. It indicates that criticisms of sociopolitical contamination constitute a legitimate reaction to the "illness" version of the model. It also reveals, however, a more restricted "disease" perspective, capable of weathering such criticism.

Clearly, this conclusion has important implications for psychiatric interventions such as psychosurgery. It strongly advises psychosurgeons to embark only from circumscribed and reasonably elaborate disease theories and not on the basis of loose and socially bound models of "mental illness". Unfortunately, as our discussion in Chapter 8 indicated, psychosurgery has frequently been undertaken without even the most modest theoretical backup. Either the disease theory tendered is primitive and rudimentary, or no disease theory is presented at all. In addition, the diagnostic labels frequently attached to surgical candidates (e.g. aggression, hyperactivity, paedophilic homosexuality) readily convey an allegiance to the expansionist "illness" model, or the application of a "disease" theory where the requirements for its application have clearly not been met (Wing, 1978); i.e. biological pathology is inferred and repair undertaken in circumstances where no "disease" theory can be usefully elaborated. While the existing genetic, biochemical and psychophysiological data (Wing, 1978) suggest that "disease" is a legitimate inference regarding schizophrenia, there would appear to be no substantial, analogous data to support the erection of general "disease" theories for such phenomena as hyperactivity, paedophilic homosexuality and aggression.

However, with regard to a disease theory, or rather theories, of schizophrenia, two points should be made. First of all, the term schizophrenia is used in both a broad and a narrow sense. In the broad sense, schizophrenia is very nearly synonymous with the social concept of "madness". American diagnostic practices often indicate an allegiance to this broader concept. In the narrow sense, schizophrenia denotes a more limited syndrome of highly discriminable core symptoms (Wing, 1978). It is this narrow concept of schizophrenia that more usually underlies diagnostic practices in the United Kingdom. This has been discussed already in Chapter 4. It is important to stress that a "disease" theory or theories would seem appropriate only with regard to this narrow syndrome of highly discriminable and reliable core symptoms. Second, the conclusion that available data seem to justify a "disease" approach in no way sanctions surgery as a treatment for schizophrenia. "Disease" theories of schizophrenia are far from complete. A specific pathological focus, if one exists, is still to be unequivocably demonstrated.

Unlike schizophrenia, some of the behavioural problems that increasingly attract psychosurgery cannot be usefully or validly conceptualized as "diseases". Let us consider one of these – the behaviours that are generally subsumed under the "hyperactivity" rubric. This particular example is chosen because it is under the umbrella of a "hyperactivity" diagnosis that psychosurgery is performed on children.

Several psychosurgical programmes have now been addressed at what is variously described as hyperactivity, hyperkinesis, hyperresponsibility or simply "behaviour disorders". (e.g. Andy, 1966, 1970; Andy & Jurko, 1972; Balasubramaniam *et al.*, 1972; Narabayashi and Uno, 1966). Whatever the label, the target behaviours are generally similar.

Balasubramaniam and his colleagues (1972) briefly revealed what they considered to be the main indications for surgery:

> There are many behavior disorders which are amenable only to stereotaxic interruption of the various parts of the limbic system. These are characterised by hyperkinesis, aggressive acts towards others, destructive tendencies, and hyperoral tendencies. (p. 156)

Amygdalectomy was the operation preferred by this group of surgeons. However, if this failed to bring these behavioural disorders under control, hypothalamotomy was subsequently performed; mesencephalic reticulotomy and unilateral temporal lobotomy were applied as additional backup procedures in some recalcitrant cases.

Andy (1966) elaborated on his target symptoms:

> Symptoms which characterise the abnormal behavior in this treatise are emotional tension, anxiety, aggressiveness, destructiveness, agitation, distractability, attack, suicidal tendencies, nervousness, mood oscillations, stealing, rage, negativism, combativeness, and explosive emotions. These various symptoms or syndromes contribute to a social maladjustment for which society demands correction or appropriate control. (p. 232)

These symptoms were subsequently summarized as the "hyperresponsive syndrome". Andy and Jurko (1972) elaborated:

> The predominating symptoms are behavioral hyperactivity, aggression, emotional instability and social maladjustment. (p. 117)

It is important to note that not all of these need be present for a "hyperresponsive" diagnosis. The syndrome would appear to be remarkably fluid and flexible in its inclusions. As Andy and Jurko stated:

> It also is of interest to note the marked difference in the composition of the hyperresponsive syndrome ... (p. 122)

In contrast to Balasubramaniam, Andy has consistently preferred thalamotomy as the initial surgical procedure. However, for both surgeons, children comprise a significant proportion of the operatees. Andy, for example, has operated on children as young as six. In the previous chapter, we offered both neuropsychological and psychological arguments against psychosurgery on children. Here, we shall focus more on the problems surrounding the diagnostic and medical status of hyperactivity and the hyperresponsive syndrome.

First of all, while Andy and Jurko (1972) have attempted some sort of quantitative analysis of the contributing behaviours, their treatment is far from satisfactory. The reliability of their ratings, for example, was never assessed. This highlights a general problem with such behaviour disorders. While substantial effort has gone into testing and refining the reliability of the diagnosis of schizophrenia, the reliability of hyperactivity phenomena across time and, in particular, across different diagnosticians has still to be established. All the indications are that it would be low on both counts.

Second, there is often little consistency or concordance of the constituent traits that comprise hyperactivity or the "hyperresponsive" syndrome. According to Wing (1978), the first requirement of a "disease" theory is the recognition of a cluster of undesirable traits or characteristics that tend to occur together. In Andy and Jurko's (1972) analysis of 30 "hyperresponsive" individuals, intra-individual consistency was far from impressive.

As indicated previously, Andy and Jurko identified three major components of the "hyperresponsive" syndrome as aggression, hyperkinesia, and patho-affect. From the composite rating data provided, it is clear that only aggression and hyperkinesia scores are significantly correlated. Patho-affect scores do not correlate significantly with either scores for aggression or scores for hyperkinesia. Further, the former significant correlation is hardly surprising given the similarity of the descriptive indices checked off to generate the overall rating. The following rating indices were included for aggression: "impulsive", "rage", "temper", "destructive", "disruptive". The hyperkinesia indices included the following: "hyperactive", "distractable", "wild", "mischievous", "uncontrollable".

Some other points should be made regarding Andy and Jurko's analysis. A quarter of the sample (i.e. seven individuals) were identified as "hyperresponsive" when their total scores on the supposed constituent components were four or less (maximum possible score was twelve). In addition, no normal control group was used, i.e. exposed to a similar behavioural rating exercise. How many of a normal control group would have scored four or less on such indices? While the inherent flaws, omissions and absurdities in this study would have certainly precluded publication in any refereed behavioural journal, it was presented as providing "a method for indicating the types of behavioural abnormality which are most amenable to specific forms of medical or surgical therapy" (p. 126).

Finally, and most importantly, hyperactivity syndromes in general and the "hyperresponsive" syndrome in particular are defined exclusively in social terms. As Wing (1978) has indicated, "... the greater the social component in the definition, the less useful a disease theory is likely to be" (p. 22). Wing continued to add the greater the recourse to social phenomena in the definition of the symptoms making up a syndrome, the less we are able to usefully hypothesize the existence and nature of some underlying biological disturbance. Hyperactivity has typically eluded biological specification. As Phyllis Breggin (1974) concluded, "There is also little evidence that the problems of hyperactive children are generally neurologic or biologic in origin" (p. 21). It is noticeable that Andy has provided absolutely no credible evidence of underlying neurological disturbance associated with "hyperresponsive" behaviour.

Hyperactivity is not the only umbrella that encourages arbitrary psychosurgical practices. Psychosurgery in the area of sexual deviance demands similar disapprobation. An example provided by Müller *et al.* (1973) serves to demonstrate the general thesis. The following profile was presented:

> One 27-year old unmarried student (Case No. 8) who had been afraid of contacts with fellows and friends (females and males) for seven years was interpreted as latent homosexuality. Since this phobia had been getting worse during 5 years of psychoanalytic treatment, he was admitted for the operation. (p. 116)

The operation was ventromedial hypothalamotomy. The authors offered the following brief postoperative summary:

> In patient No. 8 his behaviour towards women and men which prior to the operation was characterized by severe inhibition remained unchanged by hypothalamotomy. It is now obvious that his neurotic fear of human contacts, which had been getting worse during the five years of psychoanalytic treatment, was not caused by homosexuality (so called "pseudohomosexuality"). (p. 122)

In summary, we should be extremely wary of psychosurgical approaches to social and sexual deviance; they appear to be invariably founded on the application of disease theories to inapposite phenomena.

It should be appreciated, however, that advocacy of the psychosurgical approach to social "deviance" is often based on economic rather than scientific argument. Ervin (1970) illustrated the importance of the economic argument:

> We're not talking about being nice to people. I make no human argument at all. I found out 30 years ago that it didn't sell anybody. We're really talking about being cost effective. If you can work out a way to define, diagnose, treat and even prevent a problem, you're going to save a lot of money. (p. 4)

Roeder *et al.* (1972) stressed the cost-effectiveness of psychosurgery on sexual deviants:

> The treatment of such patients is at least as significant from the standpoint of the administrations for health and welfare as is that of patients with organic nervous diseases or neuroses. We need only consider the high costs incurred by the state for years, or even permanently when such an offender is consigned to jail or to a hospital for mental disease. The expenses of a stereotaxic operation on the brain which have to be spent only once or twice in any case are by no means as high. (pp. 108–109)

In a similar vein, Hunter Brown (quoted in Valenstein, 1973a) indicated the economic attraction of psychosurgery for violent criminals:

> Each violent young criminal incarcerated for 20 years to life costs taxpayers perhaps $100,000. For roughly $6,000, society can provide medical treatment which will transform him into a respectable well-adjusted citizen. (p. 255)

There is nothing new in these submissions. The early promoters of frontal operations paraded the same sort of cost benefit analyses. Freeman (1957) exemplifies:

> Lobotomy is a prime factor in abolishing "violent wards." A lobotomy project in a state hospital accomplishes notable savings in the main-

> tenance of patients. Furthermore, discharged patients earn more in a year than the total cost of the projects. (p. 943)

It is undoubtedly this apparent cost-effectiveness, coupled with the status quo orientation of the psychosurgical approach to social "deviance" (Older, 1974), that commends it to governmental funding bodies, and, ultimately, it is governments and not particular physicians that define social problems and direct the style of their treatment.

While contemporary psychosurgery is nowhere guilty of the extensive sociopolitical abuse claimed by many of its critics, the potential for abuse is sufficient to warrant constant vigilance. Further, the likelihood of misconduct increases as practitioners abandon strict and limited "disease" theories for loose and value-laden models of "mental health" and "illness". Finally, it would be naïve to dismiss as unimportant the relative cost of therapeutic interventions. However, the economic advantages of many psychosurgical procedures should not distract us from their dubious scientific merit.

12

Summary and conclusions

The recent resurgence of psychosurgery has clearly revived the same heady contrasts of opinion that greeted the first wave of operations in the 1940s and 1950s. Thus, despite the spirited efforts of many of today's proponents to dissociate present procedures from the practices of the past, psychosurgery has remained the focus of considerable controversy. Contemporary sentiments are, if anything, even more polarized.

It should be recognized, however, that psychosurgery has changed in the intervening years. Technical innovations now permit surgical incisions to be placed with somewhat greater accuracy than previously. Developments in neurophysiology, indicating the involvement of medially located brain structures in emotional behaviour and the emergence of sophisticated stereotactic procedures permitting access to these regions, have heralded a shift in surgical targets. Experience and technology have also prompted a revision in lesion extent as well as location; contemporary operations are generally more circumscribed than their predecessors.

There are exceptions to the general trend, however. The increasing advocacy of multiple target procedures and the occasional practice of expanding lesion sites often in a somewhat arbitrary and *post hoc* fashion until undesirable symptoms recede provide examples. The advocacy of subsequent operations when the initial procedures have been ineffective should also be mentioned here. Finally, to these technical and anatomical reforms must be added changes in surgical candidature. Today's operatees are generally recruited from less chronically disturbed sections of the community.

Critics have, however, tended to attach little positive significance to such procedural reforms. Our present analysis indicates that this is not an altogether unreasonable response. Increased clinical validity is not, as some enthusiasts presume, the inevitable consequence of technological advance, redirected scalpels and new clients.

Further, our present analysis reveals that many technical problems remain. For example, surgical inaccuracy has not been eliminated; individual anatomical variation and secondary lesion effects continue to conspire against surgical exactitude. In addition, problems of accuracy are clearly compounded by the absence of a consensus regarding the appropriate structures for surgical attention. Technical advance has not brought noticeable standardization. While technology and operative caution appear to have lowered the incidence of the more dramatic side effects, misfortune and misadventure are still part of the contemporary psychosurgery scene. Even with perfect accuracy, secondary anatomical disturbances, e.g. oedema, would be expected. Furthermore, there is little compelling evidence to suggest that even the most circumscribed incisions achieve changes only in designated symptoms and leave other behavioural functions unaltered. Any apparent improvement in the specificity of operative effects with more recent procedures could simply be the result of less conscientious and comprehensive investigation. Contemporary studies rarely match their predecessors in regard to the evaluation of possible adverse operative sequelae. Behavioural specificity undoubtedly remains an unrealized aspiration.

While diagnostic precision has gradually improved in some areas, e.g. schizophrenia, large regions of unreliability exist. It should also be noted that the increasing intrusion of psychiatry into arenas of human social behaviour not traditionally its concern has served to swell the catalogue of casual and unreliable diagnoses. Thus, increased standardization can only be invoked in selected instances. Further, it is possible to claim a reduction in the frequency of "diagnostic errors" subjected to psychosurgery only to the extent that surgical populations have remained constant and primarily comprise patients whose diagnostic categorization has benefited from standardization exercises. However, as indicated, surgical candidacy has changed over the years. Even if we were willing to accede to the unfounded claim that the shift from chronic to acute patient populations has inspired higher success rates, neither diagnostic refinement nor technical improvements are necessarily implicated as contributory factors. It may simply be that these more acutely disturbed patients have a better prognosis anyway; in this context, it is worth reminding the reader that today's chronic patients have a better prognosis than their predecessors in the early years of psychosurgery.

It should also be mentioned here that psychosurgery as a desperate measure of last resort for chronically incapacitated patients is a markedly different prospect from psychosurgery as an early intervention in more acutely disturbed individuals. In fact, this drift away from last-resort status has undoubtedly helped shape the character of contemporary opposition to psychosurgery.

In addition to candidature changes *per se*, it must be noted that many of the behavioural problems that currently attract psychosurgery, e.g. hyperactivity, are not furnished with anything like the same volume and tradition of research (including studies on diagnostic reliability) and theory that surround the more traditional surgical foci. For instance, the international energy that has been expended in attempting to standardize the diagnosis of schizophrenia has no counterpart in the area of hyperactivity. The suspicion that hyperactivity is nothing more than a vague and ill-defined scatter of phenomena bearing little resemblance to the traditional behavioural disturbances that engage psychiatrists can hardly be regarded as unreasonable in the circumstances.

The foregoing comparison should not be understood as implying that knowledge of schizophrenic processes is satisfyingly adequate and sufficient to justify psychosurgery. Rather, it should be taken as indicating the considerable ignorance that attends many of the behavioural targets of contemporary psychosurgery. Clearly, by itself, the shift in patient population constitutes a doubtful advance; the standardization of selective diagnostic practices may be viewed as somewhat inconsequential.

In summary, the various interim changes in procedures in no way excuse contemporary operations from the considerations that have traditionally attended psychosurgery. The fundamental empirical, conceptual and ethical issues still pertain. Questions of efficacy, validity and morality are not magically bypassed by virtue of technological innovations, changes in anatomical focus and shifts in surgical candidature. These procedural reforms can neither guarantee therapeutic success nor assure moral propriety. Thus, a properly objective analysis of psychosurgical practices, both old and new, should resolutely address their empirical, theoretical and ethical bases. Neither polemic nor the distractions of procedural revision should deflect it from that work.

While all three areas of concern have attracted considerable debate, the proponents of psychosurgery have almost invariably based their case on clinical observation. Consequently, our review embarked from a consideration of these data. At the outset, it is worth re-emphasizing that the vast majority of psychosurgical data stem from uncontrolled observations, where even the minimal attributes of good experimental design are absent; control groups, independent evaluation of treatment effects, lengthy and sophisticated postoperative assessment are frequently neglected. Thus, the available psychosurgery data have dubious scientific status and, unless supported by controlled observations, can command little confidence.

Given the range of possible biases in uncontrolled studies and our necessary reliance on non-independent sources of assessment, many of the procedures reviewed attract disappointingly low improvement rates. If, for the sake of comparison, we assume a spontaneous (i.e. without specific treatment) symptom remission rate of 40% as generally operative (see Chapter 3), a psychosurgical procedure must attract at least a 50% marked clinical improvement in order to offer a statistically significant advantage over no treatment. This estimate is based on a surgical population of 100. With 200 operatees, the percentage necessary for statistical respectability is 47%. A cursory inspection of Table 3.18 reveals that only just over half of the psychosurgical procedures reviewed meet this sort of criteria.

Further, given the casual and unstrict character of such "head-counting" modes of analysis, only capsulotomy (lesioning of fibres connecting the frontal lobes and thalamus in the internal capsule) and cingulectomy appear more than marginally impressive. Several procedures (thalamotomy, rostral leuctomy, prefrontal leucotomy and amygdalectomy) attract dismally low rates of substantive clinical improvement.

Considering psychosurgical data now from the perspective of patient populations, several disorders are poorly indicated. The most obvious of these are schizophrenia and the various behavioural disorders subsumed under headings like aggression, hyperactivity, hyperkinesis. Only obsessional neurosis and sexual deviation would seem to attract high reported percentage improvement rates.

Even here, however, some words of caution are merited. Only just over 30 "sexual deviants" have been treated with psychosurgery (most of them by Roeder and his associates). Clearly the sample is meagre. More importantly, the sophistication and objectivity of Roeder's postoperative evaluations have been severely criticized (see Chapters 7, 9 and 11). Hypothalamotomy in such cases almost certainly effects a generalized diminution in sex drive rather than the correction of specific expressions of that drive. Thus, claims of marked improvement even here should be viewed with particular suspicion.

Therefore, even the most lenient of evaluative procedures, i.e. literal acceptance of uncontrolled observations, hardly commends psychosurgery as a general approach to a wide range of psychiatric problems. While a few psychosurgical procedures may be favourably indicated, others attract improvement rates that do not exceed those that would be expected on the basis of a spontaneous remission estimate of 40%.

The onus of proof in matters of therapeutic validity lies firmly with the proposing physician. Evidence from uncontrolled studies is barely admissible; it certainly constitutes insufficient grounds on which to rest a case. Nevertheless, ambiguous data of this variety continue to guide action and policy in the area of psychosurgery. Criticisms that rehearse the shortcomings of uncontrolled studies have frequently prompted psychosurgeons to seek recourse in the curious, but not unprecedented, logic that acknowledges the legitimacy of such criticisms but simultaneously insists that they in no way undermine the intimations of therapeutic success in the data.

The critic would undoubtedly fare better if armed with negative evidence from studies employing a contemporary control group. Given the total number of psychosurgical operations performed, the proportion conducted in the context of even the most modest regimes of experimental control is abysmally small. Further, the studies using contemporary no-treatment control groups have been almost exclusively directed at the older prefrontal and transorbital procedures.

Even a cursory examination of these studies uncovers sufficient flaws to mitigate definitive pronouncements of either efficacy or ineffectiveness (see Chapter 4). There are good reasons for believing that many of the control and surgery groups were inadequately matched in a high proportion of the studies; systematic biases in favour of the psychosurgery group in terms of length of hospitalization, duration of illness and general prognostic indications are often encountered. Patients who were selected for surgery but for whom permission was not forthcoming have commonly served as control groups. However, it is likely that the reasons for withholding permission are not independent of the patient's psychiatric status, the family's attitude and expectation, and eventual outcome. Such initial biases might be substantially enhanced by exposing the two groups to markedly different rehabilitation practices.

All such factors conspire to favour the surgery group at the expense of their controls. It is perhaps not surprising, therefore, that many of the investigators reported much lower rates of symptom remission in untreated controls that have traditionally been observed. Other weaknesses existed, the most salient are the lack of sophisticated and (more crucially) independent assessment as well as the reliance on only short-term follow-ups, which are often increasingly informal and subject to the confounds of subsequent treatment.

While the control studies do not afford the satisfaction of a settled issue, some general inferences can be usefully drawn. First of all, it can be reasonably affirmed that the better the study in terms of control and design, the less the results appear to flatter psychosurgery; the better-controlled studies show either no differential clinical improvement rates for treatment and control groups or data that only marginally favour psychosurgery. Secondly, where differential improvement rates have been observed, it is usually possible to account for such effects by recourse to variables other than the lesions itself.

Apart from the shortcomings in matching control and experimental subjects, length of follow-up is undoubtedly an important factor. Initial advantages for psychosurgery frequently recede or even evaporate completely with longer-term assessment. Consequently, those studies that have employed only a modest follow-up almost certainly present an inflated picture of overall efficacy. Finally, it must be emphasized that these investigations in no way confront the placebo component of psychosurgery treatment. The evidence from other sources indicates that it is likely to be substantial in this area. By the same token, the no-treatment control studies do not reveal how psychosurgery compares directly with less intrusive therapeutic approaches.

Although the control studies do not offer the critic the definitively negative data he seeks, they may provide him with sufficient ammunition to consolidate his scepticism. To the proponents of psychosurgery they can be of little comfort; they offer neither uniform nor unequivocal indications of efficacy.

If the empirical indications for many psychosurgical procedures are unsatisfactory, the theoretical rationales offered are even more so. The conceptual models generally presented for psychosurgery betray neither substance nor consistency. In place of explicit and sophisticated physiological theory, we find loose and tenuous metaphors from technology and animal experimentation. Even when treated with care and sensitivity, such sources of information provide only approximate guidelines to the workings of the human brain; when exploited with neither caution nor subtlety, they can only mislead. In their interpretation of animal brain research, psychosurgeons have been almost invariably cavalier and highly selective; their use of technological analogies has been either naïvely simplistic or anachronistic. Further, the general schemes of brain organization implied by psychosurgeons would no longer seem acceptable. Neither narrow localization, the dominant perspective, nor equipotentiality grant the intricate and subtle character of behavioural processes; neither adequately represent the complex, concerted and dynamic operation of the cerebral functional systems that service these processes.

In addition to assessing its empirical and theoretical foundations, any comprehensive analysis of psychosurgery must also confront the wide range of ethical and sociopolitical issues generated. Although the most frequently cited reasons for according psychosurgery a special place in ethical discourse (the brain's inviolability, as well as the irreversibility of the changes produced) either do not permit or do not survive close, objective inspection, many substantive ethical problems emerge from psychosurgery's fragile scientific status.

Clearly, experimental and unproven therapies pose different ethical problems from treatments with adequate validity. The present assessment of the empirical and theoretical justification for psychosurgery leaves no doubt as to its largely experimental nature (see Chapter 9). Further, experimental activities should be construed as a continuum ranging from ideal therapeutic research at one end to purely experimental enterprises at the other. The ethical obstacles that face the experimenter undoubtedly change as he moves along this dimension. Although psychosurgeons, if they were to concede the experimental character of their business, would undoubtedly prefer the "ideal therapeutic research" classification, many psychosurgical procedures fail to conform to even the most lenient interpretation of what constitutes ideal therapeutic research. In spite of benevolent declarations of therapeutic intent, the moral propriety of such procedures is extremely doubtful.

A related issue which impinges on any therapeutic research is whether it is ever ethical to pursue such enterprises except under conditions that permit the researcher to draw unambiguous conclusions regarding validity. It is patently obvious that, with a strict application of this ethic, psychiatric practice would have had to manage without psychosurgery. The debate surrounding psychosurgery has clearly encompassed issues that extend beyond the boundaries of traditional medical deliberation. In addition to channelling ethical discourse, psychosurgery increasingly serves as a focus for related sociopolitical issues. In this respect, it is possible to discern two senses in which psychosurgery might be regarded as political.

First of all, psychosurgery might be characterized as explicitly political, as an instrument for extirpating political opposition. We are not without models of psychiatry serving such explicitly political purposes. Activities in the Soviet Union provide the clearest examples. Fortunately, there is nothing in Western psychosurgical practices to match the malevolence of Soviet psychiatry. Nevertheless, complacency would be unwarranted; psychosurgery undoubtedly still offers substantial potential for political exploitation.

In addition, psychosurgery has attracted two specific charges of actual abuse. First, it has been claimed that psychosurgery has been selectively applied to stifle racial minorities. While the available demographic data do not substantiate this claim, it is easy to see how it arises. Its foundation lies in the pronouncements of some psychosurgeons that blacks are to be preferred as surgical candidates. Mark, Sweet and Ervin's lamentably insensitive letter to the *Journal of the American Medical Association* constitutes a recent instance of this unsavoury tradition.

The second charge relates to sexual rather than racial bias. Here, the available data do reveal that more women than men are subjected to psychosurgery. However, it is important to emphasize that sex differences in surgical candidature appear to mirror closely differences apparent in the composition of the general psychiatric population. Thus, it is likely that differences in psychosurgical candidature reflect general biases in diagnosis and the pervasive social processes that result in more women than men coming to the attention of psychiatric agencies. Nevertheless, complacency would be inappropriate here; specific instances of sexual bias in psychosurgical practice are not hard to find.

The second sense in which psychosurgery can be credited with political intent is decidedly more covert and implicit. In essence, ideological factors can be uncovered in the theoretical perspectives than underlie general styles of therapeutic conduct. The perspective that governs psychosurgical practice is the medical model. According to this approach, behaviour "disorders" can be regarded as mental illnesses liable to the concepts and instruments that have proved so fruitful in countering physical illness.

It is a perspective that has attracted a range of criticisms. For example, it has been asserted that the diagnosis and attribution of mental illness represents a sociopolitical rather than a scientific judgement. Both the ease of acquisition and the often pernicious secondary consequences of such diagnoses have been well documented. Further, the medical model has been blamed for fuelling an unjustified and inappropriate expansion of psychiatric interests that has elevated the psychiatrist to the role of arbiter of all manner of human social activities. By simply labelling behaviours as "illnesses", the medical prerogative is established. Finally, the medical model has been criticized for failing to fully appreciate the social context of behaviour and, consequently, for retarding social reform, insisting on individual repair where large-scale social intervention may well be the appropriate recourse.

Following Wing's reasoned analysis, it is possible to detect two versions of the medical model; these were characterized as the "illness" and "disease" models. In contrast to "illness", "disease" here denotes much more circumscribed and socially detached phenomena. "Illness", like "health", is clearly a social construct. Accordingly, it was argued that the value-laden and stigmatizing character of many psychiatric diagnostic practices, the expansion of the psychiatric prerogative and "medical role fascism", and the socially blinkered character of much psychiatry would seem primarily to be consequences of an "illness" rather than a "disease" approach. These criticisms are much harder to sustain when psychiatric intervention embarks from a circumscribed, carefully elaborated, and logically justified theory of "disease".

Unfortunately, psychosurgery has often embarked from either a poorly-elaborated and rudimentary disease theory or no disease theory at all. The diagnostic labels attached to surgical candidates increasingly betray either an allegiance to a loose "illness" model or the application of a "disease" theory where no such theory can be usefully applied (e.g. "hyperactivity", "paedophilic homosexuality" and "aggression"). Clearly, sociopolitical neutrality is increasingly compromised as practitioners abandon strict and limited "disease" theories for vague and value-laden models of "mental illness".

Our present analysis favours the strict and formal regulation of psychosurgery. Regulation would seem advisable on several counts: to optimize patient protection; to improve the conduct of psychosurgical studies; to reflect public concern; to provide clarification on the complex social and ethical issues that surround psychosurgery. Several models of regulation were reviewed.

The peer review (i.e. the physician's peers) committee is the least intrusive and consequently has attracted the greatest support from within the medical profession. However, given the disappointing record of the profession in the area of regulating hazardous and experimental treatments, this peer review must be regarded as an insufficient arrangement. Its advocacy would seem to owe more to monopoly than reason.

With treatments such as psychosurgery, a wider perspective is essential. Thus, the multidisciplinary review committee would seem a decidedly more appropriate format, and its advocacy in several recent directives should be viewed with approval. While the optimal composition of such committees remains an unsettled issue, it should be stressed here that it is not the exact structure of the membership *per se* that is crucial (so long as it is truly broad-based) but the independence of that membership from the physicians and the institution proposing psychosurgical treatment. While multidisciplinary review panels represent a genuine advance, they do not by themselves afford a complete solution. As presently envisaged, they invariably preside only on the issue of whether an operation should or should not be performed in a specific instance. However, there is a pressing additional need to regulate the manner in which psychosurgical "experiments" are performed, i.e. to provide explicit directives on research design and assessment procedures. Further, the wisdom of their judgement in a particular case remains a function of the quality of information available to them. Accordingly, committees must be furnished with comprehensive and up-to-date summaries of the status of psychosurgical treatments.

A possible solution here is the two-tier system, where one of the two tiers comprises a central agency for the ongoing evaluation of psychosurgical procedures. The National Commission recommended such an apparatus; their National Psychosurgery Advisory Board will be charged with the ongoing compilation and assessment of available information on the nature, extent and outcomes of psychosurgical operations. Local deliberation on a particular case would only proceed after a favourable determination by the Psychosurgery Advisory Board that a specific procedure was of demonstrable benefit in this particular case. However, the National Commission's proposal suffers from two major weaknesses. First of all, the Psychosurgery Advisory Board would meet only one of the needs of local review systems – the need for information. No directives on design and assessment would be offered. Thus, in addition to evaluating psychosurgical data, the Board should also establish guidelines that standardize and optimize the quality of future data, i.e. it should regulate matters of design and assessment. Second, the Commission advocated local institutional peer review as the other tier in the system. As indicated, there are strong reasons for doubting the appropriateness of such peer review in this area.

Court review offers yet another possible regulatory strategy. Thus the National Commission, for example, advised court review as an additional safeguard for involuntarily confined patients. However, the grounds for treating involuntary and voluntary psychiatric patients differently in this respect are rather weak. Either the nature of psychosurgical procedures necessitates close control or it does not; the manner of regulation should be determined by the status of the treatment for particular patients and not by the status of the patient. As a general approach, court review would seem cumbersome. Further, there is little reason for suspecting that a lay judge and jury, exposed to a limited sample of expert testimony, are capable of better judgement in such matters than a broad-based committee serviced by centrally collated evaluations and guidelines.

Finally, some critics have advocated abolition rather than regulation. While a vociferous minority champion a total ban, the abolitionist case is more usually expressed in terms of partial or selective veto. Only certain psychosurgical operations would be permitted; or psychosurgery would be allowed only in specific classes of institution or only for certain categories of patient. Our present assessment of psychosurgery would, at the very least, commend a certain amount of selective prohibition. Let us briefly reconsider the various areas of possible veto.

First of all, psychosurgery should be prohibited in institutions unable to boast the very highest medical standards, most competent surgical personnel and the most sophisticated neurological and psychological assessment facilities. Public accountability of the institution is also a crucial consideration here.

Second, with regard to outlawing psychosurgery in certain classes of patient, several points should be re-emphasized. The case for banning psychosurgery on involuntary patients is a weak one. It is commonly based on their inferred incompetence to consent to experimental procedures (cf. the Kaimowitz case). Here, the combined or interactive effects of treatment status and patient status are considered to mitigate rationality and knowledgeability. However, the patient's legal status does not logically interact with the scientific status of the treatment. Either the application of a particular treatment to a particular patient group (as delineated by diagnostic, not legal, criteria) is too experimental, i.e. too uncertain to permit knowledgeability, or it is not. Either the patient's condition or surroundings undermine rationality or voluntariness or they do not.

However, in any discussion of this sort it is important to distinguish between different sorts of detainees: in particular, between criminal, sexual and political "deviants", and involuntary psychiatric patients. While psychosurgery might be considered as a legitimate part of the treatment package available to the latter category, it is entirely inappropriate for the former groups. There are two main reasons for this assertion. First, psychosurgery is sustained by the assumption that some latent cerebral dysfunction underlies patterns of disturbed behaviour. While it may be possible to entertain such a hypothesis with certain profiles of grossly disturbed psychotic behaviour, there is no justification for inferences of cerebral pathology in the area of criminal behaviour. On the contrary, there now exists a substantial body of evidence demonstrating the all-pervading influence of social and cultural factors.

Second, while psychosurgery on psychiatric patients can point to a build up of experience, data and debate over the years that at least offers some clues to effectiveness and risk, psychosurgery for criminal behaviour can boast no such resource. Given the existence of contrary theoretical indications and the absence of any substantial sort of data base, psychosurgery on criminals must be regarded as a purely experimental enterprise and as such should be formally prohibited. Analogous arguments apply to the psychosurgical treatment of sexual and political deviants; legislation should afford them similar protection. In summary, psychosurgery should not be performed where "disease" cannot be legitimately inferred (see Chapter 11).

Children comprise another group that warrants formal protection. Here again, there are two persuasive arguments in favour. First of all, the particularly dynamic character of cerebral organization in children ensures that the effects of operative lesions will be highly unpredictable. There always exists the possibility of stifling later, higher development by rashly disrupting through psychosurgery its necessary anatomical prerequisites. Secondly, at the behavioural level, children demonstrate a remarkable capacity for change. Highly unstable and socially maladjusted children frequently emerge as stable and responsible adults with no or substantially less drastic therapeutic intervention. With such neural and behavioural fluidity, psychosurgery must once again be considered a highly experimental activity. As with criminal behaviour, the data base pertaining to psychosurgery on children is strikingly meagre. Psychosurgery for mental handicap/retardation similarly lacks both empirical and theoretical justification. In all these cases, formal prohibition would seem the appropriate recourse.

Finally, a selective ban on particular psychosurgical procedures has much to recommend it. It rightly acknowledges that psychosurgery subsumes a range of procedures of varying scientific and clinical merit. Several of the procedures evaluated fail to satisfy even the least stringent criteria of what constitutes acceptable validity; thalamotomy, amygdalectomy, prefrontal leucotomy, rostral leucotomy and hypothalamotomy all spring immediately to mind in this context. There is much to favour explicit legislation. However, since the status of individual procedures may be subject to fairly rapid change as additional data are forthcoming, formal legislation is likely to be unwieldy and cumbersome in this context. Some central agency, such as a National Psychosurgery Advisory Board, may prove a more sensitive device.

In summary, of the models of regulation considered, broad-based, multidisciplinary review committees would seem the most appropriate. They should be guided by formal legislation prohibiting psychosurgery on social "deviants" (criminal, sexual or political) and on children, and by the deliberations of a central collating and evaluating agency on the scientific status of particular psychosurgical techniques. The latter would also furnish formal guidance on experimental design and assessment procedures. Supported in this manner, the broad-based review committee would address the scientific, clinical and ethical merits of particular psychosurgical proposals, assuring that opportunities for less drastic therapeutic intervention have been already exhausted.

It would also be charged with policing the consent procedure. Here again, formal guidelines would be provided. Given the controversy that at present surrounds consent and the lack of any clear consensus on the matter, a special commission to establish principles governing consent would seem in order. In the absence of such a body, however, the following guidance might be offered. The broad-based review committee must ensure that consent is both knowledgeable and rational. If it is deemed irrational, then a proxy should be appointed; the capacity for proxy consent would normally rest with the next of kin. Involuntarily committed patients should not be excluded from the consent process simply because of their involuntary legal status. The review committee must determine in a particular case whether the patient's circumstances are sufficiently coercive to undermine rationality. In the event of such a determination, proxy consent would again seem the appropriate recourse, and the confining institution should attract formal censure. Finally, in cases of this sort, therapy should never proceed against the patient's wishes, i.e. proxy consent should never be allowed to override patient dissent.

Our discussion of regulation clearly impinges on the matter of a prospective controlled trial of contemporary psychosurgical procedures. The present authors, it will be recalled, noted that a controlled trial would seem to be the logical corollary of the contention that the superficial indications of success from uncontrolled studies should not be trusted. However, it is necessary to add certain qualifications to this acknowledgement. First of all, any controlled trial should only be considered for those procedures whose uncontrolled exploration intimates impressive improvement rates and negligible risk. A prospective controlled trial is not the appropriate recourse when confronted with uncontrolled data indicating marginal efficacy and/or high risk. A controlled trial would be constrained by the same factors that we recommend should govern general psychosurgical practice (see above).

In addition, while clinical indications will invariably guide behaviour in such matters, theoretical indications from neurosurgery and neuropsychology should be given appropriate weighting. By the same token, a controlled trial should not be considered with procedures or patients for which strong theoretical counterindications exist. Finally, the conduct of a prospective controlled trial of a particular psychosurgical technique must permit an unequivocal and unambiguous determination, i.e. it must conform to the most rigorous principles of experimental design and control. While ensuring a clear decision constitutes the primary moral concern of a controlled trial, other ethical issues (see Chapter 7 and 9) should not be ignored.

Psychosurgery will continue to provoke intense debate. The variety, complexity and emotive force of the issues involved ensure this. Nevertheless, we would invite the reader to consider the following questions, originally posed by Dr. Paul MacLean (cited by Pines, 1973) when he addressed the National Institutes of Health in the United States on the subject of brain surgery. We hope that our account of the various psychosurgical procedures has been sufficiently definitive for the reader to answer.

> I follow a simple prescription, generally, for deciding on all elective medical procedures.... First I ask, is this a procedure I would want done to a friend? If the answer is yes, I ask myself, is this a procedure I would want done to a member of my family – my mother, my wife, my child? And if the answer is still yes, I ask, is this something I would want done to myself? (p. 207)

Bibliography

Abély, P. (1952). Enseignements d'un an de pratique des injections thérapeutiques, intracérébrales non mutilantes et non nécrosantes. *Acta Neurol. Psychiatr.*, **23**, 271–280

Achté, K. A. (1973). Depression und suizid. *Psychiatr. Fenn.*, **5**, 213–220

Andersen, R. (1972). Differences in the course of learning as measured by various memory tasks after amygdalotomy in man. In Hitchcock, E., Laitinen, L. and Vaernet, K. (eds.) *Psychosurgery*. (Springfield, IL: Charles C. Thomas)

Andy, O. J. (1966). Neurosurgical treatment of abnormal behavior. *Am. J. Med. Sci.*, **252**, 236–238

Andy, O. J. (1970). Thalamotomy in hyperactive and aggressive behavior. *Confin. Neurol.*, **27**, 322–325

Andy, O. J. (1975). Thalamotomy for psychopathic behavior. *South. Med. J.*, **68**, 437–442

Andy, O. J. (1977). Decision making in psychiatric surgery. In Sweet, W. H., Obrador, S. and Martín-Rodríguez, J. G. (eds). *Neurosurgical Treatment in Psychiatry, Pain, and Epilepsy*. (Baltimore, MD: University Park Press)

Andy, O. J. and Jurko, M. F. (1972). Thalamotomy for hyperresponsive syndrome. In Hitchcock, E., Laitinen, L. and Vaernet, K. (eds.) *Psychosurgery*. (Springfield, IL: Charles C. Thomas)

Annas, G. J. and Glantz, L. H. (1974). Psychosurgery: The law's response. *Boston Univ. Law Rev.*, **54**, 249–267

Arjona, V. E. (1974). Stereotactic hypothalamotomy in erethic children. *Acta Neurochirurg.*, **21**, (Suppl.), 185–191

Asenjo, A. (1963). *Neurosurgical Techniques*. (Springfield, IL: Charles C. Thomas)

Ash, P. (1949). The reliability of psychiatric diagnoses. *J. Abnorm. Soc. Psychol.*, **44**, 272–276

Bailey, H. R., Dowling, J. L. and Davies, E. (1973). Studies in depression, III. The control of affective illness by cingulotractotomy: A review of 150 cases. *Med. J. Aust.*, **2**, 366–371

Bailey, H. R., Dowling, J. L. and Davies, E. (1977). Studies in depression, IV. Cingulotractotomy and related procedures for severe depressive illness. In Sweet, W. H., Obrador, S. and Martin-Rodríguez, J. G. (eds.) *Neurosurgical Treatment in Psychiatry, Pain, and Epilepsy*. (Baltimore, MD: University Park Press)

Bakan, D. (1969). *On Method.* (San Francisco: Jossey-Bass)

Baker, E. F. W., Young, M. P., Gauld, D. M. and Fleming, J. F. R. (1970). A new look at bimedial prefrontal leucotomy. *Can. Med. Assoc. J.*, **102**, 37–41

Balasubramaniam, V. and Kanaka, T. S. (1975). Amygdalotomy and hypothalamotomy – A comparative study. *Confin. Neurol.*, **37**, 195–201

Balasubramaniam, V., Kanaka, T. S. and Ramamurthi, B. (1970). Surgical treatment of hyperkinetic and behavior disorders. *Int. Surg.*, **54**, 18–23

Balasubramaniam, V., Kanaka, T. S. and Ramanujam, P. B. (1973a). Stereotaxic cingulotomy for drug addiction. *Neurology, India*, **21**, 63–66

Balasubramaniam, V., Kanaka, T. S., Ramanujam, P. B. and Ramamurthi, B. (1971). Stereotaxic hypothalamotomy. *Indian J. Surg.*, **33**, 227–230

Balasubramaniam, V., Kanaka, T. S., Ramanujam, P. B. and Ramamurthi, B. (1973b). Stereotaxic hypothalamotomy. *Confin. Neurol.*, **35**, 138–143

Balasubramaniam, V., Ramanujam, P. B., Kanaka, T. S. and Ramamurthi, B. (1972). Stereotaxic surgery for behavior disorders. In Hitchcock, E., Laitinen, L. and Vaernet, K. (eds.) *Psychosurgery*. (Springfield, IL: Charles C. Thomas)

Ball, J., Klett, C. J. and Gresock, C. J. (1959). The Veterans Administration study of prefrontal lobotomy. *J. Clin. Exp. Psychopathol. Q. Rev. Psychiatry Neurol.*, **20**, 205–217

Ballantine, H. T. (1972). Quoted in: Psychosurgery returns. *Time Magazine*, April 3, p. 50

Ballantine, H. T., Levy, B. S., Dagi, T. F. and Giriunas, I. B. (1977). Cingulotomy for psychiatric illness: Report of 13 years' experience. In Sweet, W. H., Obrador, S. and Martín-Rodríguez, J. G. (eds.) *Neurosurgical Treatment in Psychiatry, Pain, and Epilepsy*. (Baltimore, MD: University Park Press)

Barahal, H. S. (1958). 1,000 prefrontal lobotomies – A five-to-10-year follow-up study. *Psychiatr. Q.*, **32**, 653–678

Bartlett, J. R. and Bridges, P. K. (1977). The extended subcaudate tractotomy lesion. In Sweet, W. H., Obrador, S. and Martín-Rodrígues, J. G. (eds.) *Neurosurgical Treatment in Psychiatry, Pain, and Epilepsy*. (Baltimore: MD: University Park Press)

Beck, E., McLardy, T. and Meyer, A. (1950). Anatomical comments on psychosurgical procedures. *J. Ment. Sci.*, **96**, 157–167

Beck, A. T., Ward, C. H., Mendelseon, M., Mock, J. E. and Erbaugh, J. K. (1962). Reliability of psychiatric diagnoses, 2. A study of consistency of clinical judgements and ratings. *Am. J. Psychiatry*, **119**, 351–357

Beecher, H. K. (1961). Surgery as placebo: A quantitative study of bias. *J. Am. Med. Assoc.*, **176**, 1102–1107

Beecher, H. K. (1962). The placebo effect and sound planning in surgery. *Surg., Gynecol. Obstet.*, **114**, 507–509

Begelman, D. A. (1973). Ethical issues in behavioral control. *J. Nerv. Ment. Dis.*, **56**, 412–419

Bernstein, I. C., Callahan, W. A. and Jaranson, J. M. (1975). Lobotomy in private practice. *Arch. Gen. Psychiatry*, **32**, 1041–1047

Billig, M. (1976). *Social Psychology and Intergroup Relations.* (London: Academic Press)

Bingley, T., Leksell, L., Meyerson, B. A. and Rylander, G. (1973). Stereotactic anterior capsulotomy in anxiety and obsessive-compulsive states. In Laitinen, L. V. and Livingston, K. E. (eds.) *Surgical Approaches in Psychiatry.* (Lancaster: MTP)

Bingley, T., Leksell, L., Meyerson, B. A. and Rylander, G. (1977). Long-term results of stereotactic anterior capsulotomy in chronic obsessive–compulsive neurosis. In Sweet, W. H., Obrador, S. and Martín-Rodrígues, J. G. (eds.) *Neurosurgical Treatment in Psychiatry, Pain, and Epilepsy.* (Baltimore, MD: University Park Press)

Birk, L. (1973). Biofeedback – Furor therapeuticus. In Birk, L. (ed.) *Biofeedback: Behavioral Medicine.* (New York: Grune & Stratton)

Black, P., Uematsu, S. and Walker, A. E. (1975). Stereotaxic hypothalamotomy for control of violent, aggressive behavior. *Confin. Neurol.*, **37**, 187–188 (Abstr.)

Blanchard, E. B. and Young, L. D. (1973). Self-control of cardiac functioning: A promise as yet unfulfilled. *Psychol. Bull.*, **79**, 145–163

Board of Control (England and Wales) (1947). *Pre-frontal Leucotomy in 1,000 Cases.* (London: HMSO)

Bockoven, J. S. and Greenblatt, M. (1950). Results of unilateral and bimedial lobotomy: A pilot study. In Greenblatt, M., Arnot, R. and Solomon, H. C. (eds.) *Studies in Lobotomy.* (New York: Grune & Stratton)

Bond, E. D. (1954). Results of psychiatric treatment in psychoses – with a control series. *Am. J. Psychiatry*, **110**, 881–887

Bond, E. D. and Braceland, F. J. (1937). Prognosis in mental disease. *Am. J. Psychiatry*, **94**, 263–274

Breggin, P. (1974). Underlying a method. Is psychosurgery an acceptable treatment for hyperactivity in children? *Ment. Health*, **58**, 19–21

Breggin, P. R. (1972a). The return of lobotomy and psychosurgery. *Congress. Rec.*, **118** (26), 5567

Breggin, P. R. (1972b). Lobotomies: An alert. *Am. J. Psychiatry*, **129**, 97–98

Breggin, P. R. (1973a). The second wave. *Ment. Health*, **57**, 10–13

Breggin, P. R. (1973b). The psychosurgery of Thomas R.: A follow-up study. *Issues Radical Ther.*, **1**, 3–5

Breggin, P. R. (1975). Psychiatry and psychotherapy as political processes. *Am. J. Psychother.*, **29**, 369–382

Brennan, M. J., Kew, J. K. and Lewis, W. D. (1955). Psychological changes following prefrontal lobotomy. *Arch. Physical Med.*, **36**, 695–698

Brickner, R. M. (1936). *The Intellectual Functions of the Frontal Lobes: A Study Based upon Observation of a Man after Partial Bilateral Frontal Lobectomy.* (New York: Macmillan)

Bridges, P. K. (1972). Psychosurgery today: psychiatric aspects. *Proc. R. Soc. Med.*, **65**, 1104–1108

Bridges, P. K. (1973). Methods of assessing patients for psychosurgery and their outcome after operation. *Psychiatr., Neurol., Neurochirurg.*, **76**, 335–344

Bridges, P. K. and Bartlett, J. R. (1973). The work of a psychosurgical unit. *Postgrad. Med. J.*, **49**, 855–859

Bridges, P. K., Göktepe, E. O. and Maratos, J. (1973). A comparative review of patients with obsessional neurosis and with depression treated by psychosurgery. *Br. J. Psychiatry*, **123**, 663–674

Brierley, J. B. and Beck, E. (1959). The significance in human stereotactic brain surgery of individual variation in the diencephalon and globus pallidus. *J. Neurol. Neurosurg. Psychiatry*, **22**, 287–298

British Medical Journal. (1971). Modified prefrontal leucotomy. *Br. Med. J.*, **3**, 595–596

Broager, B. (1947). On the technique of frontal lobotomy. *Acta Psychiatr. Neurol.*, **47**, (Suppl.), 341–347

Broca, P. (1861). Remarques sur la siège de la faculté du langage articulé. *Bull. Soc. Anat., Paris*, **6**, 330–357

Broca, P. (1867). Cas singulier de trépanation chez les Incas. *Bull. Soc. Anthropol.*, **2**, 403–408

Brodmann, K. (1909). *Vergleichende Lokalisationslehre der Grosshirnrinde.* (Leipzig: Barth)

Bromberger, B. (1977). Psychosurgery and the law in the United States of America. In Smith, J. S. and Kiloh, L. G. (eds.) *Psychosurgery and Society.* (Oxford: Pergamon)

Brothwell, D. R. (1972). *Digging up Bones.* 2nd Edn. (London: Trustees of the British Museum)

Brown, B. S., Wienckowski, L. A. and Bivens, L. W. (1975). Psychosurgery: perspective on a current issue. *Connecticut Med.*, **39**, 228–234

Brown, G. and Harris, T. (1978). *Social Origins of Depression.* (London: Tavistock)

Brown, G. W., Monck, E. M., Carstairs, G. M. and Wing, J. K. (1962). Influence of family life on the course of schizophrenic illness. *Br. J. Prevent. Soc. Med.*, **16**, 55–57

Brown, M. H. (1973). Further experience with multiple limbic targets for schizophrenia and aggression. In Laitinen, L. V. and Livingston, K. E. (eds.) *Surgical Approaches in Psychiatry.* (Lancaster: MTP)

Brown, M. H. and Lighthill, J. A. (1968). Selective anterior cingulotomy: A psychosurgical evaluation. *J. Neurosurg.*, **29**, 513–519

Bucaille, M. (1952). Infiltration novocainique préfrontale pour le traitement des douleurs irréductibles des cancéreux. *Semaine Méd Hôp. Paris*, **28**, 310–312

Burckhardt, G. (1891). Ueber Rindenexcisionen, als Beitrag zur operativen Therapie der Psychochosen. *Allgem. Z. Psychiatrie*, **47**, 463–548.

Burlingame, C. C. (1949). Rehabilitation after leucotomy. *Proc. R. Soc. Med.*, **42**, (Suppl.), 31–42.

Butler, J. (1977). *Medical Experimentation Act:* (*Unethical Experiments*). (London: HMSO)

Canadian Medical Association Journal. (1964). Standard lobotomy: The end of an era. *Canad. Med. Assoc. J.*, **91**, 1228–1229

Caplan, N. (1970). The new ghetto man: A review of recent empirical studies. *J. Soc. Iss.*, **26**, 59–74

Carmody, J. T. B. (1950). The effect of prefrontal lobotomy on peptic ulcer. *Surgical Forum*, 332–335

Carothers, J. C. (1951). Frontal lobe function in the African. *J. Ment. Sci.*, **97**, 12–48

Castelletti, V. (1951). Comportamento sessuale in schizofrenici dopo lobo o leucotomia prefrontale. *Giorn. Psichiatria Neuropatal.*, **79**, 337–347

Chapman, W. P., Rose, A. S. and Solomon, H. C. (1950). A follow-up study of motor withdrawal reaction to heat discomfort in patients before and after frontal lobotomy. *Am. J. Psychiatry*, **107**, 221–224

Chorover, S. L. (1974). Psychosurgery: A neuropsychological perspective. *Boston Univ. Law Rev.*, **54**, 231–248

Chorover, S. L. (1976). The pacification of the brain: from phrenology to psychosurgery. In Morley, T. P. (ed.) *Current Controversies in Neurosurgery*. (Philadelphia: Saunders)

Clare, A. (1976). Psychosurgery. In Clare, A. (ed.) *Psychiatry in Dissent*. (London: Tavistock)

Cohn, E. (1945). Electroencephalographic study of prefrontal lobotomy: A study of focal brain injury. *Arch. Neurol. Psychiatry*, **53**, 283–285

Coleman, L. S. (1974). Perspectives on the medical research of violence. *Am. J. Orthopsychiatry*, **44**, 675–687

Cooper, I. S. and Lee, A. St. J. (1961). Cryothalamectomy–hypothermic congelation: A technical advance in basal ganglia surgery. *J. Am. Geriatr. Soc.*, **9**, 714–718

Cooper, J. E., Kendell, R. E., Gurland, B. J., Sharpe, L., Copeland, J. R. M. and Simon, R. (1972). *Psychiatric Diagnosis in New York and London* (Maudsley Monograph 20). (London: Oxford University Press)

Copas, J. B., Fryer, M. and Robin, A. (1974). *Treatment Settings in Psychiatry*. (London: Kimpton)

Corsellis, J. A. N. and Jack, A. B. (1973). Neuropathological observations on yttrium implants and on undercutting in the orbito-frontal areas of the brain. In Laitinen, L. V. and Livingston, K. E. (eds.) *Surgical Approaches in Psychiatry*. (Lancaster: MTP)

Cox, A. W. and Brown, M. H. (1977). Results of multi-target limbic surgery in the treatment of schizophrenia and aggressive states. In Sweet, W. H., Obrador, S. and Martin-Rodríguez, J. G. (eds.) *Neurosurgical Treatment in Psychiatry, Pain, and Epilepsy*. (Baltimore, MD: University Park Press)

Craighead, W. E., Kazdin, A. E. and Mahoney, M. J. (1976). *Behavior Modification*. (Boston: Houghton-Mifflin)

Crow, H. J. (1973). Intracerebral polarisation and multifocal leucocoagulation in some psychiatric illnesses. *Psychiatr. Neurol. Neurochirurg.*, **76**, 365–381

Crow, H. (1977). The treatment of anxiety and obsessionality with chronically implanted electrodes. In Smith, J. S. and Kiloh, L. G. (eds.) *Psychosurgery and Society*. (Oxford: Pergamon)

Crow, H. J. and Cooper, R. (1972). Stimulation, polarization and coagulation using intracerebral implanted electrodes during the investigation and treatment of psychiatric and other disorders. *Med. Prog. Technol.*, **1**, 92–102

Crow, H. J., Cooper, R. and Phillips, D. G. (1961). Controlled multifocal frontal

leucotomy for psychiatric illness. *J. Neurol., Neurosurg. Psychiatry*, **24**, 353–360
Crown, S. (1951). Psychological changes following prefrontal leucotomy: A review. *J. Ment. Sci.*, **97**, 49–83
Culliton, B. J. (1976). Psychosurgery: National Commission issues surprisingly favourable report. *Science*, **194**, 299–301
Dagi, T. F. (1977). Psychiatric surgery and the ethics of uncertainty. In Sweet, W. H., Obrador, S. and Martín-Rodríguez, J. G. (eds.) *Neurosurgical Treatment in Psychiatry*. (Baltimore, MD: University Park Press)
Davison, G. C. and Neale, J. M. (1974). *Abnormal Psychology*. (New York: Wiley)
De Lange, S. A. (1973). Ethical implications of psychosurgery. *Psychiatr. Neurol. Neurochirurg.*, **76**, 383–389
Delgado, J. M. R. (1969). *Physical Control of the Mind*. (New York: Harper & Row)
Department of Health and Social Security. (1977). *In-patient Statistics for the Mental Health Enquiry for England, 1974*, Research Report Series No. 17. (London: HMSO)
Dieckmann, G. and Hassler, R. (1975). Unilateral hypothalamotomy in sexual delinquents. *Confin. Neurol.*, **37**, 177–186
Dieckmann, G. and Hassler, R. (1977). Treatment of sexual violence by stereotactic hypothalamotomy. In Sweet, W. H., Obrador, S. and Martín-Rodríguez, J. G. (eds.) *Neurosurgical Treatment in Psychiatry, Pain, and Epilepsy*. (Baltimore, MD: University Park Press)
Doering, C. R. and Raymond, A. F. (1934). Reliability of observation in psychiatric and related characteristics. *Am. J. Orthopsychiatry*, **4**, 249–257
Dohrenwend, B. P. and Dohrenwend, B. S. (1976). Sex differences and psychiatric disorders. *Am. J. Soc.*, **81**, 1447–1454
Donagio, A. (1939). In materia di discussione sulla neuropsicochirurgia. *Giorn. Psichiatria Neuropatol.*, **67**, 288–290
Drewe, E. A. (1974). The effect of type and area of brain lesion on Wisconsin Card Sorting Test performance. *Cortex*, **10**, 159–170
Drewe, E. A. (1975). Go–no-go learning after frontal lobe lesions in humans. *Cortex*, **11**, 8–16
Edgar, H. (1975). Regulating psychosurgery: issues of public policy and law. In Gaylin, W. M., Meister, J. S. and Neville, R. C. (eds.) *Operating on the Mind*. (New York: Basic Books)
Eie, N. (1954). Macroscopical investigations of twenty-nine brains subjected to frontal leukotomy. *Acta Psychiatr. Neurol. Scand.*, Suppl. 90
Ellison, G. D. and Flynn, J. P. (1968). Organized aggressive behavior in cats after surgical isolation of the hypothalamus. *Arch. Ital. Biol.*, **106**, 1–20
Ervin, F. R. (1970). Violence: As likely from faulty brain as faulty upbringing. *Boston Globe*, **Nov. 29**, 4
Ervin, F. R. (1977). The American experience. In Smith, J. S. and Kiloh, L. G. (eds.) *Psychosurgery and Society*. (Oxford: Pergamon)
Escolar, J. (1951). Presentación de un nuevo aparato estereotáxico para encéfalo humano. *Rev. Espan. Oto-Neuro-Oftamol. Neurocirurg.*, **10**, 261–264
Feinstein, A. R. (1973). The epidemiologic trohoc, the ablative risk ratio, and "retrospective" research. *Clin. Pharmacol. Ther.*, **14**, 291–307
Feldman, M. P. (1977). *Criminal Behaviour: A Psychological Analysis*. (London: Wiley)
Feldman, M. P. and Broadhurst, A. (eds.) (1978). *Theoretical and Experimental Bases of the Behaviour Therapies*. (London: Wiley)

Ferrier, D. (1886). *The Functions of the Brain*, 2nd Edn. (London: Smith, Elder)
Fiamberti, A. M. (1937). Proposta di una tecnica operatoria modificata e semplificata per gli interventi alla Moniz sur lobi prefrontali in malati di mente. *Rassegna Studi Psichiatrici*, **26**, 797–806
Fielding, A. (1978). *Blood and Consciousness*. (New York: Glucocracy)
Fleming, G. W. T. H. (1942). Some preliminary remarks on prefrontal leucotomy. *J. Ment. Sci.*, **88**, 282–284
Fleming, J. F. R. and Baker, E. F. W. (1972). Bimedial prefrontal leukotomy. In Hitchcock, E., Laitinen, L. and Vaernet, K. (eds.) *Psychosurgery*. (Springfield, IL: Charles C. Thomas)
Frank, J. (1946). Clinical survey and results of 200 cases of prefrontal leucotomy. *J. Ment. Sci.*, **92**, 497–508
Frank, J. D. (1961). *Persuasion and Healing*. (Baltimore, MD: Johns Hopkins Press)
Frankl, L. and Mayer-Gross, W. (1947). Personality change after prefrontal leucotomy. *Lancet*, **2**, 820–824
Franz, S. I. (1912). New phrenology. *Science*, **35**, 321–328
Freeman, W. (1948a). International conference on psychosurgery. *Am. J. Psychiatry*, **105**, 467–468
Freeman, W. (1948b). Transorbital leucotomy. *Lancet*, **2**, 371–373
Freeman, W. (1949). Theoretical and clinical considerations of various leucotomy techniques. *Proc. R. Soc. Med.*, **42** (Suppl.), 28–31
Freeman, W. (1953). Hazards of lobotomy: Study of two thousand operations. *J. Am. Med. Assoc.*, **152**, 487–491
Freeman, W. (1957). Transorbital lobotomy: 1936–1956. *Am. J. Psychiatry*, **113**, 877–886
Freeman, W. (1971). Frontal lobotomy in early schizophrenia: Long follow-up in 415 cases. *Br. J. Psychiatry*, **119**, 621–624
Freeman, W. (1973). Sexual behavior and fertility after frontal lobotomy. *Biol. Psychiatry*, **6**, 97–104
Freeman, W., Davis, H. W., East, I. C., Tait, H. C., Johnson, S. O. and Rogers, W. B. (1954). West Virginia Lobotomy Project *J. Am. Med. Assoc.*, **156**, 939–943
Freeman, W. and Watts, J. W. (1937). Subcortical prefrontal lobotomy in the treatment of certain psychoses. *Med. Ann. District Columbia*, **6**, 267–271
Freeman, W. and Watts, J. W. (1942). *Psychosurgery*. (Springfield, IL: Charles C. Thomas)
Freeman, W. and Watts, J. W. (1946). Psychosurgery. *Prog. Neurol. Psychiatry*, **1**, 649–661.
Freeman, W. and Watts, J. W. (1947a). Retrograde degeneration of the thalamus following prefrontal lobotomy. *J. Comp. Neurol.*, **86**, 65–93
Freeman, W. and Watts, J. W. (1947b). Psychosurgery. *Prog. Neurol. Psychiatry*, **2**, 649–661
Freeman, W. and Watts, J. W. (1950). *Psychosurgery*. 2nd Edn. (Springfield, IL: Charles C. Thomas)
Freeman, W. and Williams, J. M. (1952). Human sonar: the amygdaloid nucleus in relation to auditory hallucinations. *J. Nerv. Ment. Dis.*, **116**, 456–462
Friedman, S., Moore, B. E., Ranger, C. O. and Russman, C. (1951). A progress study of lobotomized and control patients. *Am. J. Psychiatry*, **108**, 10–18
Fry, F. J., Ades, H. W. and Fry, W. J. (1958). Production of reversible changes in the central nervous system by ultrasound. *Science*, **127**, 83–84

Fry, W. J., Mosberg, W. H., Barnard, J. W. and Fry, F. J. (1954). Production of focal destructive lesions in the central nervous system with ultrasound. *J. Neurosurg.*, **31**, 471–478

Fulton, J. F. (1947). *Howell's Textbook of Physiology*. (Philadelphia: Saunders)

Fulton, J. F. (1949). *Functional Localization in the Frontal Lobes and Cerebellum.* (Oxford: Clarendon Press)

Fulton, J. F. (1951). *Frontal Lobotomy and Affective Behaviour: A Neurophysiological Analysis*. (London: Chapman & Hall)

Fulton, J. F. (1955). Quoted in Davies, J. D. *Phrenology, Fad and Science*. (New Haven: Yale University Press)

Gaches, J., Le Beau, J. and Choppy, M. (1972). Psychosurgery in severe obsessive syndromes. In Hitchcock, E., Laitinen, L. and Vaernet, K. (eds.) *Psychosurgery*. (Springfield, IL: Charles C. Thomas)

Garrison, F. H. (1924). *An Introduction to the History of Medicine*. 3rd Edn. (Philadelphia: Saunders)

Gass, R. S. (1975). Kaimowitz v. Department of Mental Health: The Detroit psychosurgery case. In Gaylin, W. M., Meister, J. S. and Neville, R. C. (eds.) *Operating on the Mind.* (New York: Basic Books)

Gaylin, W. M. (1975). The problem of psychosurgery. In Gaylin, W. M., Meister, J. S. and Neville, R. C. (eds.) *Operating on the Mind.* (New York: Basic Books)

Gaylin, W. M., Meister, J. S. and Neville, R. C. (eds.) (1975). *Operating on the Mind.* (New York: Basic Books)

Gibson, H. B. (1965). *Manual of the Gibson Spiral Maze*. (London: University of London Press)

Göktepe, E. O., Young, L. B. and Bridges, P. K. (1975). A further review of the results of stereotactic subcaudate tractotomy. *Br. J. Psychiatry*, **126**, 270–280

Goldstein, K. (1949). Frontal lobotomy and impairment of abstract attitude. *J. Nerv. Ment. Dis.*, **110**, 93–111.

Goldstein, M. (1974). Brain research and violent behavior: A summary and evaluation of the status of biomedical research on brain and aggressive violent behavior. *Arch. Neurol.*, **30**, 1–35

Goltz, F. (1881). Ueber die Verrichtungen des Grosshirns. *Arch. Ges. Physiol.*, **26**, 1–49

Gordon, G. T. (1946). Problems of psychiatric diagnosis. *Delaware State Med. J.*, **18**, 120–122

Gove, W. R. and Tudor, J. (1973). Adult sex roles and mental illness. *Am. J. Sociol.*, **78**, 812–835

Government White Paper. (1978). *Review of the Mental Health Act, 1959*. (London: HMSO)

Grantham, E. G. (1951). Prefrontral lobotomy for relief of pain: With a report of a new operative technique. *J. Neurosurg.*, **8**, 405–410

Green, P., Glass, A. and O'Callaghan, M. A. J. (1979). Some implications of abnormal hemisphere interaction in schizophrenia. In Gruzelier, J. H. and Flor-Henry, P. (eds.) *Hemisphere Asymmetries of Function in Psychopathology*. (North Holland: Elsevier)

Greenblatt, M., Arnot, R. E., Poppen, J. L. and Chapman, W. P. (1947). Report on lobotomy studies at the Boston Psychopathic Hospital. *Am. J. Psychiatry*, **104**, 361–368

Greenblatt, M., Arnot, R. and Solomon, H. C. (eds.) *Studies in Lobotomy*. (New York: Grune & Stratton)

Greenblatt, M. and Solomon, H. C. (1953). *Frontal Lobes and Schizophrenia*. (New York: Springer)

Gurland, B. J., Fleiss, J. L., Cooper, J. E., Sharpe, L., Kendell, R. E. and Roberts, P. (1970). Cross-national study of diagnosis of mental disorders: Hospital diagnoses and hospital patients in New York and London. *Compr. Psychiatry*, **11**, 18–25

Haaijman, W. P., van Leeuwen, W. S. and van Veelen, C. W. M. (1977). Assessment of behavior modification in patients treated by psychosurgery: Five patients with severe obsessive–compulsive neurosis. In Sweet, W. H., Obrador, S. and Martín-Rodríguez, J. G. (eds.) *Neurosurgical Treatment in Psychiatry, Pain, and Epilepsy*. Baltimore, MD: University Park Press)

Halleck, S. L. (1971). Therapy as the handmaiden of the status quo. *Psychol. Today*, **4**, 30

Halpern, L. (1947). Edema of lower extremities following prefrontal lobectomy. *Harefuah*, **32**, 64–66

Halstead, W. C., Carmichael, H. T. and Bucy, P. C. (1946). Prefrontal lobotomy: A preliminary appraisal of behavioral results. *Am. J. Psychiatry*, **103**, 217–223

Hare, E. H. (1974). The changing content of psychiatric illness. *J. Psychosom. Res.*, **18**, 283–289

Harlow, J. M. (1848). Passage of an iron through the head. *Boston Med. Surg. J.*, **39**, 389–393

Harlow, J. M. (1866–1868). Recovery after severe injury to head. *Mass. Med. Soc. Publ.*, **2**, 329–346

Harris, A. and Norris, V. (1954). Changes in duration of stay of mental hospital patients suffering from functional psychoses during the past 20 years. *J. Ment. Sci.*, **100**, 241

Hassler, R. and Dieckmann, G. (1973). Relief of obsessive–compulsive disorders, phobias, and tics by stereotactic coagulation of the rostral intralaminar and medial–thalamic nuclei. In Laitinen, L. V. and Livingston, K. E. (eds.) *Surgical Approaches in Psychiatry*. (Lancaster: MTP)

Heath, R. G. and Cox, A. W. (1976). Surgical treatment of psychological disease: Historical review, 1950 to 1974. In Morley, T. P. (ed.) *Current Controversies in Neurosurgery*. (Philadelphia: Saunders)

Heath, R. G., Weber, J. J. and Crandell, A. (1949). Psychiatry. In Mettler, F. A. (ed.) *Selective Partial Ablation of the Frontal Cortex*. (New York: Hoeber)

Heimburger, R. F., Small, I. F., Small, J. G., Milstein, V. and Moore, D. (1978). Stereotactic amygdalotomy for convulsive and behavioral disorders. *Appl. Neurophysiol.*, **41**, 43–51

Heimburger, R. F., Whitlock, C. C. and Kalsbeck, J. E. (1966). Stereotaxic amygdalotomy for epilepsy with aggressive behavior. *J. Am. Med. Assoc.*, **198**, 741–745

Herner, T. (1961). Treatment of mental disorders with frontal stereotaxic thermolesions: A follow-up of 116 cases. *Acta Psychiatr. Neurol. Scand.*, **36** (Suppl. 159), 1–140

Hetherington, R. F., Haden, P. and Craig, W. J. (1972). Neurosurgery in affective disorder: Criteria for selection of patients. In Hitchcock, E., Laitinen, L. V. and Vaernet, K. (eds.) *Psychosurgery*. (Springfield, IL: Charles C. Thomas)

Hirose, S. (1965). Orbito-ventromedial undercutting 1957–1963: Follow-up study of 77 cases. *Am. J. Psychiatry*, **121**, 1194–1202
Hirose, S. (1973). Long-term evaluation of orbito-ventromedial undercutting in "atypical" schizophrenic patients. In Laitinen, L. V. and Livingston, K. E. (eds.) *Surgical Approaches in Psychiatry*. (Lancaster: MTP)
Hirose, S. (1977). Psychiatric evaluation of psychosurgery. In Sweet, W. H., Obrador, S. and Martín-Rodríguez, J. G. (eds.) *Neurosurgical Treatment in Psychiatry, Pain, and Epilepsy*. (Baltimore, MD: University Park Press)
Hirose, S. and Inugami, K. (1958). Studies on selective critical undercutting. *Fol. Psychiatr. Neurol. Japon.*, **10** (Suppl. 5), 55–57
Hitchcock, E., Ashcroft, G. W., Cairns, V. M. and Murray, L. G. (1972). Preoperative and postoperative assessment and management of psychosurgical patients. In Hitchcock, E., Laitinen, L. V. and Vaernet, K. (eds.) *Psychosurgery*. (Springfield, IL: Charles C. Thomas)
Hitchcock, E. and Cairns, V. (1973). Amygdalectomy. *Postgrad. Med.*, **49**, 894–904
Hitchcock, E. R., Ashcroft, G. W., Cairns, V. M. and Murray, L. G. (1973). Observations on the development of an assessment scheme for amygdalectomy. In Laitinen, L. V. and Livingston, K. E. (eds.) *Surgical Approaches in Psychiatry*. (Lancaster: MTP)
Hoch, P. H. (1951). Personality changes after topectomy. *Psychiatr. Q.*, **25**, 402–408
Hoch, P. H., Cattell, J. P., Pennes, H. H. and Glaser, G. H. (1956). In Landis, N. D. C., Landis, C. and King, H. E. (eds.) *Studies in Topectomy*. (New York: Grune & Stratton)
Hofstatter, L., Smolik, E. A. and Busch, A. K. (1945). Prefrontal lobotomy in treatment of chronic psychoses, with special reference to section of orbital areas only. *Arch. Neurol. Psychiatry*, **53**, 125–130
Hohman, L. B., Odom, G. L., Suitt, R. B., Wilson, W. P., Carroll, R. C., Glass, S. E. and Murdoch, J. P. (1951). Preliminary report on the follow-up of prefrontal lobotomies performed by the Duke neurosurgical staff. *NC Med. J.*, **12**, 529–534
Horsley, V. and Clarke, R. H. (1908). The structure and functions of the cerebellum examined by a new method. *Brain*, **31**, 45–124
Hunt, W. A., Wittson, C. L. and Hunt, E. B. (1953). A theoretical and practical analysis of the diagnostic process. In Hoch, P. H. and Zubin, J. (eds.) *Current Problems in Psychiatric Diagnosis*. (New York: Grune & Stratton)
Hunter, W. S. (1930). A consideration of Lashley's theory of equipotentiality of cerebral action. *J. Gen. Psychol.*, **3**, 455–468
Hutton, E. L., Fleming, G. W. T. H. and Fox, F. E. (1941). Early results of prefrontal leucotomy. *Lancet*, **2**, 3–7
Ingram, I. M. (1961). Obsessional illness in mental hospital patients. *J. Ment. Sci.*, **107**, 382–402
Jackson, C. L. and Jaco, E. G. (1954). Some prognostic factors in 538 transorbital lobotomy cases. *Am. J. Psychiatry*, **111**, 353–357
Jackson, H. (1954). Leucotomy – A recent development. *J. Ment. Sci.*, **100**, 62–65
Jackson, J. H. (1932). Selected writings of John Hughlings Jackson (Vol. 2) (Taylor, J. ed.). (London: Hodder & Stoughton)
Jacobsen, C. F., Wolfe, J. B. and Jackson, T. A. (1935). An experimental analysis of

the functions of the frontal association areas in primates. *J. Nerv. Ment. Dis.*, **82**, 1–14

Jenkins, R. L. and Holsopple, J. Q. (1953). Criteria and experimental design for evaluating results of lobotomy. *Res. Publ. Assoc. Nerv. Ment. Dis.*, **31**, 319–327

Jenkins, R. L., Holsopple, J. Q. and Lorr, M. (1954). Effects of prefrontal lobotomy on patients with severe chronic schizophrenia. *Am. J. Psychiatry*, **111**, 84–90

Jennett, W. B. (1964). *An Introduction to Neurosurgery*. (London: Heinemann)

Jones, C. H. and Shanklin, J. G. (1950). Transorbital lobotomy in institutional practice. *Am. J. Psychiatry*, **107**, 120–127

Kalinowsky, L. B. (1973). Attempt at localization of psychological manifestations observed in various psychosurgical procedures. In Laitinen, L. V. and Livingston, K. E. (eds.) *Surgical Approaches in Psychiatry*. (Lancaster: MTP)

Kalinowsky, L. B. and Hoch, P. H. (1952). *Shock Treatments, Psychosurgery and other Somatic Treatments in Psychiatry*, 2nd Edn. (New York: Grune & Stratton)

Kandel, E. and Chebotaryova, N. M. (1972). Conray ventriculography in stereotaxic surgery: Experience with 320 operations. *Confin. Neurol.*, **34**, 34–40

Kazdin, A. E. and Wilcoxon, L. A. (1976). Systematic desensitization and non-specific treatment effects: A methodological evaluation. *Psychol. Bull.*, **83**, 729–758

Kelly, D. (1973). Therapeutic outcome in limbic leucotomy in psychiatric patients. *Psychiatr., Neurol. Neurochirurg.*, **76**, 353–363

Kelly, D. (1975). What's new in psychosurgery. In Arieti, S. and Chrzanowski, G. (eds.) *New Dimensions in Psychiatry: A World View*. (New York: Wiley)

Kelly, D. and Mitchell-Heggs, N. (1973). Stereotactic limbic leucotomy – A follow-up study of thirty patients. *Postgrad. Med. J.*, **49**, 865–882

Kelly, D., Richardson, A. and Mitchell-Heggs, N. (1973a). Stereotactic limbic leucotomy: Neurophysiological aspects and operative technique. *Br. J. Psychiatry*, **123**, 133–140

Kelly, D., Richardson, A. and Mitchell-Heggs, N. (1973b). Technique and assessment of limbic leucotomy. In Laitinen, L. V. and Livingston, K. E. (eds.) *Surgical Approaches in Psychiatry*. (Lancaster: MTP)

Kelly, D., Richardson, A., Mitchell-Heggs, N., Greenup, J., Chen, C. and Hafner, R. J. (1973c). Stereotactic limbic leucotomy: A preliminary report on 40 patients. *Br. J. Psychiatry*, **123**, 141–148

Kendell, R. E. (1973). The influence of the 1968 glossary on the diagnoses of English psychiatrists. *Br. J. Psychiatry*, **123**, 527–530

Kendell, R. E. (1975). *The Role of Diagnosis in Psychiatry*. (Oxford: Blackwell)

Kiloh, L. G., Gye, R. S., Rushworth, R. G., Bell, D. S. and White, R. T. (1974). Stereotactic amygdaloidotomy for aggressive behaviour. *J. Neurol., Neurosurg. Psychiatry*, **37**, 437–444

King, P. A. (1977). Dissenting statement of Commissioner Patricia A. King. In *National Commission for the Protection of Human Subjects of Biomedical and Behavioral Research*. (Washington: US Dept. Health, Education and Welfare)

Kisker, G. W. (1943). Psychological factors in bilateral prefrontal lobotomy. *Ohio State Med. J.*, **39**, 913–916

Kisker, G. W. (1944). Abstract and categorical behavior following therapeutic brain surgery. *Psychosom. Med.*, **6**, 146–150

Kleist, K. (1934). *Gehirnpathologie*. (Leipzig: Barth)

Kling, A. (1972). Effects of amygdalectomy on social-affective behavior in non-human primates. In Eleftheriou, B. E. (ed.) *The Neurobiology of the Amygdala.* (New York: Plenum)

Klotz, M., Ritchie, W. P. and Schiele, B. C. (1952). Prefrontal leukotomy: A clinical survey of 100 cases given an active retraining program in a mental hospital. *Psychiatr. Q.*, **26**, 54–72

Klüver, H. and Bucy, P. C. (1937). "Psychic blindness" and other symptoms following bilateral temporal lobectomy in rhesus monkeys. *Am. J. Physiol.*, **119**, 352–353

Klüver, H. and Bucy, P. C. (1938). An analysis of certain effects of bilateral temporal lobectomy in the rhesus monkey with special reference to "psychic blindness". *J. Psychol.*, **5**, 33–54

Knight, G. (1964). The orbital cortex as an objective in the surgical treatment of mental illness. *Br. J. Surg.*, **51**, 114–124

Knight, G. (1965). Stereotactic tractotomy in the surgical treatment of mental illness. *J. Neurol., Neurosurg. Psychiatry*, **28**, 304–310

Knight, G. G. (1972). Bifrontal stereotaxic tractotomy in the substantia innominata: An experience of 450 cases. In Hitchcock, E., Laitinen, L. and Vaernet, K. (eds.) *Psychosurgery*. (Springfield, IL: Charles C. Thomas)

Knight, G. (1973). Further observations from an experience of 660 cases of stereotactic tractotomy. *Postgrad. Med. J.*, **49**, 845–854

Knight, G. G. and Tredgold, R. F. (1955). Orbital leucotomy – A review of 52 cases. *Lancet*, **1**, 981–986

Kolb, L. C. (1949). An evaluation of lobotomy and its potentialities for future research in psychiatry and the basic sciences. *J. Nerv. Ment. Dis.*, **110**, 112–148

Kolb, L. C. (1973). Psychosurgery – justifiable? *N. Engl. J. Med.*, **289**, 1141–1142

Kramer, M. (1969). Cross-national study of diagnosis of the mental disorders: Origin of the problem. *Am. J. Psychiatry*, **125** (Suppl.), 1–11

Krapf, E. E. and Lyonnet, J. H. (1951). Lobotomia química "de prueba": Bloqueo prefrontal novocaínico: Comunicación previa. *Prensa Méd. Argentina*, **38**, 2866–2868

Kreitman, N., Sainsbury, P., Morrissey, J., Towers, J. and Scrivener, J. (1961). The reliability of psychiatric assessment: An analysis. *J. Ment. Sci.*, **107**, 887–908

Kullberg, G. (1977). Differences in effect of capsulotomy and cingulotomy. In Sweet, W. H., Obrador, S. and Martín-Rodríguez, J. G. (eds.) *Neurosurgical Treatment in Psychiatry, Pain, and Epilepsy*. (Baltimore, MD: University Park Press)

Lader, M. (1977). *Psychiatry on Trial.* (Harmondsworth: Penguin)

Laing, R. D. (1967). *The Politics of Experience* and *The Bird of Paradise.* (Harmondsworth: Penguin)

Laitinen, L. (1971). A new stereoencephalotome. *Zeit. Neurochirurg.*, **32**, 67–73

Laitinen, L. V. (1972). Stereotactic lesions in the knee of the corpus callosum in the treatment of emotional disorders. *Lancet*, **1**, 472–475

Laitinen, L. V. and Vílkki, J. (1972). Stereotaxic ventral anterior cingulotomy in some psychological disorders. In Hitchcock, E., Laitinen, L. and Vaernet, K. (eds.) *Psychosurgery*. (Springfield, IL: Charles C. Thomas)

Laitinen, L. V. and Vílkki, J. (1973a). Observations on the transcallosal emotional connections. In Laitinen, L. V. and Livingston, K. E. (eds.) *Surgical Approaches in Psychiatry*. (Lancaster: MTP)

Laitinen, L. V. and Vilkki, J. (1973b). Electrophysiological and psychological studies on the function of the rostral cingulum and the knee of the corpus callosum in man. *Psychiatr. Fenn.*, **5**, 249–259

Landis, C. (1951). Psychological observations on psychosurgery patients. *Psychiatr. Q.*, **25**, 409–417

Landis, C., Zubin, J. and Mettler, F. A. (1950). The functions of the human frontal lobe. *J. Psychol.*, **30**, 123–138

Lashley, K. S. (1929). *Brain Mechanisms and Intelligence*. (Chicago: University of Chicago Press)

Lashley, K. S. (1952). Functional interpretation of anatomic patterns. *Res. Publ. Assoc. Nerv. Ment. Dis.*, **30**, 529–547

Le Beau, J. (1954a). Anterior cingulectomy in man. *J. Neurosurg.*, **11**, 268–276

Le Beau, J. (1954b). *Psycho-chirurgie et Fonctions Mentales*. (Paris: Masson)

Le Beau, J. and Pecker, J. (1950). Psycho-chirurgie: Contrôle radiologique post-opératoire par la gélatine lipiodalée. *Presse Méd.*, **58**, 777–778

Leksell, L. (1949). A stereotaxic apparatus for intracerebral surgery. *Acta Chirurg. Scand.*, **99**, 229–233

Leksell, L. (1974). Advances in stereotactic and functional neurosurgery: Opening address. *Acta Neurochirurg.*, Suppl. **21**, 1–3

Leriche, R. (1949). *La Chirurgie de la Douleur*, 3rd Edn. (Paris: Masson)

Levine, J. and Alpert, H. (1951). Sexual behavior after lobotomy. *J. Nerv. Ment. Dis.*, **113**, 332–341

Lewis, A. J. (1946). Ageing and senility: A major problem of psychiatry. *J. Ment. Sci.*, **92**, 150–170

Lewis, A. J. (1967). *The State of Psychiatry*. (London: Routledge & Kegan Paul)

Lewis, N. D. C. (1947). Review of psychiatric progress, 1946. *Am. J. Psychiatry*, **103**, 535–538

Lindstrom, P. A. (1954). Prefrontal ultrasonic irradiation – a substitute for lobotomy. *Arch. Neurol. Psychiatry*, **72**, 399–425

Lindstrom, P. A. (1972). Prefrontal sonic treatment – sixteen years' experience. In Hitchcock, E., Laitinen, L. and Vaernet, K. (eds.) *Psychosurgery*. (Springfield, IL: Charles C. Thomas)

Livingston, K. E. (1953). Cingulate cortex isolation for the treatment of psychoses and psychoneuroses. *Res. Publ. Assoc. Nerv. Ment. Dis.*, **31**, 374–378

Livingston, K. E. (1969). The frontal lobes revisited: The case for a second look. *Arch. Neurol.*, **20**, 90–95

Logothetis, J. (1976). A long-term evaluation of convulsive seizures following prefrontal lobotomy. In Suinn, R. M. and Weigel, R. G. (eds.) *Innovative Medical–psychiatric Therapies*. (Baltimore, MD: University Park Press)

López Ibor, J. J. and López-Ibor Aliño, J. J. (1977). Selection criteria for patients who should undergo psychiatric surgery. In Sweet, W. H., Obrador, S. and Martín-Rodríguez, J. G. (eds.) *Neurosurgical Treatment in Psychiatry, Pain, and Epilepsy*. (Baltimore, MD: University Park Press)

López-Ibor Aliño, J. J. and Burzaco, J. (1972). Stereotaxic anterior limb capsulotomy in selected psychiatric patients. In Hitchcock, E., Laitinen, L. and Vaernet, K. (eds.) *Psychosurgery*. (Springfield, IL: Charles C. Thomas)

Lorr, M., Holsopple, Q., Jenkins, R. L. and O'Connor, J. P. (1955). Factors of change in lobotomised chronic schizophrenic patients. *J. Consult. Psychol.*, **19**, 39–43

Love, J. G. (1943). Prefrontal lobotomy in treatment of mental diseases: Surgical technic. *Proc. Staff Meet. Mayo Clin.*, **18**, 372–376

Luria, A. R. (1973). *The Working Brain.* (Harmondsworth: Penguin)

Lyerly, J. G. (1938). Prefrontal lobotomy in involutional melancholia. *J. Fl. Med. Assoc.*, **25**, 225–229

Lyerly, J. G. (1939). Transection of the deep association fibers of the prefrontal lobes in certain mental disorders. *South. Surg.*, **123**, 426–434

Lykken, D. T. (1968). Statistical significance in psychological research. *Psychol. Bull.*, **70**, 151–159

McCaughey, J. D. (1977). Civil liberties and patient rights. In Smith, J. S. and Kiloh, L. G. (eds.) *Psychosurgery and Society.* (Oxford: Pergamon)

Macedo, C. M. (1917). La trepanación del cráneo y su representación en la cerámica peruana. *Proc. 2nd Pan Am. Scient. Congr., Section 1. Anthropology*, **1**, 265–267

McGregor, J. S. and Crumbie, J. R. (1941). Surgical treatment of mental diseases. *Lancet*, **2**, 7–8

McKenzie, K. G. (1944). Results of bilateral frontal leucotomies. *Am. J. Psychiatry*, **101**, 281

McKenzie, K. G. and Kaczanowski, G. (1964). Prefrontal leukotomy: A five-year controlled study. *Canad. Med. Assoc. J.*, **91**, 1193–1196

McKissock, W. (1943). The technique of pre-frontal leucotomy. *J. Ment. Sci.*, **89**, 194–198

McKissock, W. (1951). Rostral leucotomy. *Lancet*, **2**, 91–94

Macklay, W. S. (1953). Death due to treatment. *Proc. R. Soc. Med.*, **46**, 13–20

MacLean, P. D. (1949). Psychosomatic disease and the "visceral brain": Recent developments bearing on the Papez theory of emotion. *Psychosom. Med.*, **11**, 338–353

Maddison, J. C. (1977). The legal aspects of psychosurgery in New South Wales. In Smith, J. S. and Kiloh, L. G. (eds.) *Psychosurgery and Society.* (Oxford: Pergamon)

Malmo, R. B. (1948). Psychological aspects of frontal gyrectomy and frontal lobotomy in mental patients. *Res. Publ. Assoc. Nerv. Ment. Dis.*, **27**, 537–563

Mandl, F. (1951). Kann die Lobotomie bei Schmerzkranken durch eine intrakranielle Injektion ersetzt werden? *Wiene Klin. Wochenschr.*, **63**, 13–16

Mark, V. H. (1973). Social and ethical issues: Brain surgery in aggressive epileptics. *Hastings Cent. Rep.*, **3**, 1–5

Mark, V. H. (1974). A psychosurgeon's case *for* psychosurgery. *Psychol. Today*, **8**, 28; 30; 33; 84; 86; 94

Mark, V. H. and Ervin, F. R. (1970). *Violence and the Brain.* (New York: Harper & Row)

Mark, V. H. and Neville, R. (1973). Brain surgery in aggressive epileptics: Social and ethical implications. *J. Am. Med. Assoc.*, **226**, 765–772

Mark, V. H. and Ordia, I. J. (1976). The controversies over the use of neurosurgery in aggressive states and an assessment of the critics of this kind of surgery. In Morley, T. P. (ed.) *Current Controversies in Neurosurgery.* (Philadelphia: Saunders)

Mark, V. H. and Sweet, W. H. (1974). The role of limbic brain dysfunction in

aggression. In Frazier, S. H. (ed.) *Aggression*. (Baltimore: Williams & Wilkins)
Mark, V. H., Sweet, W. H. and Ervin, F. R. (1967). Role of brain disease in riots and urban violence. *J. Am. Med. Assoc.*, **201**, 895
Mark, V. H., Sweet, W. H. and Ervin, F. R. (1972). The effect of amygdalotomy on violent behavior in patients with temporal lobe epilepsy. In Hitchcock, E., Laitinen, L. and Vaernet, K. (eds.) *Psychosurgery*. (Springfield, IL: Charles C. Thomas)
Marks, I. M., Birley, J. L. T. and Gelder, M. G. (1966). Modified leucotomy in severe agoraphobia: A controlled serial enquiry. *Br. J. Psychiatry*, **112**, 757–769
Martin, W. L., McElhaney, M. L. and Meyer, G. A. (1977). Stereotactic cingulotomy: Results of psychological testing and clinical evaluation preoperatively and postoperatively. In Sweet, W. H., Obrador, S. and Martín-Rodríguez, J. G. (eds.) *Neurosurgical Treatment in Psychiatry, Pain, and Epilepsy*. (Baltimore, MD: University Park Press)
Marzillier, J. S. and Birchwood, M. J. (1980). Behavioral treatment of cognitive disorders. In Michelson, L., Hersen, M. and Turner, S. (eds.) *Future Perspectives in Behavior Therapy*. (New York: Plenum)
Mason, D. (1973). New threat to blacks. Brain surgery to control behavior. *Ebony*, February, **28**, 62; 63; 64; 66; 69; 72
Masserman, J. H. and Carmichael, H. T. (1938). Diagnosis and prognosis in psychiatry: With a follow-up study of the results of short-term general hospital therapy of psychiatric cases. *J. Ment. Sci.*, **84**, 893–946
May, P. R. A. (1974). Treatment of schizophrenia: III. A survey of the literature on prefrontal leucotomy. *Compr. Psychiatry*, **15**, 375–388
May, P. R. A. and Van Putten, T. (1974). Treatment of schizophrenia: II. A proposed rating scale of design and outcome for use in literature surveys. *Compr. Psychiatry*, **15**, 267–275
Medina, R. F., Pearson, J. S. and Buchstein, H. F. (1954). The long-term evaluation of prefrontal lobotomy in chronic psychotics. *J. Nerv. Ment. Dis.*, **119**, 23–30
Meister, J. (1974). Violence and the safe society. *Hastings Cent. Rep.*, **4**, 5–7
Meister, J. S. (1975). The need for policy. In Gaylin, W. M., Meister, J. S. and Neville, R. C. (eds.) *Operating on the Mind*. (New York: Basic Books)
Mempel, E. (1971). The effect of partial amygdalectomy on emotional disturbances and epileptic seizures. *Polish Med. J.*, **10**, 967–974
Mettler, F. A. (ed.) (1949). *Selective Partial Ablation of the Frontal Cortex*. (New York: Hoeber)
Mettler, F. A. (ed.) (1952). *Columbia-Greystone Associates-Second Group: Psychological problems*. (London: Routledge & Kegan Paul)
Meyer, A. and Beck, E. (1954). *Prefrontal Leucotomy and Related Operations: Anatomical Aspects of Success and Failure*. (Edinburgh: Oliver & Boyd)
Meyer, G., McElhaney, M., Martin, W. and McGraw, C. P. (1973). Stereotactic cingulotomy with results of acute stimulation and serial psychological testing. In Laitinen, L. V. and Livingston, K. E. (eds.) *Surgical Approaches in Psychiatry*. (Lancaster: MTP)
Meyer, V. (1960). Psychological effects on brain damage. In Eysenck, H. J. (ed.) *Handbook of Abnormal Psychology*. (London: Pitman)
Miller, A. (1967). The lobotomy patient – a decade later. *Canad. Med. Assoc. J.*, **96**, 1095–1103

Miller, H. R. and Spiegel, E. A. (1940). Sleep induced by subthalamic lesions with the hypothalamus intact. *Proc. Soc. Exp. Biol. Med.*, **43**, 300–302
Miller, M. R. (1948). The vocational needs of prefrontal lobotomy patients. *J. Indiana Med. Assoc.*, **41**, 1184–1186
Mingrino, S. and Schergna, E. (1972). Stereotaxic anterior cingulotomy in the treatment of severe behavior disorders. In Hitchcock, E., Laitinen, L. and Vaernet, K. (eds.) *Psychosurgery*. (Springfield, IL: Charles C. Thomas)
Mirsky, A. F. and Orzak, M. H. (1977). Final report on psychosurgery pilot study. In *National Commission for the Protection of Human Subjects of Biomedical and Behavioral Research*. (Washington: US Dept. Health, Education and Welfare)
Mitchell-Heggs, N., Kelly, D. and Richardson, A. (1976). Stereotactic limbic leucotomy: A follow-up at 16 months. *Br. J. Psychiatry*, **128**, 226–240
Mitchell-Heggs, N., Kelly, D. and Richardson, A. E. (1977). Stereotactic limbic leucotomy: clinical, psychological, and physiological assessment at 16 months. In Sweet, W. H., Obrador, S. and Martín-Rodríguez, J. G. (eds.) *Neurosurgical Treatment in Psychiatry, Pain, and Epilepsy*. (Baltimore, MD: University Park Press)
Moniz, E. (1936a). *Tentatives Opératoires dans le Traitement de Certaines Psychoses*. (Paris: Masson)
Moniz, E. (1936b). Les premières tentatives opératoires dans le traitement de certaines psychoses. *Encéphale*, **31**, 1–29
Moniz, E. (1948). Mein Weg zür Leukotomie. *Dtsch. Med. Wochenschr.*, **73**, 581–583
Moniz, E. (1956). How I succeeded in performing the prefrontal leukotomy. In Sackler, A., Sackler, M., Sackler, R. and Marti-Ibanez, F. (eds.) *The Great Psychodynamic Therapies in Psychiatry*. (New York: Harper & Row)
Moniz, E. and Lima, A. (1936). Premiers essais de psycho-chirurgie: Technique et résultats. *Lisboa Méd.*, **13**, 152–161
Moore, J. N. P. (1952). Prefrontal leucotomy: A follow-up study of 71 cases. *J. Irish Med. Assoc.*, **30**, 120–127
Morley, T. P. (ed.) (1976). *Current Controversies in Neurosurgery*. (Philadelphia: Saunders)
Müller, D., Roeder, F. and Orthner, H. (1973). Further results of stereotaxis in human hypothalamus in sexual deviations: First use of this operation in addiction to drugs. *Neurochirurgia*, **16**, 113–126
Munk, H. (1877–1880). *Die Functionen der Grosshirnrinde*, p. 1881. Berlin
Nádvorník, P., Pogády, J. and Šramka, M. (1973). The results of stereotactic treatment of the aggressive syndrome. In Laitinen, L. V. and Livingston, K. E. (eds.) *Surgical Approaches in Psychiatry*. (Lancaster: MTP)
Nádvorník, P., Šramka, M. and Patoprstá, G. (1977). Transventricular anterior hypothalamotomy in stereotactic treatment of hedonia. In Sweet, W. H., Obrador, S. and Martín-Rodríguez, J. G. (eds.) *Neurosurgical Treatment in Psychiatry, Pain, and Epilepsy*. (Baltimore, MD: University Park Press)
Narabayashi, H. (1972). Stereotaxic amygdalotomy. In Eleftheriou, B. E. (ed.) *The Neurobiology of the Amygdala*. (New York: Plenum)
Narabayashi, H. (1979). Long-range results of medial amygdalotomy on epileptic traits in adult patients. In Rasmussen, T. and Marino, R. (eds.) *Functional Neurosurgery*. (New York: Raven Press)
Narabayashi, H. and Uno, M. (1966). Long range results of stereotaxic amygdalotomy for behavior disorders. *Confin. Neurol.*, **27**, 168–171

Narabayashi, H., Nagao, T., Saito, T., Yoshida, M. and Nagahata, M. (1963). Stereotaxic amygdalotomy for behavior disorders. *Arch. Neurol.*, **9**, 1–25
National Commission for the Protection of Human Subjects of Biomedical and Behavioral Research (1977). *Report and Recommendations: Psychosurgery*. (Washington: US Department of Health Education and Welfare)
Neville, R. C. (1975). Zalmoxis or the morals of ESB and psychosurgery. In Gaylin, W. M., Meister, J. S. and Neville, R. C. (eds.) *Operating on the Mind*. (New York: Basic Books)
Newcombe, R. L. (1973). Anatomical placement of lesions in the ventromedial segment of the frontal lobe. In Laitinen, L. V. and Livingston, K. E. (eds.) *Surgical Approaches in Psychiatry*. (Lancaster: MTP)
Newcombe, R. (1975). The lesion in stereotactic subcaudate tractotomy. *Br. J. Psychiatry*, **126**, 478–481
Nicholas, M. (1967). The rehabilitation of long-stay schizophrenic patients who have had a leucotomy. *Br. J. Psychiatry*, **113**, 153–154
Nielson, J. M. (1946). *Agnosia, Apraxia, Aphasia.* (New York: Hoeber)
Nobel Foundation. (1964). *Nobel Lectures – Physiology and Medicine*. (Amsterdam: Elsevier)
Oakley, K. P., Brooke, W. M. A., Akester, A. R. and Brothwell, D. R. (1959). Contributions on trepanning or trephination in ancient and modern times. *Man*, **59**, 93–96
Obrador, S. (1947). Temporal lobotomy, *J. Neuropathol. Exp. Neurol.*, **6**, 185–193
Obrador, S. (1972). Observations and reflections on psychosurgery at different levels. In Hitchcock, E., Laitinen, L. and Vaernet, K. (eds.) *Psychosurgery*. (Springfield, IL: Charles C. Thomas)
Obrador, S., Dierssen, G. and Pelaz, E. (1967). Psicocirugía en el nivel diencéfalo-hipotalámico. *Arch. Neurobiol.*, **30**, 275–286
Ody, F. (1938). Le traitement de la démence précoce pour résection du lobe préfrontal. *Arch. Ital. Chirurg.*, **53**, 321–330
Offir, C. W. (1974). Psychosurgery and the law. *Psychol. Today*, **7**, 69–70
Older, J. (1974). Psychosurgery: Ethical issues and a proposal for control. *Am. J. Orthopsychiatry*, **44**, 661–674
Oltman, J. E. and Friedman, S. (1961). Long-term results of frontal lobotomy in schizophrenic patients. *Am. J. Psychiatry*, **118**, 70–71
Otenasek, F. J. (1948). Prefrontal lobotomy for the relief of intractable pain. *Bull. John Hopkins Hosp.*, **83**, 229–236
Paganini, A. E. and Zlotlow, M. (1960). Denial of lobotomy as a continuation of the defense mechanism of denial in schizophrenics. *Psychiatr. Q.*, **34**, 260–268
Paillas, J. E., Chabert, G., Alliez, B., and Masquin, L. (1971). Réflexions sur la psychochirurgie dans le traitement des névroses obsessionnelles. *Semaines Hôp. Paris*, **15**, 944–949
Papez, J. W. (1937). A proposed mechanism of emotion. *Arch. Neurol. Psychiatry*, **38**, 725–743
Partridge, M. (1950). *Pre-frontal Leucotomy*. (Oxford: Blackwell)
Paul, N. L., Fitzgerald, M. A. and Greenblatt, M. (1956). Five-year follow-up of patients subjected to three different lobotomy procedures. *J. Am. Med. Assoc.*, **161**, 815–819
Penfield, W. and Rasmussen, T. (1950). *The Cerebral Cortex of Man: A Clinical Study*

L

of Localization of Function. (New York: Macmillan)
Penrose, L. S. (1944). *Results of Special Therapies in the Ontario Hospitals: Coma, Convulsions and Leucotomy up to November, 1944*. Ontario Department of Health
Peraita, P. and Lopez de Lerma, J. (1977). Frontal psychosurgery – a review of 424 cases. In Sweet, W. H., Obrador, S. and Martín-Rodríguez, (eds.) *Neurosurgical Treatment in Psychiatry, Pain, and Epilepsy*. (Baltimore, MD: University Park Press)
Petersen, M. C. and Buchstein, H. H. (1942). Prefrontal lobotomy in chronic psychoses. *Am. J. Psychiatry*, **99**, 426–430
Petrie, A. (1949). Personality changes after prefrontal leucotomy. *Br. J. Med. Psychol.*, **22**, 206–207
Petrie, A. (1952). *Personality and the Frontal Lobes*. (London: Routledge & Kegan Paul)
Peyton, W. T., Noran, H. H. and Miller, E. (1948). Prefrontal lobectomy (excision of the anterior areas of the cerebrum): a new form of psychosurgery. *Am. J. Psychiatry*, **104**, 513–523
Pickett, J. M. (1952). Nonequipotential cortical function in maze learning. *Am. J. Psychol.*, **65**, 177–195
Piggott, S. (1940). A trepanned skull of the Beaker Period from Dorset and the practice of trepanning in prehistoric Europe. *Proc. Prehist. Soc.*, **6**, 112–132
Pines, M. (1973). *The Brain Changers*. (New York: Harcourt, Brace, Jovanovich)
Pippard, J. (1955a). Rostral leucotomy: A report of 240 cases personally followed up after 1½ to 5 years. *J. Ment. Sci.*, **101**, 756–773
Pippard, J. (1955b). Personality changes after rostral leucotomy: A comparison with standard prefrontal leucotomy. *J. Ment. Sci.*, **101**, 774–787
Pippard, J. (1956). Reflections on leucotomy. *Br. Med. J.*, **1**, 1402–1405
Pirovano, A. (1952). Sul comportamento della funzionalità gastrica dopo leucotomia prefrontale. *Minerva Chirurg.*, **7**, 400–404
Pokorny, A. D. (1964). Suicide rates in various psychiatric disorders. *J. Nerv. Ment. Dis.*, **139**, 499–506
Pokorny, A. D. and Faibish, G. M. (1968). Criteria of outcome in schizophrenia. *Hosp. Community Psychiatry*, **19**, 341–346
Pollitt, J. D. (1960). Natural history studies in mental illness. *J. Ment. Sci.*, **106**, 93–113
Pomeroy, W. B. (1956). Psychosurgery and sexual behavior. In Lewis, N. D. C., Landis, C. and King, H. E. (eds.) *Studies in Topectomy*. (New York: Grune & Stratton)
Pool, J. L. (1949). Topectomy. *Proc. R. Soc. Med.*, **42** (Suppl.), 1–3
Pool, J. L. (1951). Topectomy, 1946–1951: Report on 106 consecutive non-project topectomy operations. *Trans. Stud. Coll. Physicians Philadelphia*, **19**, 49–67
Poppen, J. L. (1948). Technic of prefrontal lobotomy. *J. Neurosurg.*, **5**, 514–520
Poppen, J. L., Dynes, J. B. and Weadon, P. S. (1948). Prefrontal lobotomy. *Surg. Clin. N. Am.*, **23**, 811–816
Poppen, R. L., Pribram, K. H. and Robinson, R. S. (1965). Effects of frontal lobotomy in man on the performance of a multiple choice task. *Exp. Neurol.*, **11**, 217–229
Porteus, S. D. and Kepner, R. de M. (1944). Mental changes after bilateral prefrontal lobotomy. *Genet. Psychol. Monogr.*, **29**, 4–115
Post, F. and Schurr, P. H. (1977). Changes in the pattern of diagnosis of patients subjected to psychosurgical procedures, with comments on their use in the treatment

of self-mutilation and anorexia nervosa. In Sweet, W. H., Obrador, S. and Martín-Rodríguez, J. G. (eds.) *Neurosurgical Treatment in Psychiatry, Pain, and Epilepsy.* (Baltimore, MD: University Park Press)

Pötzl, O. (1950). Leukotomie und Vegetativum. *Acta Neuroveg.*, **1**, 317–341

Powell, C. W. (1955). An evaluation of results in 71 transorbital lobotomy cases. *W. Virginia Med. J.*, **51**, 287–290

Puusepp, L. (1937). Alcune considerazioni sugli interventi chirurgici nelle malattie mentali. *Giorn. Accad. Med. Torino*, **100**, 3–16

Quaade, F., Vaernet, K. and Larsson, S. (1974). Stereotaxic stimulation and electro-coagulation of the lateral hypothalamus in obese humans. *Acta Neurochirurg.*, **30**, 111–117

Rada, R. T. (1974). Psychosurgery and the psychiatric implications of the Kaimowitz case. *Bull. Am. Acad. Psychiatry Law*, **11**, 96–100

Ranson, S. W. (1934). On the use of the Horsley–Clarke stereotaxic instrument. *Psychiatr. Neurol. Bladen*, **38**, 534–543

Ranson, S. W. (1939). Somnolence caused by hypothalamic lesions in the monkey. *Arch. Neurol. Psychiatry*, **41**, 1–23

Rao, B. N. B. and Govindaswamy, M. V. (1944). Prefrontal leucotomy in schizophrenia with report of 25 cases. *Indian Med. Gaz.*, **79**, 212–219

Rawlings, E. E. (1972/3). The doctor's potential for doing harm. *Psychother. Psychosom.*, **21**, 105–106

Reed, J. A. (1948). A study of gastric acid in prefrontal lobotomy. *Gastroenterology*, **10**, 118–119

Rees, W. L. L. (1978). *A Short Textbook of Psychiatry*, 2nd Edn. (London: Hodder & Stoughton)

Reiss, S. (1972). A critique of Thomas S. Szasz's "Myth of Mental Illness." *Am. J. Psychiatry*, **128**, 1081–1085

Reitman, F. (1946). Neurologic complications following prefrontal leucotomy. *Br. Med. J.*, **1**, 235–236

Reitman, F. (1947). Leucotomy as an instrument of research. *Proc. R. Soc. Med.*, **40**, 147–149

Reitman, F. (1948). Evaluation of leucotomy results. *Am. J. Psychiatry*, **106**, 86–89

Richardson, A. (1975). Cryosurgery in neurosurgery. *Br. J. Hosp. Med.*, **14**, 39; 44; 46

Richardson, D. E. (1972). Stereotaxic cingulunotomy and prefrontal lobotomy in mental disease. *South. Med. J.*, **65**, 1221–1224

Robin, A. A. (1958a). A retrospective controlled study of leucotomy in schizophrenia and affective disorders. *J. Ment. Sci.*, **104**, 1025–1042

Robin, A. A. (1958b). A controlled study of the effects of leucotomy. *J. Neurol., Neurosurg. Psychiatry*, **21**, 262–269

Robin, A. A. (1959). The value of leucotomy in relation to diagnosis. *J. Neurol., Neurosurg. Psychiatry*, **22**, 132–136

Robin, A. and MacDonald, D. (1975). *Lessons of Leucotomy*. (London: Henry Kimpton)

Rodin, E. A. (1973). Psychomotor epilepsy and aggressive behavior. *Arch. Gen. Psychiatry*, **28**, 210–213

Roeder, F. and Müller, D. (1969). The stereotaxic treatment of paedophilic homosexuality. *German Med. Mon.*, **14**, 265–271

Roeder, F., Orthner, H. and Müller, D. (1972). The stereotaxic treatment of paedophilic homosexuality and other sexual deviations. In Hitchcock, E., Laitinen, L. and Vaernet, K. (eds.) *Psychosurgery*. (Springfield, IL: Charles C. Thomas)

Rollin, H. (1973). Saints and sinners. *Br. Med. J.*, **2**, 594–595

Rosenhan, D. L. (1973). On being sane in insane places. *Science*, **179**, 250–258

Rosenthal, R. (1966). *Experimenter Bias in Behavioural Research*. (New York: Appleton-Century-Crofts)

Rosvold, H. E. and Mishkin, M. (1950). Evaluation of the effects of prefrontal lobotomy on intelligence. *Canad. J. Psychol.*, **4**, 122–126

Rosvold, H. E., Mirsky, A. F. and Pribram, K. H. (1954). Influence of amygdalectomy on social behavior in monkeys, *J. Comp. Physiol. Psychol.*, **47**, 173–178

Roth, M. (1959). Mental health problems of ageing and the aged. *Bull. WHO*, **21**, 527–561

Roussy, G. (1907). *La Couche Optique*. (Paris: Steinheil)

Rowbotham, G. F., Haigh, A. L. and Leslie, W. G. (1959). Cooling cannula for use in the treatment of cerebral neoplasms. *Lancet*, **1**, 12–15

Royal College of Psychiatrists, Research Committee. (1977). Evaluation of the surgical treatment of functional mental illness: Proposal for a prospective controlled trial. In Sweet, W. H., Obrador, S. and Martín-Rodríguez, J. G. (eds.) *Neurosurgical Treatment in Psychiatry, Pain, and Epilepsy*. (Baltimore, MD: University Park Press)

Rubio, E., Arjona, V. and Rodriguez-Burgos, F. (1977). Stereotactic cryohypothalamotomy in aggressive behavior. In Sweet, W. H., Obrador, S. and Martín-Rodríguez, J. G. (eds.) *Neurosurgical Treatment in Psychiatry, Pain, and Epilepsy*. (Baltimore, MD: University Park Press)

Rylander, G. (1939). *Personality Changes after Operations on the Frontal Lobes: A Clinical Study of 32 Cases*. (London: Oxford University Press)

Rylander, G. (1947). Psychological tests and personality analyses before and after frontal lobotomy. *Acta Psychiatr. Neurol.*, **47** (Suppl.), 383–398

Rylander, G. (1973). The renaissance of psychosurgery. In Laitinen, L. and Livingston, K. E. (eds.) *Surgical Approaches in Psychiatry*. (Lancaster: MTP)

Sandifer, M. G., Pettus, C. and Quade, D. (1964). A study of psychiatric diagnosis. *J. Nerv. Ment. Dis.*, **139**, 350–356

Sands, S. L. and Malamud, W. (1949). A rating scale analysis of the clinical effects of lobotomy. *Am. J. Psychiatry*, **106**, 760–766

Sano, K. (1962). Sedative neurosurgery: With special reference to postero-medial hypothalamotomy. *Neurol. Medico-Chirurg.*, **4**, 112–142

Sano, K., Sekino, H. and Mayanagi, Y. (1972). Results of stimulation and destruction of the posterior hypothalamus in cases with violent aggressive, or restless behaviors. In Hitchcock, E., Laitinen, L. and Vaernet, K. (eds.) *Psychosurgery*. (Springfield, IL: Charles C. Thomas)

Sargant, W. (1951). Leucotomy in psychosomatic disorders. *Lancet*, **2**, 87–91

Sargant, W. and Slater, E. (1972). *An Introduction to Physical Methods of Treatment in Psychiatry*. (Edinburgh: Livingstone)

Sawa, M., Ueki, Y., Arita, M. and Harada, T. (1954). Preliminary report on the amygdaloidectomy on the psychotic patients, with interpretation of oral–emotional manifestation in schizophrenics. *Fol. Psychiatr. Neurol. Japon.*, **7**, 309–329

Scarff, J. E. (1948). Unilateral prefrontal lobotomy with relief of ipsilateral, contralateral, and bilateral pain: A preliminary report. *J. Neurosurg.*, **5**, 288–293

Scarff, J. E. (1950). Reaction to life stresses following unilateral prefrontal lobectomy

or lobotomy. *Res. Publ. Assoc. Nerv. Ment. Dis.*, **29**, 121–126
Schaltenbrand, G. and Bailey, P. (1959). *Introduction to Stereotaxis, with an Atlas of the Human Brain.* (New York: Grune & Stratton)
Schaltenbrand, G., Spuler, H., Prucker, G. and Wahren, W. (1974). Electroanatomical observations on the ventrocaudal parts of the thalamus according to the facts of stereotactic stimulation in man. *Z. Neurol.*, **206**, 287–308
Scheff, T. J. (1966). *Being Mentally Ill: A Sociological Theory.* (Chicago: Aldine)
Scheflin, A. W. and Opton, E. M. Jr. (1978). *The Mind Manipulators.* (New York: Paddington Press)
Scherer, I. W. and Trehub, A. (1957). Effects of physiodynamic treatments in a hospital over a ten year period. *Dis. Nerv. Syst.*, **18**, 55–88
Scherer, I. W., Klett, C. J. and Winnie, J. F. (1957). Psychological changes over a five year period following bilateral prefrontal lobotomy. *J. Consult. Psychol.*, **21**, 291–295
Schmidt, H. O. and Fonda, C. P. (1956). The reliability of psychiatric diagnosis: A new look. *J. Abnorm. Soc. Psychol.*, **52**, 262–267
Schneider, H. (1977). Psychic changes in sexual delinquency after hypothalamotomy. In Sweet, W. H., Obrador, S. and Martín-Rodríguez, J. G. (eds.) *Neurosurgical Treatment in Psychiatry, Pain, and Epilepsy.* (Baltimore, MD: University Park Press)
Schreiner, L. and Kling, A. (1953). Behavioral changes following rhinencephalic injury in cat. *J. Neurophysiol.*, **16**, 643–659
Schreiner, L. and Kling, A. (1956). Rhinencephalon and behavior. *Am J. Physiol.*, **184**, 486–490
Schvarcz, J. R. (1977). Results of stimulation and destruction of the posterior hypothalamus: A long-term evaluation. In Sweet, W. H., Obrador, S. and Martín-Rodríguez, J. G. (eds.) *Neurosurgical Treatment in Psychiatry, Pain, and Epilepsy.* (Baltimore, MD: University Park Press)
Schvarcz, J. R., Driollet, R., Rios, E. and Betti, O. (1972). Stereotactic hypothalamotomy for behavior disorders. *J. Neurol., Neurosurg. Psychiatry*, **35**, 356–359
Scoville, W. B. (1949). Selective cortical undercutting. *Proc. R. Soc. Med.*, **42** (Suppl.), 3–8
Scoville, W. B. (1971). The effect of surgical lesions of the brain on psyche and behavior in man. In Winter, A. (ed.) *The Surgical Control of Behavior: A Symposium.* (Springfield, IL: Charles C. Thomas)
Scoville, W. B. (1972). Psychosurgery and other lesions of the brain affecting human behavior. In Hitchcock, E., Laitinen, L. and Vaernet, K. (eds.) *Psychosurgery.* (Springfield, IL: Charles C. Thomas)
Scoville, W. B. (1973). Surgical locations for psychiatric surgery with special reference to orbital and cingulate operations. In Laitinen, L. V. and Livingston, K. E. (eds.) *Surgical Approaches in Psychiatry.* (Lancaster: MTP)
Scoville, W. B. and Bettis, D. B. (1977). Results of orbital undercutting today: A personal series. In Sweet, W. H., Obrador, S. and Martín-Rodríguez, J. G. (eds.) *Neurosurgical Treatment in Psychiatry, Pain, and Epilepsy.* (Baltimore, MD: University Park Press)
Sellier, J. and Verger, H. (1898). Application de l'électrolyse bipolaire à la destruction de parties limitées de l'encéphale. *Soc. Anat. Physiol. Bordeaux, Bull.*, 68–71

Shapiro, A. K. (1971). Placebo effects in medicine, psychotherapy, and psychoanalysis. In Bergin, A. E. and Garfield, S. L. (eds.) *Handbook of Psychotherapy and Behavior Change*. (New York: John Wiley)

Shepherd, M. (1957). *A Study of the Major Psychoses in an English County*: Maudsley monograph No. 3. (London: Chapman & Hall)

Shevitz, S. A. (1976). Psychosurgery: Some current observations. *Am. J. Psychiatry*, **133**, 266–270

Shuman, S. I. (1977). *Psychosurgery and the Medical Control of Violence: Autonomy and Deviance*. (Detroit: Wayne State University Press)

Siegfried, J. and Ben-Shmuel, A. (1973). Long-term assessment of stereotactic amygdalotomy for aggressive behaviour. In Laitinen, L. V. and Livingston, K. E. (eds.) *Surgical Approaches in Psychiatry*. (Lancaster: MTP)

Sims, A. (1973). Mortality in neurosis. *Lancet*, **2**, 1072–1076

Smith, A. (1960). Changes in porteus maze scores of brain-operated schizophrenics after an eight-year interval. *J. Ment. Sc.*, **106**, 967–978

Smith, A. (1964). Changing effects of frontal lesions in man. *J. Neurol., Neurosurg. Psychiatry*, **27**, 511–515

Smith, W. K. (1945). The functional significance of the rostral cingular cortex as revealed by its responses to electrical excitation. *J. Neurophysiol.*, **8**, 241–255

Smolik, E. A. (1950). Lobotomy in the management of intractable pain and narcotic addiction. *Dis. Nerv. Syst.*, **11**, 327–331

Snodgrass, V. (1973). Debate over benefits and ethics of psychosurgery involves public. *J. Am. Med. Assoc.*, **225**, 913–920

Somerhoff, G. (1974). *Logic of the Living Brain*. (New York: Wiley)

Soupault, R. and Bucaille, M. (1955). Procaine injection of the prefrontal lobe of the brain: technic and present indications. *Ann. Surg.*, **141**, 388–397

Spiegel, E. A. and Wycis, H. T. (1949). Physiological and psychological results of thalamotomy. *Proc. R. Soc. Med.*, **42** (Suppl.), 84–92

Spiegel, E. A., Wycis, H. T. and Baird, H. W. (1952). Studies in stereoencephalotomy: I. Topical relationships of subcortical structure to the posterior commissure. *Confin. Neurol.*, **12**, 121–133

Spiegel, E. A., Wycis, H. T. and Freed, H. (1949). Thalamotomy: neuropsychiatric aspects. *NY State J. Med.*, **49**, 2273–2274

Spiegel, E. A., Wycis, H. T., Freed, H. and Orchinik, C. (1953). Thalamotomy and hypothalamotomy for the treatment of psychoses. *Res. Publ. Assoc. Nerv. Ment. Disord.*, **31**, 379–391

Spiegel, E. A., Wycis, H. T., Marks, M. and Lee, A. J. (1947). Stereotaxic apparatus for operations on the human brain. *Science*, **106**, 349–350

Spitzer, R. L. and Fleiss, J. L. (1974). A re-analysis of the reliability of psychiatric diagnosis. *Br. J. Psychiatry*, **125**, 341–347

Spitzer, R. L. and Wilson, P. T. (1968). A guide to the American Psychiatric Association's new diagnostic nomenclature. *Am. J. Psychiatry*, **124**, 1619–1629

Spitzer, R. L. and Wilson, P. T. (1975). Nosology and the official psychiatric nomenclature. In Freedman, A. M., Kaplan, H. I. and Sadock, B. J. (eds.) *Comprehensive Textbook of Psychiatry*, 2nd Edn., Vol. 1. (Baltimore, MD: Williams & Wilkins)

Squier, E. G. (1877). *Peru: Incidents of Travel and Exploration in the Land of the Incas*. (London: Macmillan)

Stanford Law Review. (1949). Editorial. *Stanford Law Rev.*, **474**

Staudt, V. M. and Zubin, J. (1957). A biometric evaluation of the somatotherapies in schizophrenia. *Psychol. Bull.*, **54**, 171–196

Stender, A. (1950). Über die transorbitale Leukotomie und eine neue Variante: Intrafrontale Eigenblutinjektion. *Nervenarzt*, **21**, 514–517

Stevens, H. and Mosovich, A. (1947). Clinical and EEG investigation of prefrontal lobotomy patients. *Am. J. Psychiatry*, **104**, 73–80

Stevens, J. R., Mark, V. H., Ervin, F., Pacheco, P. and Suematsu, K. (1969). Deep temporal stimulation in man: Long latency, long lasting psychological changes. *Arch. Neurol.*, **21**, 157–169

Stjernberg, F. (1947). Pneumoencephalographic findings in some cases of leucotomy. *Acta Psychiatr. Neurol.*, **47** (Suppl.), 400–415

Stone, A. A. (1975). Psychosurgery in Massachusetts: A task force report. *Mass. J. Ment. Health*, **5**, 26–46

Strauss, M. B. (1973). Ethics of experimental therapeutics. *N. Engl. J. Med.*, **288**, 1183–1184

Ström-Olsen, R. and Carlisle, S. (1971). Bi-frontal stereotactic tractotomy: A follow-up study of its effects on 210 patients. *Br. J. Psychiatry*, **118**, 141–154

Ström-Olsen, R. and Carlisle, S. (1972). Bifrontal stereotaxic tractotomy. In Hitchcock, E., Laitinen, L. and Vaernet, K. (eds.) *Psychosurgery*. (Springfield, IL: Charles C. Thomas)

Strom-Olsen, R., Last, S. L., Brody, M. B. and Knight, G. C. (1943). Results of prefrontal leucotomy in thirty cases of mental disorder. *J. Ment. Sci.*, **89**, 165–181

Ström-Olsen, R. and Northfield, D. W. C. (1955). Undercutting of orbital cortex in chronic neurotic and psychotic tension states. *Lancet*, **1**, 986–991

Sykes, M. K. and Tredgold, R. F. (1964). Restricted orbital undercutting. *Br. J. Psychiatry*, **110**, 609–640

Szasz, T. S. (1961). *The Myth of Mental Illness*. (New York: Harper & Row)

Tan, E., Marks, I. M. and Marset, P. (1971). Bimedial leucotomy in obsessive–compulsive neurosis: A controlled serial enquiry. *Br. J. Psychiatry*, **118**, 155–164

Teuber, H. L., Cortin, S. H. and Twitchell, T. E. (1977). Study of cingulotomy in man: A summary. In Sweet, W. H., Obrador, S. and Martín-Rodríguez, J. G. (eds.) *Neurosurgical Treatment in Psychiatry, Pain, and Epilepsy*. (Baltimore, MD: University Park Press)

Tooth, G. C. and Newton, M. P. (1961). Leucotomy in England and Wales 1942–1954. *Great Britain Ministry of Health Reports on Public Health and Medical Subjects*, No. 104 (London: HMSO)

Tow, P. M. and Armstrong, R. W. (1954). Anterior cingulectomy in schizophrenia and other psychiatric disorders. *Br. J. Psychiatry*, **100**, 46–61

Tow, P. M. and Lewin, W. (1953). Orbital leucotomy. *Lancet*, **2**, 644–649

Tsuang, M. T. and Woolson, R. F. (1978). Excess mortality in schizophrenia and affective disorders. *Arch. Gen. Psychiatry*, **35**, 1181–1185

Tuma, A. H., May, P. R. A., Yale, C. and Forsythe, A. B. (1978). Therapist characteristics and the outcome of treatment in schizophrenia. *Arch. Gen. Psychiatry*, **35**, 81–85

Turner, E. (1972). Operations for aggression: Bilateral temporal lobotomy and posterior cingulectomy. In Hitchcock, E., Laitinen, L. and Vaernet, K. (eds.) *Psychosurgery*. (Springfield, IL: Charles C. Thomas)

Turner, E. (1973). Custom psychosurgery. *Postgrad. Med. J.*, **49**, 834–844

Ukena, T. E. and Nichols, T. R. (1972). Psychosurgery. *Lancet*, **2**, 434–435

Ullman, L. P. and Krasner, L. (1975). *A Psychological Approach to Abnormal Behavior*, 2nd Edn. (Englewood Cliffs, NJ: Prentice-Hall)

Vaernet, K. (1972). Stereotaxic amygdalotomy in temporal lobe epilepsy. *Confin. Neurol.*, **34**, 176–180

Vaernet, K. and Madsen, A. (1970). Stereotaxic amygdalotomy and basofrontal tractotomy in psychotic with aggressive behaviour. *J. Neurol., Neurosurg. Psychiatry*, **33**, 858–863

Valenstein, E. S. (1973a). *Brain Control: A Critical Examination of Brain Stimulation and Psychosurgery*. (New York: Wiley)

Valenstein, E. S. (1973b). *Brain Stimulation and Motivation: Research and Commentary*. (Glenview, IL: Scott, Foresman)

Valenstein, E. S. (1977). The practice of psychosurgery: A survey of the literature (1971–1976). In *National Commission for the Protection of Human Subjects of Biomedical and Behavioral Research: Appendix*. (Washington: US Dept. Health, Education and Welfare)

Van Wagenen, W. P. and Liu, C. T. (1952). Procaine block of frontal lobe white fibers as a means of predicting the effect of prefrontal lobotomy. II. Clinical evaluation. *J. Neurosurg.*, **9**, 30–51

Vargha, M., Benkó, S. and Hetényi, G. (1951). The effect of prefrontal leukotomy on gastric acid secretion. *Acta Med. Acad. Scient. Hung.*, **2**, 229–242

Vílkki, J. (1977). Late psychological and clinical effects of subrostral cingulotomy and anterior mesoloviotomy in psychiatric illness. In Sweet, W. H., Obrador, S. and Martín-Rodríguez, J. G. (eds.) *Neurosurgical Treatment in Psychiatry, Pain, and Epilepsy*. (Baltimore, MD: University park Press)

Von Economo, C. and Koskinas, G. N. (1925). *Die Cytoarchitektonik der Hirnrinde des erwachsenen Menschen*. (Berlin: Springer)

Walder, H. A. D. (1976). The role of local tissue freezing in neurosurgery. In Morely, T. P. (ed.) *Current Controversies in Neurosurgery*. (Philadelphia: Saunders)

Walder, H. A. D. and Jaspar, H. H. J. (1970). The type of lesion produced in stereotactic operations. *Psychiatr., Neurol., Neurochirurg.*, **73**, 353–364

Walker, A. E. (1944). Psychosurgery: A collective review. *Int. Abstr. Surg.*, **78**, 1–11

Walker, A. E. (1951). *A History of Neurological Surgery*. (London: Baillière, Tindall & Cox)

Walsh, K. W. (1978). *Neuropsychology: A Clinical Approach*. (Edinburgh: Churchill Livingstone)

Ward, A. A., Jr. (1948). The anterior cingular gyrus and personality. *Res. Publ. Assoc. Nerv. Ment. Dis.*, **27**, 438–445

Watts, J. W. and Murphy, J. P. (1949). Psychosurgery: surgical aspects. *Prog. Neurol. Psychiatry*, **4**, 395–404

Whitman, R. L. (1948). Prefrontal leucotomy: Aftercare and rehabilitation. *Northwest Med.*, **47**, 419–420

Whitty, C. W. M., Duffield, J. E., Tow, P. M. and Cairns, H. (1952). Anterior cingulectomy in the treatment of mental disease. *Lancet*, **1**, 475–481

Willet, R. A. (1960). The effects of psychosurgical procedures on behaviour. In Eysenck, H. J. (ed.) *Handbook of Abnormal Psychology*. (London: Pitman)

Williams, J. M. and Freeman, W. (1951). Amygdaloidectomy for the suppression of auditory hallucinations. *Med. Ann. DC*, **20**, 192–196

Wilson, W. W., Pittman, A. R., Bennett, R. E. and Garber, R. S. (1953). Results of transorbital lobotomy in 400 state hospital patients. *Neurology*, **3**, 879–885

Wing, J. K. (1966). Five-year outcome in early schizophrenia. *Proc. R. Soc. Med.*, **59**, 17–18

Wing, J. K. (1978). *Reasoning about Madness*. (Oxford: Oxford University Press)

Winkler, R. (1977). Current psychosurgery in Australia: Local concerns. In Smith, J. S. and Kiloh, L. G. (eds.) *Psychosurgery and Society*. (Oxford: Pergamon)

Witton, K. and Ellsworth, R. B. (1962). Social and psychological (MMPI) changes 5–10 years after lobotomy. *Dis. Nerv. Syst.*, **23**, 440–444

Woltman, H. W., Smith, B. F., Moersch, F. P. and Love, J. G. (1941). Prefrontal lobotomy in the treatment of certain mental disorders. *Proc. Staff Meet. Mayo Clin.*, **16**, 200–201

Woods, J. W. (1956). "Taming" of the wild Norway rat by rhinencephalic lesions. *Nature (London)*, **178**, 869

Worchel, P. and Lylerly, J. G. (1941). Effects of prefrontal lobotomy on depressed patients. *J. Neurophysiol.*, **4**, 62–67

World Health Organization (1977). *Manual of the International Statistical Classification of Diseases, Injuries, and Causes of Death*, Vol. 1. (Geneva: WHO)

Worthing, H. J., Brill, H. and Widgerson, H. (1951). Evaluation of immediate and late results of prefrontal lobotomy in 600 cases, including a case of post-encephalitis and other organic states. *Am. J. Psychiatry*, **108**, 328–336

Wortis, J. (1972). Lobotomy and the law. *Biol. Psychiatry*, **5**, 99–100

Wycis, H. T. (1972). The role of stereotaxic surgery in the compulsive state. In Hitchcock, E., Laitinen, L. and Vaernet, K. (eds.) *Psychosurgery*. (Springfield, IL: Charles C. Thomas)

Wycis, H. T. and Spiegel, E. A. (1949). Thalamotomy – neurological aspects. *Proc. R. Soc. Med.*, **42** (Suppl.), 12–13

Wycis, H. T., Soloff, L. and Spiegel, E. A. (1950). Facial pain, persisting after retrogasserian rhizotomy, relieved by mesencephalothalamotomy. *Surgery*, **27**, 115–121

Yacorzynski, G. H., Boshes, B. and Davis, L. (1948). Psychological changes produced by frontal lobotomy. *Res. Publ. Assoc. Nerv. Ment. Dis.*, **27**, 642–657

Yakolev, P. I. (1965). Discussion of: Cassidy, W. L., Ballantine, H. T., and Flanagan, N. B. Frontal cingulotomy for affective disorders. *Rec. Adv. Biol. Psychiatry*, **8**, 269–275

Year Book of Neurology and Neurosurgery. (1976). de Jong, R. N. and Sugar, O. (eds.) (Chicago: Year Book Medical Publishers)

Ziegler, L. H. and Osgood, C. W. (1945). Edema and trophic disturbances of lower extremities complicating prefrontal lobotomy. *Arch. Neurol. Psychiatry*, **53**, 262–268

Zlotlow, M. and Paganini, A. E. (1959). Auto and homoerotic manifestations in hospitalized male postlobotomy patients. *Psychiatr. Q.*, **33**, 490–497

Zubin, J. (1958). Discussion of "1,000 prefrontal lobotomies": III. *Psychiatr. Q.*, **32**, 683–690

Zubin, J. (1967). Classification of the behavior disorders. *Annu. Rev. Psychol.*, **18**, 373–406

L

Zubin, J. (1969). Cross-national study of diagnosis of the mental disorders: Methodology and planning. *Am. J. Psychiatry*, **125** (Suppl.), 12–20

Zuckerman, M. (1972). Physiological measures of sexual arousal in the human. In Greenfield, N. S. and Sternback, R. A. (eds.) *Handbook of Psychophysiology*. (New York: Holt, Rinehart & Winston)

Author index

Subject index

GPSR Compliance

The European Union's (EU) General Product Safety Regulation (GPSR) is a set of rules that requires consumer products to be safe and our obligations to ensure this.

If you have any concerns about our products, you can contact us on ProductSafety@springernature.com

In case Publisher is established outside the EU, the EU authorized representative is:

Springer Nature Customer Service Center GmbH
Europaplatz 3
69115 Heidelberg, Germany

Batch number: 10607220

Printed by Printforce, the Netherlands